09-BTN-461

Resounding acclaim for T. Colin Campbell and *The China Study*

"Backed by well-documented, peer-reviewed studies and overwhelming statistics, the case for a vegetarian diet as a foundation for a healthy lifestyle has never been stronger."

—BRADLEY SAUL, OrganicAthlete.com

"*The China Study* is the most important book on nutrition and health to come out in the last seventy-five years. Everyone should read it, and it should be the model for all nutrition programs taught at universities. The reading is engrossing if not astounding. The science is conclusive. Dr. Campbell's integrity and commitment to truthful nutrition education shine through."

—DAVID KLEIN, Publisher/Editor *Living Nutrition Magazine*

"*The China Study* describes a monumental survey of diet and death rates from cancer in more than 2,400 Chinese counties and the equally monumental efforts to explore its significance and implications for nutrition and health. Dr. Campbell and his son, Thomas, have written a lively, provocative, and important book that deserves widespread attention."

—FRANK RHODES, PhD, President (1978–1995)
Emeritus, Cornell University

"Colin Campbell's *The China Study* is an important book, and a highly readable one. With his son, Tom, Colin studies the relationship between diet and disease, and his conclusions are startling. *The China Study* is a story that needs to be heard."

—ROBERT C. RICHARDSON, PhD, Nobel Prize Winner, Professor of
Physics and Vice Provost of Research, Cornell University

"*The China Study* is the account of a ground-breaking research that provides the answers long sought by physicians, scientists, and health-conscious readers. Based on painstaking investigations over many years, it unearths surprising answers to the most important nutritional questions of our time: What really causes cancer? How can we extend our lives? What will turn around the obesity epidemic? *The China Study* quickly and easily dispenses with fad diets, relying on solid and convincing evidence. Clearly and beautifully written by one of the world's most respected nutrition authorities, *The China Study* represents a major turning-point in our understanding of health."

—NEAL BARNARD, MD, President, Physician's
Committee for Responsible Medicine

"All concerned with the obesity epidemic, their own health, and the staggering environmental and social impacts of the Western diet will find wise and practical solutions in Dr. Campbell's *The China Study*."

—ROBERT GOODLAND, Lead Advisor on the Environment,
The World Bank Group (1978–2001)

"Everyone in the field of nutrition science stands on the shoulders of T. Colin Campbell, who is one of the giants in the field. This is one of the most important books about nutrition ever written—reading it may save your life."

—DEAN ORNISH, MD, Founder & President, Preventative Medicine
Research Institute, Clinical Professor of Medicine University of
California, San Francisco, Author, *Dr. Dean Ornish's
Program for Reversing Heart Disease and Love & Survival*

"*The China Study* is the most convincing evidence yet on preventing heart disease, cancer, and other Western diseases by dietary means. It is the book of choice both for economically developed countries and for countries undergoing rapid economical transition and lifestyle change."

—JUNSHI CHEN, MD, PHD, Senior Research Professor, Institute of Nutrition
and Food Safety, Chinese Center for Disease Control and Prevention

"Dr. Campbell's book *The China Study* is a moving and insightful history of the struggle—still ongoing—to understand and explain the vital connection between our health and what we eat. Dr. Campbell knows this subject from the inside: he has pioneered the investigation of the diet-cancer link since the days of the seminal China Study, the NAS report, *Diet, Nutrition and Cancer*, and AICR's expert panel report, *Food, Nutrition and the Prevention of Cancer: A Global Perspective*. Consequently, he is able to illuminate every aspect of this question. Today, AICR advocates a *predominantly plant-based diet* for lower cancer risk because of the great work Dr. Campbell and just a few other visionaries began twenty-five years ago."

—MARILYN GENTRY, President, American Institute for Cancer Research

"*The China Study* is a well-documented analysis of the fallacies of the modern diet, lifestyle, and medicine and the quick fix approach that often fails. The lessons from China provide compelling rationale for a plant-based diet to promote health and reduce the risk of the diseases
of affluence."

—SUSHMA PALMER, PHD, Former Executive Director Food and
Nutrition Board, U.S. National Academy of Sciences

"*The China Study* is extraordinarily helpful, superbly written, and profoundly important. Dr. Campbell's work is revolutionary in its implications and spectacular in its clarity. I learned an immense amount from this brave and wise book. If you want to eat bacon and eggs for breakfast and then take cholesterol-lowering medication, that's your right. But if you want to truly take charge of your health, read *The China Study* and do it soon! If you heed the counsel of this outstanding guide, your body will thank you every day for the rest of your life."

—JOHN ROBBINS, Author of the Best-Selling Books
Diet for a New America and *The Food Revolution*

"*The China Study* is a rare treat. Finally, a world-renowned nutritional scholar has explained the truth about diet and health in a way that everyone can easily understand—a startling truth that everyone needs to know. In this superb volume, Dr. Campbell has distilled, with his son Tom, for us the wisdom of his brilliant career. If you feel any confusion about how to find the healthiest path for yourself and your family, you will find precious answers in *The China Study*. Don't miss it!"

—DOUGLAS J. LISLE, PHD, & ALAN GOLDHAMMER, DC Authors of *The Pleasure Trap: Mastering the Hidden Force That Undermines Health and Happiness*

"So many diet and health books contain conflicting advice, but most have one thing in common—an agenda to sell something. Dr. Campbell's only agenda is truth. As a distinguished professor at Cornell University, Dr. Campbell is the Einstein of nutrition. *The China Study* is based on hardcore scientific research, not the rank speculation of a Zone, Atkins, SugarBusters, or any other current fad. Dr. Campbell lays out his lifetime of research in an accessible, entertaining way. Read this book and you will know why."

—JEFF NELSON, President, VegSource.com
(most visited food website in the world)

"If you are looking to enhance your health, performance, and your success, read *The China Study* immediately. Finally, scientifically valid guidance on how much protein we need and where we should get it. The impact of these findings is enormous."

—JOHN ALLEN MOLLENHAUER, Founder,
MyTrainer.com and NutrientRich.com

"You want to live a longer, healthier, happier life but don't know where to start? This book gives you much more than a million statements reminding you to 'preserve your health!' It will certainly initiate new discussions, but more than that it will open new horizons to anyone who wants to embark upon different kind of living."

—Dr. Vytenis Andriukaitis, Commissioner for Health and Food Safety, European Commission

THE
CHINA STUDY

— REVISED AND EXPANDED EDITION —

THE CHINA STUDY

— REVISED AND EXPANDED EDITION —

The Most Comprehensive Study *of* Nutrition
Ever Conducted *and the* Startling Implications
for Diet, Weight Loss, *and* Long-Term Health

T. COLIN CAMPBELL, PhD
THOMAS M. CAMPBELL II, MD

BenBella Books, Inc.
Dallas, TX

BenBella Books, Inc.
10440 N. Central Expressway, Suite 800
Dallas, Texas 75231
www.benbellabooks.com
Send feedback to feedback@benbellabooks.com

Printed in the United States of America
10 9 8 7 6 5 4 3 2 1

Library of Congress has cataloged the hardcover edition as follows:
Campbell, T. Colin, 1934–
    The China study : the most comprehensive study of nutrition ever conducted and the
    startling implications for diet, weight loss, and long-term health / by T. Colin Campbell
    and Thomas M. Campbell II.
        p. cm.
    ISBN 1-932100-38-5
    1. Nutrition. 2. Nutritionally induced diseases. 3. Diet in disease.
    I. Campbell, Thomas M. II. Title.
RA784.C235 2004
613.2—dc22

This paperback edition: 978-1-941631-56-0
E-book edition: 978-1-942952-90-9

Editing by Leah Wilson
Copyediting by James Fraleigh
Proofreading by Michael Fedison
Text design and composition by Aaron
    Edmiston

Front cover design by Faceout Studio,
    Emily Weigel
Full cover design by Sarah Dombrowsky
Printed by Lake Book Manufacturing

Distributed by Perseus Distribution
www.perseusdistribution.com

To place orders through Perseus Distribution:
Tel: (800) 343-4499
Fax: (800) 351-5073
E-mail: orderentry@perseusbooks.com

To Karen Campbell, whose incredible love and caring made this book possible.

And to Thomas McIlwain Campbell and Betty DeMott Campbell for their incredible gifts.

ACKNOWLEDGMENTS
(FIRST EDITION)

This book, from its original conception to its final form, was in the making for many years. But it was the last three that gave the book form. And this happened because Karen, my lifelong love and wife of forty-three years, made it so. I wanted to do it, but she wanted it even more. She said it had to be done for the children of the world. She cajoled, she pushed, and she insisted that we keep our nose to the grindstone. She read every word, those kept and those discarded—some several times.

Most importantly, Karen first suggested that I work with Tom, the youngest of our five children. His writing skills, his persistence in keeping integrity with the message, and his exceptionally quick learning of the subject matter made the project possible. He wrote several chapters in this book himself and rewrote many more, bringing clarity to my message.

And our other children (Nelson and wife Kim, LeAnne, Keith, Dan) and grandchildren (Whitney, Colin, Steven, Nelson, Laura) could not have been more encouraging. Their love and support cannot be measured in mere words.

I also am indebted to another family of mine: my many undergraduate honors students, postgraduate doctoral students, postdoctoral research associates, and my fellow professorial colleagues who worked in my research group and who were the gems of my career. Regretfully, I could only cite in this book a small sample of their findings, but far, far more could have been included.

Yet more friends, associates, and family contributed mightily, through their meticulous reading of various versions of the manuscript and their detailed feedback. Alphabetically, they include Nelson Campbell, Ron Campbell, Kent Carroll, Antonia Demas, Mark Epstein, John and Martha Ferger, Kimberly Kathan, Doug Lisle, John Robbins, Paul Sontrop, and Glenn Yeffeth. Advice, support, and generous help also came in many other forms from Neal Barnard, Jodi Blanco, Junshi Chen, Robert Goodland, Michael Jacobson, Ted Lange, Howard Lyman, Bob Mecoy, John Allen Mollenhauer,

Jeff Nelson, Sushma Palmer, Jeff Prince, Frank Rhodes, Bob Richardson, and Kathy Ward.

Of course, I am grateful to all those at BenBella Books, including Glenn Yeffeth, Shanna Caughey, Meghan Kuckelman, Laura Watkins, and Leah Wilson for turning a messy Word document into the book you now have. In addition, Kent Carroll added professionalism, understanding, and a clear vision with his valuable editing work.

The heart of this book is the China Study itself. It was not the whole story, of course, but it was the "tipping point" in the development of my ideas. The actual study in China could not have happened without the extraordinary leadership and dedicated hard work of Junshi Chen and Li Junyao in Beijing; Sir Richard Peto and Jillian Boreham at the University of Oxford in England; and Linda Youngman, Martin Root, and Banoo Parpia in my own group at Cornell. Dr. Chen directed more than 200 professional workers as they carried out the nationwide study in China. His professional and personal characteristics have been an inspiration to me; it is his kind of work and persona that makes this world a better place.

Similarly, Drs. Caldwell Esselstyn, Jr., and John McDougall (and Ann and Mary, respectively) generously agreed to participate in this book. Their dedication and courage are inspiring.

All of this was possible, of course, because of the exceptional start given to me by my parents, Tom and Betty Campbell, to whom this book is dedicated. Their love and dedication created for me and my siblings more opportunities than they ever dreamed of having.

I must also credit my colleagues who have worked to discredit my ideas and, not infrequently, me personally. They inspire in a different way. They compel me to ask why there is so much unnecessary hostility to ideas that should be part of the scientific debate. In searching for answers, I have gained a wiser, more unique perspective that I could not have considered otherwise.

Lastly, I must thank you, the taxpaying American public. You funded my work for more than four decades, and I hope that in telling you the lessons I've learned, I can begin to repay my debt to you.

—T. Colin Campbell

In addition to all those listed previously, I acknowledge my parents. My involvement in this book was, and still is, a gift from them I shall cherish for the rest of my life. Words cannot describe my good fortune in having parents who are such wonderful teachers, supporters, and motivators.

—Thomas M. Campbell, II

ACKNOWLEDGMENTS
(SECOND EDITION)

Among those acknowledged in the first edition, I would like to re-acknowledge those "who have worked to discredit my ideas and, not infrequently, me personally." Little did I know, when I wrote that previous acknowledgment, how real their contribution would be.

Their hostility to this book's message about the role of food in our health is palpable and so passionate that I have often been surprised. They often are quite articulate, and in some ways scientifically competent, although among those I have observed, most are more adept at language than science. Some of these have even availed themselves of others more skilled in science to edit their draft documents. Bottom line? They are often quite deft at fooling the public into believing they have crafted a credible second opinion.

Then there are those critics who are the most hostile and who use language that is not acceptable for this book. I have been curious about their passion and am of the opinion that they often represent the interests of major companies who believe that this message will cost them market share, if not more. But I am also convinced that there are some who honestly believe their critiques. They and their families and friends are accustomed to their traditional diets, having eaten them for a long time, perhaps for generations. Old habits die hard and the future may be too uncertain for them to contemplate.

Still, some of these critiques, no matter their sharp edges, have substance, and they must be answered. These critiques will be addressed in this book.

I also must acknowledge the innumerable people who have attended the 500-plus lectures I have given since publication of the first edition. Their questions matter and, without doubt, they have helped me learn to better articulate my comments and thoughts. I consider this to be my good fortune.

My wife, Karen, and our family (Tom, Dan, Keith, LeAnne, Nelson, Erin, Lisa, and Kim) continue to be more than supportive and creative in advancing this book's message. I could not expect more. Then, too, I acknowledge the production of the movie documentary *Forks Over Knives*, produced by Brian Wendel and John Corry and directed by Lee Fulkerson. Its theater and DVD runs featuring *The China Study* have been unusually successful in advancing this message.

Tom co-authored the first edition of this book and then, with a new enthusiasm, chose to change his career from theater to medicine (he is now board certified in family medicine). In doing so, he since has acquired an unusually informed knowledge of this topic. I am convinced that, thanks to him and other young medical practitioners, the message of this book will be adopted on a wide scale in the future.

—T. Colin Campbell

Since the first edition of *The China Study*, I immersed myself fully in the medical system, becoming a practicing, board-certified family physician. It was a remarkable experience to see the four years of work we put into writing *The China Study* change so many lives while being immersed in a very separate world of medical education.

I want to thank my mentors and educators from that immense and consuming journey. In particular, I want to thank those faculty and staff at the University of Rochester Medical Center Department of Family Medicine who offered support and education during my residency. The UR Primary Care Network, my current employer, has also been remarkably supportive over the past several years. By allowing me and my wife to bring a diet and lifestyle intervention to patients in the UR Program for Nutrition in Medicine (URNutritionInMedicine.com), they are proving themselves to be among a very small group of forward-thinking national leaders in health care.

Of course, as many doctors will tell you, perhaps the most valuable teachers have been my patients. There is no greater satisfaction than to help a patient heal himself or herself, and this book is intended to help its readers do just that.

I want to also acknowledge my wife, Erin Campbell, MD, MPH, who is co-founder of our Nutrition in Medicine program. Her personal and professional support and interest, along with her skills and abilities, make all of this possible.

Last, I want to acknowledge the staff at the nonprofit T. Colin Campbell Center for Nutrition Studies (nutritionstudies.org), who have propelled our plant-based certificate program to be among the most popular programs at eCornell. Having been the executive director for over a year and half, and now as the medical director, I can confidently say that Jenny Miller, Anne Ledbetter, Sarah Dwyer, Juan Lube, Jeremy Rose, Jill Edwards, Michael Ledbetter, and all the center's instructors and past employees have worked as much as anyone in the world to help the message of *The China Study* reach as broad an audience as possible.

—THOMAS M. CAMPBELL, II

CONTENTS

PREFACE
(FROM THE FIRST EDITION)

T. Colin Campbell, at his core, is still a farm boy from northern Virginia. When we spend time together, we inevitably share our stories from the farm. Whether it is spreading cow manure, driving tractors, or herding cattle, both of us share a rich history in farming.

But from these backgrounds, both he and I went on to other careers. It is for his other career accomplishments that I came to admire Colin. He was involved in the discovery of a chemical later called dioxin, and he went on to direct one of the most important diet and health studies ever conducted, the China Study. In between, he authored hundreds of scientific papers, sat on numerous government expert panels, and helped shape national and international diet and health organizations, like the American Institute for Cancer Research/World Cancer Research Fund. As a scientist, he has played an instrumental role in how our country views diet and health.

And yet, as I have gotten to know Colin on a personal level, I have come to respect him for reasons other than just his list of professional accomplishments. I have come to respect him for his courage and integrity.

Colin seriously questions the status quo, and even though the scientific evidence is on his side, going against the grain is never easy. I know this well because I have been a co-defendant with Oprah Winfrey when a group of cattlemen decided to sue her after she stated her intention not to eat beef. I have been in Washington, D.C., lobbying for better agricultural practices and fighting to change the way we raise and grow food in this country. I have taken on some of the most influential, well-funded groups in the country and I know that it's not easy.

Because of our parallel paths, I feel connected to Colin's story. We started on the farm, learning independence, honesty, and integrity in small communities, and went on to become established in mainstream careers. Although we both had success (I still remember the first seven-figure check I wrote for my massive cattle operation in Montana), we came to realize that the system we lived in could use some improvements.

Challenging the system that provided us with such rewards has demanded an iron will and steadfast integrity. Colin has both, and this book is a brilliant capstone to a long and dignified career. We would do well to learn from Colin, who has reached the top of his profession and then had the courage to reach even higher by demanding change.

Whether you have interest in your personal health or in the wretched state of health in the United States, this book will richly reward you. Read it carefully, absorb its information, and apply it to your life.

—HOWARD LYMAN, AUTHOR OF *MAD COWBOY*

FOREWORD
(FROM THE FIRST EDITION)

I f you are like most Americans today, you are surrounded by fast-food chain restaurants. You are barraged by ads for junk foods. You see other ads, for weight-loss programs, that say you can eat whatever you want, not exercise, and still lose weight. It's easier to find a Snickers bar, a Big Mac, or a Coke than it is to find an apple. And your kids eat at a school cafeteria whose idea of a vegetable is the ketchup on the burgers.

You go to your doctor for health tips. In the waiting room, you find a glossy 243-page magazine titled *Family Doctor: Your Essential Guide to Health and Well-being*. Published by the American Academy of Family Physicians and sent free to the offices of all 50,000 family doctors in the United States, it's filled with full-page color ads for McDonald's, Dr Pepper, chocolate pudding, and Oreo cookies.

You pick up an issue of *National Geographic Kids*, a magazine published by the National Geographic Society "for ages six and up," expecting to find wholesome reading for youngsters. The pages, however, are filled with ads for Twinkies, M&Ms, Frosted Flakes, Froot Loops, Hostess Cup Cakes, and Xtreme Jell-O Pudding Sticks.

This is what scientists and food activists at Yale University call a toxic food environment. It is the environment in which most of us live today.

The inescapable fact is that certain people are making an awful lot of money today selling foods that are unhealthy. They want you to keep eating the foods they sell, even though doing so makes you fat, depletes your vitality, and shortens and degrades your life. They want you docile, compliant, and ignorant. They do not want you informed, active, and passionately alive, and they are quite willing to spend billions of dollars annually to accomplish their goals.

You can acquiesce to all this, you can succumb to the junk-food sellers, or you can find a healthier and more life-affirming relationship with your body and the food you eat. If you want to live with radiant health, lean and clear and alive in your body, you'll need an ally in today's environment.

Fortunately, you have in your hand just such an ally. T. Colin Campbell, PhD, is widely recognized as a brilliant scholar, a dedicated researcher, and a great humanitarian. Having had the pleasure and privilege to be his friend, I can attest to all of that, and I can also add something else. He is also a man of humility and human depth, a man whose love for others guides his every step.

Dr. Campbell's new book—*The China Study*—is a great ray of light in the darkness of our times, illuminating the landscape and the realities of diet and health so clearly, so fully, that you need never again fall prey to those who profit from keeping you misinformed, confused, and obediently eating the foods they sell.

One of the many things I appreciate about this book is that Dr. Campbell doesn't just give you his conclusions. He doesn't preach from on high, telling what you should and shouldn't eat, as if you were a child. Instead, like a good and trusted friend who happens to have learned, discovered, and done more in his life than most of us could ever imagine, he gently, clearly, and skillfully gives you the information and data you need to fully understand what's involved in diet and health today. He empowers you to make informed choices. Sure, he makes recommendations and suggestions, and terrific ones at that. But he always shows you how he has arrived at his conclusions. The data and the truth are what are important. His only agenda is to help you live as informed and healthy a life as possible.

I've read *The China Study* twice already, and each time I've learned an immense amount. This is a brave and wise book. *The China Study* is extraordinarily helpful, superbly written, and profoundly important. Dr. Campbell's work is revolutionary in its implications and spectacular in its clarity.

If you want to eat bacon and eggs for breakfast and then take cholesterol-lowering medication, that's your right. But if you want to truly take charge of your health, read *The China Study*, and do it soon! If you heed the counsel of this outstanding guide, your body will thank you every day for the rest of your life.

—JOHN ROBBINS, AUTHOR OF *DIET FOR A NEW AMERICA*, *RECLAIMING OUR HEALTH*, AND *THE FOOD REVOLUTION*

INTRODUCTION

The public's hunger for nutrition information never ceases to amaze me, even after devoting my entire working life to conducting experimental research into nutrition and health. Diet books are perennial best sellers. Almost every popular magazine features nutrition advice, newspapers regularly run articles, and TV and radio programs constantly discuss diet and health. On the internet, you can shop for health advice of any persuasion that suits your fancy.

Given the barrage of information, are you confident that you know what you should be doing to improve your health?

Should you buy food that is labeled organic to avoid pesticide exposure? Are environmental chemicals a primary cause of cancer? Or is your health "predetermined" by the genes you inherited when you were born? Do carbohydrates really make you fat? Should you be more concerned about the total amount of fat you eat, or just saturated fats and trans fats? What vitamins, if any, should you be taking? Do you buy foods that are fortified with extra fiber? Should you eat fish, and, if so, how often? Will eating soy foods prevent heart disease?

My guess is that you're not really sure of the answers to these questions. If this is the case, then you aren't alone. Even though information and opinions are plentiful, very few people truly know what they should be doing to improve their health.

This isn't because the research hasn't been done. It has. We know an enormous amount about the links between nutrition and health. But the real science has been buried beneath a clutter of irrelevant or even harmful information—junk science, fad diets, and food industry propaganda.

I want to change that. I want to give you a new framework for understanding nutrition and health, a framework that eliminates confusion, prevents and treats disease, and allows you to live a more fulfilling life.

I have been "in the system" for almost sixty years, often at the very highest levels, designing and directing large research projects, deciding which research gets funded, and translating massive amounts of scientific research into national expert-panel reports.

After a long career in research, policy making, and lecturing to a wide variety of public and professional audiences, I now understand why Americans are so confused. As a taxpayer who foots the bill for research and health policy in America, you deserve to know that many of the common notions you have been told about food, health, and disease are wrong:

- Synthetic chemicals in the environment and in your food, as problematic as they may be, are not the main cause of cancer.
- The genes that you inherit from your parents are not the most important factors in determining whether you fall prey to any of the ten leading causes of death.
- The hope that genetic research will eventually lead to drug cures for diseases ignores more powerful solutions that can be employed today.
- Obsessively controlling your intake of any one nutrient, such as carbohydrates, fat, cholesterol, or omega-3 fats, will not result in long-term health.
- Vitamins and nutrient supplements do not give you long-term protection against disease.
- Drugs and surgery don't cure the diseases that kill most Americans.
- Your doctor probably does not know what you need to do to be the healthiest you can be.

I propose to do nothing less than redefine what we think of as good nutrition. The provocative results of my four decades of experimental research, including the findings from a twenty-seven-year laboratory program (funded by the most reputable funding agencies), prove that eating right can save your life.

I will not ask you to believe conclusions based on my personal observations, as some popular authors do. There are over 800 references in this book, and the vast majority of them are primary sources of information, including hundreds of scientific publications from other researchers that point the way to less cancer, less heart disease, fewer strokes, less obesity, less diabetes, less autoimmune disease, less osteoporosis, less Alzheimer's, fewer kidney stones, and less blindness.

Some of the findings, published in the most reputable scientific journals, show that:

- Dietary change can enable diabetic patients to go off their medication.
- Heart disease can be reversed with diet alone—and in doing so, reducing animal protein is more significant than reducing saturated fat.
- Breast cancer is related to levels of female hormones in the blood, which are determined by the food we eat.
- Consuming dairy foods can increase the risk of prostate cancer.
- Antioxidants, found in fruits and vegetables, are linked to better mental performance in old age.
- Kidney stones can be prevented by a healthy diet.
- Type 1 diabetes, one of the most devastating diseases that can befall a child, is convincingly linked to infant feeding practices.

These findings demonstrate that a good diet is the most powerful weapon we have against disease and sickness. An understanding of this scientific evidence is not only important for improving health; it also has profound implications for our society as well as societies around the world. We must know why misinformation dominates our cultural conversation and why we are grossly mistaken in how we investigate diet and disease, how we promote health, and how we treat illness.

By any number of measures, America's health is failing. We spend far more, per capita, on health care than any other society in the world, yet two-thirds of Americans are overweight, and over 25 million Americans have diabetes, an increase of about 10 million since the first edition of this book. Heart disease is still the number one cause of death, just as it was forty years ago, and the War on Cancer, launched in the 1970s, has been a miserable failure. Half of Americans have a health problem that requires taking a prescription drug every week. Though the number of Americans with high cholesterol has been on a mysterious downward trend over the last few decades, there are still over 70 million who are living with this condition.

To make matters worse, we are leading our youth down a path of disease earlier and earlier in their lives. One-third of the young people in this country are overweight or at risk of becoming overweight. Increasingly, they are falling prey to a form of diabetes that used to be seen only in adults, and these young people now take more prescription drugs than ever before.

These issues all come down to three things: breakfast, lunch, and dinner.

Sixty years ago, at the beginning of my career, I would have never guessed that food is so closely related to health problems. For years I never gave much thought to which foods were best to eat. I just ate what everyone else did: what I was told was good food. We all eat what is tasty or what is convenient or what our parents taught us to prefer. Most of us live within cultural boundaries that define our food preferences and habits.

So it was with me. I was raised on a dairy farm where milk was central to our existence. We were told in school that cow's milk made strong, healthy bones and teeth. It was nature's most perfect food. On our farm, we produced most of our own food in the garden or in the livestock pastures.

I was the first in my family to go to college. I studied pre-veterinary medicine at Penn State and then attended veterinary school at the University of Georgia for a year when Cornell University beckoned with scholarship money for me to do graduate research in "animal nutrition." I transferred, in part, because they were going to pay me to go to school instead of me paying them. There I did a master's degree. I was the last graduate student of Professor Clive McCay, a Cornell professor famed for extending the lives of rats by feeding them much less food than they would otherwise eat. My PhD research at Cornell was devoted to finding better ways to make cows and sheep grow faster. I was attempting to improve on our ability to produce animal protein, the cornerstone of what I was told was "good nutrition."

I was on a trail to promote better health by advocating the consumption of more meat, milk, and eggs. It was an obvious sequel to my own life on the farm and I was happy to believe that the American diet was the best in the world. Through these formative years, I encountered a recurring theme: we were supposedly eating the right foods, especially plenty of high-quality animal protein.

Much of my early career was spent working with two of the most toxic chemicals ever discovered, dioxin and aflatoxin. I initially worked at MIT, where I was assigned a chicken feed puzzle. Millions of chicks a year were dying from an unknown toxic chemical in their feed, and I had the responsibility of isolating and determining the structure of this chemical. After two and one-half years, I helped discover dioxin, arguably the most toxic chemical ever found. This chemical has since received widespread attention, especially because it was part of the herbicide 2,4,5-T, or Agent Orange, then being used to defoliate forests in the Vietnam War.

After leaving MIT and taking a faculty position at Virginia Tech, I began coordinating technical assistance for a nationwide project in the Philippines working with malnourished children. Part of the project became an investigation of the unusually high prevalence of liver cancer, usually an adult disease, in Filipino children. It was thought that high consumption of aflatoxin, a mold toxin found in peanuts and corn, caused this problem. Aflatoxin has been called one of the most potent carcinogens ever discovered.

For ten years our primary goal in the Philippines was to improve childhood malnutrition among the poor, a project funded by the U.S. Agency for International Development. Eventually, we established about 110 nutrition "self-help" education centers around the country.

The aim of these efforts in the Philippines was simple: make sure that children were getting as much protein as possible. It was widely thought that much of the childhood malnutrition in the world was caused by a lack of protein, especially from animal-based foods. Universities and governments around the world were working to alleviate a perceived "protein gap" in the developing world.

In this project, however, I uncovered a dark secret. Children who ate the highest-protein diets were the ones most likely to get liver cancer! They were the children of the wealthiest families.

I then noticed a research report from India that had some very provocative, relevant findings. Indian researchers had studied two groups of rats. In one group, they administered the cancer-causing aflatoxin, then fed a diet that was composed of 20% protein, a level near what many of us consume in the West. In the other group, they administered the same amount of aflatoxin, but then fed a diet that was only composed of 5% protein. Incredibly, every single animal that consumed the 20% protein diet had evidence of liver cancer, and every single animal that consumed a 5% protein diet avoided liver cancer. It was a 100 to 0 score, leaving no doubt that nutrition trumped chemical carcinogens, even very potent carcinogens, in controlling cancer.

This information countered everything I had been taught. It was heretical to say that protein wasn't healthy, let alone say it promoted cancer. It was a defining moment in my career. Investigating such a provocative question so early in my career was not a very wise choice. Questioning protein and animal-based foods in general ran the risk of my being labeled a heretic, even if it passed the test of "good science."

But I never was much for following directions just for the sake of following directions. When I first learned to drive a team of horses or herd cattle, to hunt animals, to fish our creek, or to work in the fields, I came to accept that independent thinking was part of the deal. It had to be. Encountering problems in the field meant that I had to figure out what to do next. It was a great classroom, as any farm boy can tell you. That sense of independence has stayed with me until today.

So, faced with a difficult decision, I decided to start an in-depth laboratory program that would investigate the role of nutrition, especially protein, in the development of cancer. My colleagues and I were cautious in framing our hypotheses, rigorous in our methodology, and conservative in interpreting our findings. I chose to do this research at a very basic science level, studying the biochemical details of cancer formation. It was important to understand not only whether but also how protein might promote cancer. It was the best of all worlds. By carefully following the rules of good science, I was able to study a provocative topic without provoking knee-jerk responses that arise with radical ideas. Eventually, this research became handsomely funded for twenty-seven years by the best-reviewed and most competitive funding sources (mostly the National Institutes of Health [NIH], the American Cancer Society, and the American Institute for Cancer Research). Then our results were reviewed (a second time) for publication in many of the best scientific journals.

What we found was shocking. Low-protein diets inhibited the initiation of cancer by aflatoxin, regardless of how much of this carcinogen was administered to these animals. After cancer initiation was completed, low-protein diets also dramatically blocked subsequent cancer growth. In other words, the cancer-producing effects of this highly carcinogenic chemical were rendered insignificant by a low-protein diet. In fact, dietary protein proved to be so powerful in its effect that we could turn on and turn off cancer growth simply by changing the level consumed.

Furthermore, the amounts of protein being fed were those that we humans routinely consume. We didn't use extraordinary levels, as is so often the case in carcinogen studies.

But that's not all. We found that not all proteins had this effect. What protein consistently and strongly promoted cancer? Casein, which makes up 87% of cow's milk protein, promoted all stages of the cancer process. What type of protein did not promote cancer, even at high levels of intake? The safe proteins were from plants, including wheat and soy. As this picture came into view, it began to challenge and then to shatter some of my most cherished assumptions.

These experimental animal studies didn't end there. I went on to direct what was, at the time, the most comprehensive study of diet, lifestyle, and disease ever done with humans in the history of biomedical research. It was a massive undertaking jointly arranged through Cornell University, Oxford University, and the Chinese Academy of Preventive Medicine. The *New York Times* called it the "Grand Prix of Epidemiology." This project surveyed a vast range of diseases and diet and lifestyle factors in rural China and, six year later, in Taiwan. More commonly known as the China Study, this project eventually produced more than 8,000 statistically significant associations between various dietary factors and disease!

What made this project especially remarkable is that, among the many associations that are relevant to diet and disease, so many pointed to the same finding: people who ate the most animal-based foods got the most chronic disease. Even relatively small intakes of animal-based food were associated with adverse effects. People who ate the most plant-based foods were the healthiest and tended to avoid chronic disease. These results could not be ignored. From the initial experimental animal studies on animal protein effects to this massive human study on dietary patterns, the findings proved to be consistent. The health implications of consuming either animal- or plant-based nutrients were remarkably different.

I could not, and did not, rest on the findings of our animal studies and the massive human study in China, however impressive they may have been. I sought out the findings of other researchers and clinicians. The findings of these individuals have proved to be some of the most exciting findings of the past fifty years.

These findings—the contents of Part II of this book—show that heart disease, diabetes, and obesity can be reversed by a healthy diet. Other research shows that various cancers, autoimmune diseases, bone health, kidney health, vision and brain disorders in old age (like cognitive dysfunction and Alzheimer's) are convincingly influenced by diet. Most importantly, the diet that has time and again been shown to reverse and/or prevent these diseases is the same whole foods, plant-based (WFPB) diet that I had found to promote optimal health in my laboratory research and in the China Study. The findings are consistent.

Yet, despite the power of this information, despite the hope it generates, and despite the urgent need for this understanding of nutrition and health, people are still confused. I have friends with heart disease who are resigned and despondent about being at the mercy of what they consider to be an inevitable disease. I've talked with women who are so terrified of breast cancer that they wish to have their own breasts, even their daughters' breasts, surgically removed, as if that's the only way to minimize risk. So many of the people I have met have been led down a path of illness, despondency, and confusion about their health and what they can do to protect it.

Americans are confused, and I will tell you why. The answer, discussed in Part IV, has to do with how health information is generated and communicated and who controls such activities. Because I have been behind the scenes generating health information for so long, I have seen what really goes on—and I'm ready to tell the world what is wrong with the system. The distinctions between government, industry, science, and medicine have become blurred. The distinctions between making a profit and promoting health have become blurred. The problems with the system do not come in the form of Hollywood-style corruption. The problems are much more subtle, and yet much more dangerous. The result is massive amounts of misinformation, for which average American consumers pay twice. They provide the tax money to do the research, and then they provide the money for their health care to treat their largely preventable diseases.

This story, starting from my personal background and culminating in a new understanding of nutrition and health, is the subject of this book. After spending time at MIT and Virginia Tech, then coming back to Cornell over forty years ago, I was charged with the task of integrating the concepts and principles of chemistry, biochemistry, physiology, and toxicology in an upper-level course in nutritional biochemistry. Twenty years ago at Cornell University, I organized and taught a new elective course called Vegetarian Nutrition. It was the first such course on an American university campus and proved far more successful than I could have imagined. The course focused on the health value of a plant-based diet. This course is now organized online by a nonprofit organization that I founded and that has partnered with the Cornell University program that does online courses for faculty. Headed by a long-time associate of mine, Jenny Miller, under the medical direction of my son and co-author, Thomas Campbell, MD, it has emerged among the most popular of the 200-plus courses offered by the Cornell online group.

After more than four decades of scientific research, education, and policy making at our society's highest levels, I had gained considerable confidence that I could adequately integrate my research findings and experiences into a cogent story. Many readers of the first edition of this book and viewers of three especially successful documentary movies in which our work was featured—*Forks Over Knives* and *PlantPure Nation* in the United States (directed by my son Nelson), and *Planeat* in England—have told me that their lives have been changed for the better. In many cases, the information was life saving. That's what I and Tom intend to keep doing in this second edition. I hope your life is changed as well.

PART I

THE CHINA STUDY

PROBLEMS WE FACE, SOLUTIONS WE NEED

"He who does not know food, how can he understand the diseases of man?"
—Hippocrates, the father of medicine (460–357 BC)

On a golden morning in 1946, when summer was all tuckered out and fall wanted to be let in, all you could hear on my family's dairy farm was quiet. There was no growl from cars driving by or airplanes burning trails overhead. Just quiet. There were the songbirds, of course, and the cows, and the roosters who would chime in once in a while, but these noises merely filled out the quiet, the peace.

Standing on the second floor of our barn, with the immense brown doors gaping open, allowing the sun to soak through, I was a happy twelve-year-old. I had just finished a big country breakfast of eggs, bacon, sausage, fried potatoes, and ham with a couple of glasses of whole milk. My mom had cooked a fantastic meal. I had been working up my appetite since 4:30 AM, when I had gotten up to milk the cows with my father, Tom, and my brother Jack.

My father, then forty-five, stood with me in the quiet sun. He opened a fifty-pound sack of alfalfa seed, dumped all the tiny seeds on the wooden barn floor in front of us, and then opened a box containing fine black powder. The powder, he explained, was bacteria that would help the alfalfa grow. They would attach themselves to the seeds and become part of the roots of the growing plant throughout its life. Having had only two years of formal education, my father was proud of knowing that the bacteria helped the alfalfa convert nitrogen from the air into protein. The protein, he explained, was good for the cows that would eventually eat it. So our work that morning was to mix the bacteria and the alfalfa seeds before planting. Always curious, I asked my dad why it worked and how. He was glad to explain it, and I was glad to hear it. This was important knowledge for a farm boy.

Seventeen years later, in 1963, my father had his first heart attack. He was sixty-one. At age seventy, he died from a second massive coronary. I was devastated. My father, who had stood with my siblings and me for so many days in the quiet countryside, teaching us the things that I still hold dear in life, was gone.

Now, after decades of doing experimental research on diet and health, I know that the very disease that killed my father, heart disease, can be prevented, even reversed. Vascular (arteries and heart) health is possible without life-threatening surgery and without potentially lethal drugs. I have learned that it can be achieved simply by eating the right food.

This is the story of how food can change our lives. I have spent my career in research and teaching unraveling the complex mystery of why health eludes some and embraces others, and I now know that food primarily determines the outcome. This information could not come at a better time. Our health care system costs too much, excludes far too many people, and neither promotes health nor prevents disease. Volumes have been written on how the problem might be solved, but progress has been painfully slow.

SICKNESS, ANYONE?

If you are male in this country, the American Cancer Society says that you have a 47% lifetime chance of getting cancer. If you are female, you fare a little better, but you still have a whopping 38% lifetime chance of getting cancer.[1] The rates at which we die from cancer are among the highest in the world and, except for continuing declines in some cancers[2] due to preventing exposure to well-known cancer initiators (avoiding tobacco for lung cancer and brine-preserved food for stomach cancer), it has been getting worse (Chart 1.1). Despite forty-seven years of the massively funded War on Cancer, we have made only a small amount of progress beyond controlling these exposures or finding better cancer treatments.

Contrary to what many believe, cancer is not a natural event. Adopting a healthy diet and lifestyle can prevent a sizable number of cancers in the United States. Old age can and should be graceful and peaceful.

Chart 1.1: Cancer Death Rates (Per 100,000 People)[1]

But cancer is only part of a larger picture of disease and death in America. Looking elsewhere, we see that there is an overall pattern of poor health. For example, we are rapidly becoming the heaviest people on earth. Overweight Americans now significantly outnumber those who maintain a healthy weight. As shown in Chart 1.2, our rates of obesity have been skyrocketing over the past several decades.[3]

According to the National Center for Health Statistics, as of 2015, more than a third of the adults twenty years of age and over in this country are obese! One is considered obese if he or she is carrying more than a third of a person above and beyond a healthy weight. Similarly frightening trends have been occurring in children as young as two years of age.[4]

Chart 1.2: Percent Obese Population[3]

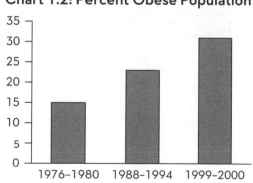

Chart 1.3: What is Obese (Both Sexes)?

Height	Weight in Excess of (lbs)
5'0"	153
5'2"	164
5'4"	174
5'6"	185
5'8"	197
5'10"	209
6'0"	221
6'2"	233

But cancer and obesity are not the only epidemics casting a large shadow over American health. Diabetes has also increased in unprecedented proportions. One out of eleven Americans now has diabetes, and that ratio continues to rise. If we don't heed the importance of diet, millions of additional Americans will unknowingly develop diabetes and suffer its consequences, including blindness, limb amputation, cardiovascular disease, kidney disease, and premature death. Despite this, fast-food restaurants that serve nutritionally defunct foods are now fixtures in almost every town. We eat out more than ever[5] and speed has taken precedence over quality. As we spend more time watching TV, playing video games, and using the computer, we are less physically active.

Both diabetes and obesity are merely symptoms of poor health in general. They rarely exist in isolation of other diseases and often forecast deeper, more serious health problems, such as heart disease, cancer, and stroke. In our first edition, we reported two frightening statistics: that diabetes among people in their thirties had increased 70% in less than ten years and that the percentage of obese people had nearly doubled in the past thirty years. Such an incredibly fast increase in these "signal" diseases in America's young to middle-age population forecasted a health care catastrophe on the horizon that may become an unbearable burden on a health system that is already strained in countless ways.

Diabetes Statistics

Percent Increase in Incidence from 1990 to 1998[6]: Age 30–39 (70%) • Age 40–49 (40%) • Age 50–59 (31%)
Percent of Diabetics Who Aren't Aware of Their Illness[6]: 34%
Diabetes Outcomes[7]: Heart Disease and Stroke; Blindness; Kidney Disease; Nervous System Disorders; Dental Disease; Limb Amputation
Annual Economic Cost of Diabetes[8]: $98 Billion

Since that ominous forecast, the latest (2012) American Diabetes Association figures now show that the total cost for diabetes is even higher, at $245 billion, with more than 20% of total health care costs being "directly attributable to diabetes."[9] In just two recent years, between 2010 and 2012, the number of people with diabetes increased 13%, from 25.8 million to 29.1 million. We're well on the way to that catastrophe.

But the most pervasive killer in our culture is not obesity, diabetes, or cancer. It still is heart disease. Heart disease will kill one out of every three Americans. According to the American Heart Association, over 60 million Americans currently suffer from some form of cardiovascular disease, including high blood pressure, stroke, and heart disease.[10] Like me, you undoubtedly have known someone who died of heart disease. But since my own father died from a heart attack almost fifty years ago, a great amount of knowledge has been uncovered in understanding this disease. The most dramatic recent finding is that very close to 100% of heart disease can be prevented and even reversed by a healthy diet.[11,12]

People who cannot perform the most basic physical activity because of severe angina can find a new life simply by changing their diets. By embracing this revolutionary information, we could collectively defeat the most dangerous disease in this country.

OOPS . . . WE DIDN'T MEAN TO HAVE THAT HAPPEN!

As increasing numbers of Americans fall victim to chronic diseases, we hope that our hospitals and doctors will do all that they can to help us. Unfortunately, in recent decades, both the newspapers and the courts have been filled with stories and cases that tell us that inadequate care has become the norm—although, since the first edition of this book, I have seen increasing interest within the medical community in the role that diet and nutrition might play in health care.

One of the most well-regarded voices representing the medical community, the *Journal of the American Medical Association*, had, as of the writing of the first edition, published an article by Barbara Starfield, MD, stating that physician error, medication error, and adverse events from drugs or surgery were killing 225,400 people per year (Chart 1.5),[13] thus making our health care system the third leading cause of death in the United States, behind only cancer and heart disease (Chart 1.4).[14]

Chart 1.4: Leading Causes of Death[14]

Cause of Death	Deaths
Disease of the Heart	710,760
Cancer (Malignant Neoplasms)	553,091
Medical Care[13]	225,400
Stroke (Cerebrovascular Diseases)	167,661
Chronic Lower Respiratory Diseases	122,009
Accidents	97,900
Diabetes Mellitus	69,301
Influenza and Pneumonia	65,313
Alzheimer's Disease	49,558

Chart 1.5: Death by Health Care[13]

Number of Americans Per Year Who Die From:	
Medication Errors[15]	7,400
Unnecessary Surgery[16]	12,000
Other Preventable Errors in Hospitals[13]	20,000
Hospital Borne Infections[13]	80,000
Averse Drug Effects[17]	106,000

The last and largest category of deaths in this group were the hospitalized patients who were dying from the "noxious, unintended, and undesired effect of a drug,"[17] when administered at normal doses.[18] Even with the use of approved medicines and correct medication procedures, over 100,000 people were dying every year from unintended reactions to the "medicine" that was intended to revive their health.[17] Incidentally, this same report, which summarized and analyzed thirty-nine separate studies, found that almost 7% (one out of fifteen) of all hospitalized patients had experienced a serious adverse drug reaction, one that "requires hospitalization, prolongs hospitalization, is permanently disabling, or results in death."[17] These are people who took their medicine as directed. This number does not include the tens of thousands of people who suffered from the incorrect administration and use of these drugs. Nor does it include adverse drug events that are labeled "possible" effects, or drugs that do not accomplish their intended goal. In other words, one out of fifteen was a conservative number.[17]

Has anything changed in the past ten years? No. By all indications, it has, if anything, become worse. In 2013, a new assessment[19] found that "a lower limit of 210,000 deaths per year was associated with preventable harm in hospitals [but] the true number of premature deaths associated with preventable harm to patients was estimated at more than 400,000 per year." It also found that "serious harm seems to be 10- to 20-fold more common than lethal harm." This assessment was based on four key studies published between 2008 and 2011, and the methodology appears to be more thorough and reliable than that of the previous report.

No one can doubt this trend in increasingly poor performance in health care in hospitals. Indeed, the most recent report calls for "an outcry of overdue changes and increased vigilance in medical care,"[19] especially by systematic listening to the harmed patients and their survivors. One thing is certain: official health agencies continue to turn a deaf ear. The U.S. Centers for Disease Control and Prevention, which publishes the government's list of top ten causes of death, still fails to list deaths from medical care at all, much less where it belongs, as the third leading cause of death in this country.

If nutrition were better understood, and prevention and natural treatments were more accepted in the medical community, we would not be pouring so many toxic, potentially lethal drugs into our bodies at the last stage of disease. We would not be frantically searching for the new medicine that alleviates the symptoms but often does nothing to address the fundamental causes of our illnesses. We would not be spending our money developing, patenting, and commercializing "magic bullet" drugs that often cause additional health problems. The current system has not lived up to its Hippocratic Oath to do no harm. It is time to shift our thinking toward a broader perspective on health, one that includes a proper understanding and use of good nutrition.

As I look back on what I've learned, I am appalled that the circumstances surrounding the way in which Americans die are often unnecessarily early, painful, and costly.

AN EXPENSIVE GRAVE

We pay more for our health care than any other country in the world (Chart 1.6).

In 1997, we spent over a trillion dollars on health care.[20] As we wrote in 2005, the cost of our "health" was spiraling so far out of control that the Health Care Financing Administration had predicted that our system would cost 16 trillion dollars by 2030.[20] Costs so consistently outpaced inflation that we were spending one out of every seven dollars the economy produced on health care (Chart 1.7). We had seen almost a 300% increase in expenditures, as a percentage of GDP, in less than forty years! What was all the extra financing buying? Was it creating health? I say no, and many serious commentators agree.

In 2013, the health status of 34 countries including the U.S., Canada, Australia, and several Western European countries was compared using a variety of different indicators of health care efficacy.[22] Other countries spent one-half or less of what the U.S. spent per capita on health care—making it seem reasonable, therefore, for us to expect our system to rank above theirs. Unfortunately, among these countries, the U.S. system was consistently among the worst performers.[13] In a separate analysis, as reported in the first edition of this book, the World Health Organization ranked the United States thirty-seventh best in the world according to health care system performance.[23] As of this writing, our life expectancy is less than average—4.2 fewer years for men and 4.8 fewer years less for women compared to Switzerland. Our health care system is clearly not the best in the world, even though we spend far more money per capita on it.

Chart 1.6: Health Care Expenditures Per Person, 1997 $US[20]

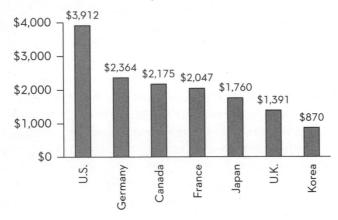

Chart 1.7: Percentage of U.S. GDP Spent on Health Care[20, 21]

Also during this last decade, we suffered a substantial economic recession, in the midst of which we debated how to reconstruct our health care system. In October 2013, the Affordable Care Act (also known as Obamacare) went into effect, and it is not yet clear what effect it may have on trends in health care spending. Therefore, it is difficult to predict what costs might be in the next few years.

However, in 2013, the U.S. still spent more money per capita "by a wide margin" than any of the 34 OECD countries. It also should be noted that, except for Greece and Poland, both of which have suffered economic difficulties, all the OECD countries have universal health coverage except for the U.S. The projected total health care spending in the U.S. for 2015 is now at $2.8 trillion, more than doubling the 1997 estimate cited above.[24]

Additionally, and even more alarmingly, we are spending a higher and higher proportion of our disposable income on health care. According to de Rugy, "the share of American GDP devoted to health spending grew from 9% in the 1980s to about 18% of GDP in 2011."[25] The government's Centers for Medicare & Medicaid Services now estimate that health care spending will be 19.9% of GDP by 2022.[26] Using this much of our income for our health care was unsustainable when we wrote the first edition; now it is even more so. How far can this go?

There also has been curiosity in recent years as to what effect the recession has had on escalating health care costs. PricewaterhouseCoopers, a professional services company, claims that the five-year (2007–2011) slowdown in the customary inflation of health care costs has ended and the upward trend has resumed. Health care cost inflation rates were 6.5% in 2014 and 6.8% in 2015. By comparison, overall inflation was only 1.58% in 2014 and -0.09% in 2015.[27] In other words, health care costs during the period from 2007 to 2015 have been eating up a larger and larger share of our income and continued to grow even when the overall economy was contracting. This is unsustainable.

What I find peculiar about these various trends and projections is the unusual attention given to the more detailed properties of the health care cost program—issues like trends in development and costs of specialty drugs, location of physician practices inside and outside hospital settings, streamlining of administrative matters, and consumer shopping for more cost-effective health care plans—while discussion of the larger perspective has been minimized.[28] Namely, we are arguing over the minutiae of who is going to pay for health care services rather than implementing the public health, nutrition, and lifestyle measures we already know will significantly reduce our need for services to begin with. To use a metaphor, a fire is starting in the foundation of our house, and instead of putting the fire out, we are fixated on buying low-cost fire retardant for the upstairs bedrooms.

Too often in the United States, a doctor's treatment decisions are made based on what will be reimbursed by health insurance rather than what is best for the patient's health. The consequences of not having health insurance, I suspect, have never been more terrifying. As of the writing of the first edition, close to 44 million Americans were uninsured.[29] This number continued to rise since until 2013 when it was 14.4% of the total population (45.4 million), before dropping to 11.5% in 2014 (36.8 million) and 9.2% in 2015 (29.4 million) in response to the adoption of the Affordable Care Act.[30] It's unacceptable to me that we have been spending more money on health care than any other country on this planet, and we still have tens of millions of people without access to basic care.

From three perspectives—disease prevalence, medical care efficacy, and economics—we have a deeply troubled medical system. But I do not do justice to this topic simply by recounting figures and statistics. Many of us have spent awful times in hospitals or in nursing homes watching a loved one succumb to disease. Perhaps you've been a patient yourself and you know firsthand how poorly the system sometimes functions. Isn't it paradoxical that the system that is supposed to heal us too often hurts us?

WORKING TO LESSEN CONFUSION

The American people need to know the truth. They need to know what we have uncovered in our research. People need to know why we are unnecessarily sick, why too many of us die early despite the billions spent on research. The irony is that the solution is simple and inexpensive. The answer to the American health crisis is the food that each of us chooses to put in our mouths each day. It's as simple as that.

Although many of us think we're well informed on nutrition, we're not. We tend to follow one faddish diet after another. We disdain saturated fats, butter, or carbohydrates, and then embrace vitamin E, calcium supplements, aspirin, or zinc and focus our energy and effort on extremely specific food components, as if this will unlock the secrets of health. All too often, fancy outweighs fact. Perhaps you remember the protein diet fad that gripped the country in the late 1970s. The promise was that you could lose weight by replacing real food with a protein shake. In a very short while, almost sixty women died from the diet. In recent decades, millions have adopted high-protein, high-fat diets based on books such as *Dr. Atkins' New Diet Revolution*; *Protein Power*; *The South Beach Diet*; *Good Calories, Bad Calories*; and *The Paleo Diet*. There is increasing evidence that these modern protein fads continue to inflict a great variety of dangerous health disorders. What we don't know—what we don't understand—about nutrition can hurt us.

I've been wrestling with this public confusion for more than two decades. In 1988, I was invited before the U.S. Senate Governmental Affairs Committee, chaired by Senator John Glenn, to give my views on why the public is so confused about diet and nutrition. After examining this issue both before and since that testimony, I can confidently state that one of the major sources of confusion is this: far too often, we scientists focus on details while ignoring the larger context. For example, we pin our efforts and our hopes on one isolated nutrient at a time, whether it is vitamin A to prevent cancer or vitamin E to prevent heart attacks. We oversimplify and disregard the infinite complexity of nature. Often, investigating minute biochemical parts of food and trying to reach broad conclusions about diet and health leads to contradictory results. Contradictory results lead to confused scientists and policy makers, and to an increasingly confused public.

A DIFFERENT KIND OF PRESCRIPTION

Most of the authors of several best-selling "nutrition" books claim to be researchers, but I am not aware that their "research" involves original, professionally developed experimentation. That is, they have not designed and conducted studies under the scrutiny of fellow colleagues or peers. They have few or no publications in peer-reviewed scientific journals; they have virtually no formal training in nutritional science; they belong to no professional research societies; they have not participated as peer review-ers. They do, nonetheless, often develop very lucrative projects and products that put money in their pockets while leaving the reader with yet another short-lived and useless diet fad.

If you are familiar with the "health" books at your nearby bookstore, you have likely heard of *Dr. Atkins' New Diet Revolution*, *The South Beach Diet*, *Sugar Busters*, *The Zone*, *Eat Right for Your Type*, or other like-minded titles proposing "low carb" diets—not so subtly meaning diets high in pro-tein and fat. These titles have made health information more confusing, more difficult to grasp, and ultimately more elusive. If you aren't fatigued, constipated, or half-starved by these quick-fix plans, your head is spinning from counting calories and measuring grams of carbohydrates, protein, and fat. What's the real problem, anyway? Is it fat? Is it carbohydrates? What's the ratio of nutrients that provides greatest weight loss? Are cruciferous vegetables good for my blood type? Am I taking the right supplements? How much vitamin C do I need every day? Am I in ketosis? How many grams of protein do I need?

You get the picture. This is not health. These are fad diets that embody the worst of medicine, science, and the popular media.

If you are only interested in a two-week menu plan to lose weight, then this book is not for you. I am appealing to your intelligence, not to your ability to follow a recipe or menu plan. I want to offer you a more profound and more beneficial way to view health. I have a prescription for maximum health that is simple, easy to follow, and offers more benefits than any drug or surgery, without any of the side effects. This prescription isn't merely a menu plan, it doesn't require daily charts or calorie counting, and it doesn't exist to serve my own financial interests; I am selling no products or ser-vices. Most importantly, the supporting evidence is overwhelming. This is about changing the way you eat and live and the extraordinary health that will result.

So, what is my prescription for good health? In short, it is about the multiple health benefits of consuming whole, plant-based foods, and the largely unappreciated health dangers of consuming animal-based foods, including all types of meat, dairy, and eggs. I did not begin with precon-ceived ideas, philosophical or otherwise, to prove the worthiness of whole foods, plant-based diets. I started at the opposite end of the spectrum: as a meat-loving dairy farmer in my personal life and an "establishment" scien-tist in my professional life. I even used to lament the views of vegetarians as I taught nutritional biochemistry to pre-med students.

My only interest now is to explain the scientific basis for my views in the clearest way possible. Changing dietary practices will only occur and be maintained when people believe the evidence and experience the benefits. People decide what to eat for a number of reasons, health considerations being only one. My task is only to present the scientific evidence in a form that can be understood. The rest is up to you.

The scientific basis for my views is largely empirical, obtained through observation and measurement. It is not illusory, hypothetical, or anecdotal; it is from legitimate research findings. It is a type of science originally advocated 2,400 years ago by the Father of Medicine, Hippocrates, who said, "There are, in effect, two things: to know and to believe one knows. To know is science. To believe one knows is ignorance." I plan to show you what I have come to know.

Much of my evidence comes from human studies done by myself and by my students and colleagues in my research group. These studies were diverse both in design and in purpose. They included an investigation of liver cancer in Philippine children and their consumption of a mold toxin, aflatoxin[31,32]; a nationwide program of self-help nutrition centers for malnourished preschool children in the Philippines[33]; a study of dietary factors affecting bone density and osteoporosis in 800 women in China[34–36]; a study of biomarkers that characterize the emergence of breast cancer[37,38]; and a nationwide, comprehensive study of dietary and lifestyle factors associated with disease mortality in 170 villages in mainland China and Taiwan (widely known as the China Study).[39–42]

These studies, exceptionally diverse in scope, dealt with diseases thought to be related to varied dietary practices, thus providing the opportunity to investigate diet and disease associations comprehensively. Our project in China, of which I was director, began in 1983. In addition to these human studies, I maintained a twenty-seven-year laboratory research program in experimental animal studies. Begun in the late 1960s, this NIH-funded research investigated the link between diet and cancer in considerable depth. Our findings, which were published in the highest-quality scientific journals, brought into question some widely assumed fundamental principles of cancer causation.

When all was said and done, my colleagues and I were honored to have received a total of seventy-four grant-years of funding. In other words, because we had more than one research program being conducted at once, my colleagues and I did seventy-four years' worth of funded research in less than thirty-five years. From this research I have authored or co-authored over 350 scientific articles. Numerous awards were extended to me and to my students and colleagues for this long series of studies and publications. They included, among others, the 1998 American Institute for Cancer Research award "in recognition of a lifetime of significant accomplishments in scientific research . . . in diet, nutrition and cancer," a 1998 award as one of the "Top 25 Food Influentials" by *Self* magazine, and the 2004 Burton Kallman Scientific Award by the Natural Nutrition Food Association. Moreover, invitations to lecture at research and medical institutions in more than forty states and several foreign countries attested to the interest in these findings from the professional communities. My appearance before congressional committees and federal and state agencies also indicated substantial public interest in our findings. Interviews on the *McNeil-Lehrer News Hour* program, at least twenty-five other TV programs, lead stories in *USA Today*, the *New York Times*, and the *Saturday Evening Post,* and widely publicized TV documentaries on our work have also been a part of our public activities.

Since publication of the first edition of this book in early 2005, I have presented at hundreds of lectures here in the U.S. and abroad, often to medical institutions and their sponsored conferences. Tom has completed seven years of medical training, including residency, and is a board-certified family physician. Presently he is an instructor of clinical family medicine at the University of Rochester Medical School; is medical director of our nonprofit organization, the T. Colin Campbell Center for Nutrition Studies (nutritionstudies.org); and is co-founder and clinical director of the Program for Nutrition in Medicine at the University of Rochester Medical Center (URNutritionInMedicine.com). He is presenting lectures to the same professional audiences as I am, and has also published a "how-to" companion to this book, *The China Study Solution.*

THE PROMISE OF THE FUTURE

Through all of this, both Tom and I have come to see that the benefits produced by eating a plant-based diet are far more diverse and impressive than any drug or surgery used in medical practice. Heart diseases, cancers, diabetes, stroke and hypertension, arthritis, cataracts, Alzheimer's disease, impotence, and all sorts of other chronic diseases may often be prevented. These diseases, which generally occur with aging and tissue degeneration, kill the majority of us before our time.

Additionally, impressive evidence now exists to show that advanced heart disease, cancers of certain types, diabetes, and a few other degenerative diseases might be *reversed* by diet. I remember when my superiors were only reluctantly accepting the evidence of nutrition being able to prevent heart disease, for example, but vehemently denying its ability to reverse such a disease when already advanced. But the evidence can no longer be ignored. Those in science or medicine who shut their minds to such an idea are being more than stubborn; they are being irresponsible.

During the past decade, it has become abundantly clear that this message is exceptionally powerful, now attracting a wide public audience in addition to a rapidly growing group of medical professionals. Its time has come and there is no doubt that it will gradually wend its way into public consciousness. It is the only dietary message that can sustain our future.

One of the more exciting benefits of good nutrition is the prevention of diseases that are thought to be due to genetic predisposition. We now know that we can largely avoid these "genetic" diseases even though we may harbor one or more genes responsible for the disease. But funding of genetic research continues to spiral upwards in the belief that specific genes account for the occurrence of specific diseases, in the hope that we somehow will be able to "turn off" these nasty genes. Drug company public relations programs now depict a future where each of us will have a personal ID card cataloging all of our good and bad genes. Using this card, we will be expected to go to our doctor, who will prescribe a single pill to suppress our bad genes. I strongly suspect these miracles will never be realized, or if tried, they will have serious, unintended consequences. These futuristic pipe dreams obscure the affordable, efficacious health solutions that currently exist: solutions based in nutrition.

In my own laboratory we have shown in experimental animals that cancer growth can be turned on and off by nutrition, despite very strong genetic predisposition. We have studied these effects in great detail and have published our findings in the very best scientific journals. As you will see later, these findings are nothing short of spectacular, and the same effects have been indicated over and over again in humans.

Eating the right way not only prevents disease but also generates health and a sense of well-being, both physically and mentally. Some world-class athletes, such as six-time Ironman champion Dave Scott, track stars Carl Lewis and Edwin Moses, tennis great Martina Navratilova, world champion wrestler Chris Campbell (no relation), and seventy-eight-year-old marathoner Ruth Heidrich, have discovered that consuming a low-fat, plant-based diet gives them a significant edge in performance. In the laboratory, we fed experimental rats a diet similar to the usual American fare—rich in animal-based protein—and compared them with other rats fed a diet low in animal-based protein. Guess what happened when both sets of rats had an opportunity to voluntarily use exercise wheels? Those fed the low-animal-protein diet exercised substantially more, with less fatigue, than those fed the type of diet that most of us eat. This was the same effect observed by these world-class athletes.

This shouldn't be news to the medical establishment. A century ago, Professor Russell Chittenden, a famous, well-established nutrition researcher at Yale University Medical School, investigated whether eating a plant-based diet affected students' physical capacities.[43,44] He fed some students, fellow faculty, and himself a low-protein, mostly plant-based diet and measured their physical performance tests. He got the same results as our rats almost a century later—and they were equally spectacular.

Then there is the question of our excessive dependence on drugs and surgery to control our health. In its simplest form, eating the right way would largely obviate the enormous costs of using drugs, as well as their side effects. Fewer people would need to wage lengthy, expensive battles with chronic disease in hospitals over their last years of life. Health care costs would drop and medical mistakes would wane as premature death plummeted. In essence, our health care system would finally protect and promote our health as it is meant to do.

SIMPLE BEGINNINGS

As I look back, I often think about life on the farm and how it shaped my thinking in so many ways. My family was immersed in nature every waking moment. In the summer, from sunrise to sunset, we were outdoors planting and harvesting the crops and taking care of the animals. My mother had the best garden in our part of the country and toiled day in and day out during the summer to keep our family well fed with fresh food, all produced on our own farm.

I've had an amazing journey, to be sure. I have been startled time and time again by what I have learned. I wish that my family and others around us had had the same information back in the mid-1900s that we now have about food and health. If we had, my father could have prevented, or reversed, his heart disease. He could have met my youngest son, Tom, his namesake. He might have lived for several more years with a higher quality of health. My journey in science over the past six decades has convinced me that it is now more urgent than ever to show how people can avoid these tragedies. The science is there and it must be made known. We cannot let the status quo go unchallenged and watch our loved ones suffer unnecessarily. It is time to stand up, clear the air, and take control of our health.

A HOUSE OF PROTEINS

My entire professional career in biomedical research has centered on protein. Like an invisible leash, protein tethered me wherever I went, from the basic research laboratory to the practical programs of feeding malnourished children in the Philippines, to the government boardrooms where our national health policy was being formulated. Protein, often regarded with unsurpassed awe, is the common thread tying together past and present knowledge about nutrition, and its supposed importance has permeated the practice of diet and health, even on the professional level, in ways that have suffused our very beings.

The story of protein is part science, part culture, and a good dose of mythology. I am reminded of the words of Goethe, first brought to my attention by my friend Howard Lyman, a prominent lecturer, author, and former cattle rancher: "We are best at hiding those things which are in plain sight." Nothing has been so well hidden as the untold story of protein. The dogma surrounding protein censures, reproaches, and guides, directly or indirectly, almost every thought we have in biomedical research.

Ever since the discovery of this nitrogen-containing chemical in 1839 by the Dutch chemist Gerhard Mulder,[1] protein has loomed as the most sacred of all nutrients. The word protein comes from the Greek word *proteios*, which means "of prime importance." This begs the question of why there was such irrational exuberance for this nutrient in the first place, especially given the belief that protein was only present in animal flesh and products. Some have speculated that it was due to people's belief that eating animals might impart strength, endurance, and agility to the consumer. Or, perhaps, it was related to the human desire to dominate other sentient beings. Whatever the motivation, in the nineteenth century, protein was synonymous with meat, and this connection has stayed with us for well over a hundred years, and has had enormous consequences for our dietary beliefs and practices. Many people today still equate protein with animal-based food. If you were to name the first food that comes to mind when I say protein, you might say beef. If you did, you aren't alone.

Confusion reigns on many of the most basic questions about protein:

- What are good sources of protein?
- How much protein should one consume?
- Is plant protein as good as animal protein?
- Is it necessary to combine certain plant foods in a meal to get complete proteins?
- Is it advisable to take protein powders or amino acid supplements, especially for someone who does vigorous exercise or plays sports?
- Should one take protein supplements to build muscle?
- Some protein is considered high quality, some low quality; what does this mean?
- Where do vegetarians and vegans get protein?
- Can vegetarian and vegan children grow properly without animal protein?

Fundamental to many of these common questions and concerns is the belief that meat is protein and protein is meat. This belief comes from the fact that the "soul" of animal-based foods is protein. In many meat and dairy products, we can selectively remove the fat but we are still left with recognizable meat and dairy products. We do this all the time, with lean cuts of meat and skim milk. But if we selectively remove the protein from animal-based foods, we are left with nothing like the original. A non-protein steak, for example, would be a puddle of water, fat, and a small amount of micronutrients. Who would eat that? In brief, for a food to be recognized as an animal-based food, it must have protein. Protein is the core element of animal-based foods.

Early scientists like Carl Voit (1831–1908), a prominent German scientist, were staunch champions of protein. Voit found that "man" needed only 48.5 grams per day, but nonetheless he recommended a whopping 118 grams per day because of the cultural bias of the time. Protein equaled meat, and everyone aspired to have meat on his or her table, just as we aspire to have bigger houses and faster cars. Voit figured you can't get too much of a good thing.

Voit went on to mentor several well-known nutrition researchers of the early 1900s, including Max Rubner (1854–1932) and W. O. Atwater

(1844–1907). Both students closely followed the advice of their teacher. Rubner stated that protein intake, meaning meat, was a symbol of civilization itself: "A large protein allowance is the right of civilized man." Atwater went on to organize the first nutrition laboratory at the United States Department of Agriculture (USDA). As director of the USDA, he recommended 125 grams per day (only about 55 grams per day is now recommended). Later, we will see how important this early precedent was to this government agency.

A cultural bias had become firmly entrenched. If you were civilized, you ate plenty of protein. If you were rich, you ate meat, and if you were poor, you ate staple plant foods, like potatoes and bread. The lower classes were considered by some to be lazy and inept as a result of not eating enough meat, or protein. Elitism and arrogance dominated much of the burgeoning field of nutrition in the nineteenth century. The entire concept that bigger is better, more civilized, and perhaps even more spiritual permeated every thought about protein.

Major McCay, a prominent English physician in the early twentieth century, provided one of the more entertaining, but most unfortunate, moments in this history. Physician McCay was stationed in the English colony of India in 1912 to identify good fighting men in the Indian tribes. Among other things, he said that people who consumed less protein were of a "poor physique, and a cringing effeminate disposition is all that can be expected."

PRESSING FOR QUALITY

Protein, fat, carbohydrate, and alcohol provide virtually all of the calories that we consume. Fat, carbohydrate, and protein, as macronutrients, make up almost all the weight of food, aside from water, with the remaining small amount being the vitamin and mineral micronutrients. The amounts of these latter micronutrients needed for optimum health are tiny (milligrams to micrograms).

Protein, the most sacred of all nutrients, is a vital component of our bodies, and there are hundreds of thousands of different kinds. They function as enzymes, hormones, structural tissue, and transport molecules, all of which make life possible. Proteins are constructed as long chains of hundreds or thousands of amino acids, of which there are fifteen to twenty different kinds, depending on how they are counted. Proteins wear out on a regular basis and must be replaced. This is accomplished by consuming foods that contain protein. When digested, these proteins give us a whole new supply of amino acid building blocks to use in making new protein replacements for those that wore out. Various food proteins are said to be of different quality, depending on how efficiently they provide the needed amino acids used to replace our body proteins.

This process of disassembling and reassembling the amino acids of proteins is like someone giving us a multicolored string of beads to replace an old string of beads that we lost. However, the colored beads on the string given to us are not in the same order as the string we lost. So, we break the string and collect its beads. Then, we reconstruct our new string so that the colored beads are in the same order as our lost string. But if we are short of blue beads, for example, making our new string is going to be slowed down or stopped until we get more blue beads. This is the same concept as in making new tissue proteins to match our old worn-out proteins.

About eight amino acids ("colored beads") that are needed for making our tissue proteins must be provided by the food we eat. They are called "essential" because our bodies cannot make them. If, like our string of beads, our food protein lacks enough of even one of these eight essential amino acids, then the synthesis of the new proteins will be slowed down or stopped. This is where the idea of protein quality comes into play. Food proteins of the highest quality are, very simply, those that provide, upon digestion, the right kinds and amounts of amino acids needed to efficiently synthesize our new tissue proteins. This is what that word *quality* really means: it is the ability of food proteins to provide the right kinds and amounts of amino acids to make our new proteins and to do so efficiently.

Can you guess what food we might eat to most efficiently provide the building blocks for our replacement proteins? The answer is human flesh. Its protein has just the right proportionate amounts of the needed amino acids. But while our fellow men and women are not for dinner, we do get the next "best" protein by eating other animals. The proteins of other animals are very similar to our proteins because they mostly have the right proportionate amounts of each of the needed amino acids. These proteins can be used very efficiently and therefore are called "high quality." Among animal foods, the proteins of milk and eggs represent the best amino acid matches for our proteins, and thus are considered the highest quality. While the "lower quality" plant proteins may be lacking in one or more of the essential amino acids, as a group they do contain all of them.

The concept of quality really means the efficiency with which food proteins are used to promote growth. This would be well and good if the greatest efficiency equaled the greatest health, but it doesn't, and that's why the terms *efficiency* and *quality* are misleading. In fact, to give you a taste of what's to come, there is a mountain of compelling research showing that "low-quality" plant protein, which allows for slow but steady synthesis of new proteins, is the healthiest type of protein. Slow but steady wins the race. The quality of protein found in a specific food is determined by seeing how fast animals grow while consuming it. Some foods, namely those from animals, emerge with a very high protein efficiency ratio and value.[2]

This focus on efficiency of body growth, as if it were good health, encourages the consumption of protein with the highest "quality." As any marketer will tell you, a product that is defined as being high quality instantly earns the trust of consumers. For well over 100 years, we have been captive to this misleading language and have oftentimes made the unfortunate leap to thinking that more quality equals more health.

The basis for this concept of protein quality was not well known among the public, but its impact was—and still is—highly significant. People who choose, for example, to consume a plant-based diet will often ask, even today, "Where do I get my protein?" as if plants don't have protein. Even if it is known that plants have protein, there is still the concern about its perceived poor quality. This has led people to believe that they must meticulously combine proteins from different plant sources during each meal so that they can mutually compensate for each other's amino acid deficits. However, this is overstating the case. We now know that through enormously complex metabolic systems, the human body can derive all the essential amino acids from the natural variety of plant proteins that we encounter every day. It doesn't require eating higher quantities of plant protein or meticulously planning every meal. Unfortunately, the enduring concept of protein quality has greatly obscured this information.

THE PROTEIN GAP

The most important issue in nutrition and agriculture during my early career was figuring out ways to increase the consumption of protein, making sure it was of the highest possible quality. My colleagues and I all believed in this common goal. From my early years on the farm to my graduate education, I accepted this virtual reverence for protein. As a youngster, I remember that the most expensive part of farm animal feed was the protein supplements that we fed to our cows and pigs. Then, at graduate school, I spent three years (1958–1961) doing my PhD research trying to improve the supply of high-quality protein by growing cows and sheep more efficiently so we could eat more of them.[3,4]

I went all the way through my graduate studies with a profound belief that promoting high-quality protein, as in animal-based foods, was a very important task. My graduate research, although cited a few times over the next decade or so, was only a small part of much larger efforts by other research groups to address a protein situation worldwide. During the 1960s and 1970s, I was to hear over and over again about a so-called protein gap in the developing world.[5]

The protein gap stipulated that world hunger and malnutrition among children in the developing world was a result of not having enough protein to consume, especially high-quality (i.e., animal) protein.[1,5,6] According to this view, those in the developing world were especially deficient in "high-quality" protein, or animal protein. Projects were springing up all over the place to address this protein gap. A prominent MIT professor and his younger colleague concluded in 1976 that "an adequate supply of protein is a central aspect of the world food problem"[6] and further that "unless . . . desirably [supplemented] by modest amounts of milk, eggs, meat or fish, the predominantly cereal diets [of poor nations] are . . . deficient in protein for growing children." To address this dire problem:

- MIT was developing a protein-rich food supplement called INCAPARINA.
- Purdue University was breeding corn to contain more lysine, the "deficient" amino acid in corn protein.
- The U.S. government was subsidizing the production of dried milk powder to provide high-quality protein for the world's poor.
- Cornell University was providing a wealth of talent to the Philippines to help develop both a high-protein rice variety and a livestock industry.
- Auburn University and MIT were grinding up fish to produce "fish protein concentrate" to feed the world's poor.

The United Nations, the U.S. Government Food for Peace Program, major universities, and countless other organizations and universities were taking up the battle cry to eradicate world hunger with high-quality protein. I knew most of the projects firsthand, as well as the individuals who organized and directed them.

The Food and Agriculture Organization (FAO) of the United Nations exerts considerable influence in developing countries through their agriculture development programs. Two of its staffers[7] declared in 1970 that "by and large, the lack of protein is without question the most serious qualitative deficiency in the nutrition of developing countries. The great mass of the population of these countries subsists mainly on foods derived from plants frequently deficient in protein, which results in poor health and low productivity per man." M. Autret, a very influential man from the FAO, added that "owing to the low-animal protein content of the diet and lack of diversity of supplies [in developing countries], protein quality is unsatisfactory."[5] He reported on a very strong association between consumption of animal-based foods and annual income. Autret strongly advocated increasing the production and consumption of animal protein to meet the growing "protein gap" in the world. He also advocated that "all resources of science and technology must be mobilized to create new protein-rich foods or to derive the utmost benefits from hitherto insufficiently utilized resources to feed mankind."[5]

Bruce Stillings at the University of Maryland and the U.S. Department of Commerce, another proponent of consuming animal-based diets, admitted in 1973 that "although there is no requirement for animal protein in the diet *per se*, the quantity of dietary protein from animal sources is usually accepted as being indicative of the overall protein quality of the diet."[1] He went on to say that the "supply of adequate quantities of animal products is generally recognized as being an ideal way to improve world protein nutrition."

Of course, it's quite correct that a supply of protein can be an important way of improving nutrition in the developing world, particularly if populations are getting all of their calories from one plant source. But it's not the only way, and, as we shall see, it isn't necessarily the way most consistent with long-term health.

FEEDING THE CHILDREN

So this was the climate at that time, and I was a part of it as much as anyone else. I left MIT to take a faculty position at Virginia Tech in 1965. Professor Charlie Engel, who was then the head of the Department of Biochemistry and Nutrition at Virginia Tech, had considerable interest in developing an international nutrition program for malnourished children. He was interested in implementing a "mothercraft" self-help project in the Philippines. This project was called "mothercraft" because it focused on educating mothers of malnourished children. The idea was that if mothers were taught that the right kinds of locally grown foods can make their children well, they would not have to rely on scarce medicines and the mostly nonexistent doctors. Engel started the program in 1967 and invited me to be his Campus Coordinator and to come for extended stays in the Philippines while he resided full-time in Manila.

Consistent with the emphasis on protein as a means of solving malnutrition, we had to make this nutrient the centerpiece of our educational mothercraft centers and thereby help to increase protein consumption. Fish as a source of protein was mostly limited to the seacoast areas. Our own preference was to develop peanuts as a source of protein because this crop could be grown most anywhere. The peanut is a legume, like alfalfa, soybeans, clover, peas, and other beans. Like these other nitrogen "fixers," peanuts are rich in protein.

There was, however, a nagging problem with these tasty legumes. Considerable evidence had been emerging, first from England[8-10] and later from MIT (the same lab that I had worked in),[11,12] to show that peanuts often were contaminated with a fungus-produced toxin called aflatoxin (AF). It was an alarming problem because AF was being shown to cause liver cancer in rats. It was said to be the most potent chemical carcinogen ever discovered.

So we had to tackle two closely related projects: alleviate childhood malnutrition and resolve the AF contamination problem.

Prior to going to the Philippines, I had traveled to Haiti to observe a few experimental mothercraft centers organized by my colleagues at Virginia Tech, Professors Ken King and Ryland Webb. It was my first trip to an underdeveloped country, and Haiti certainly fit the bill. Papa Doc Duvalier, president of Haiti, extracted what little resources the country had for his own rich lifestyle. In Haiti at that time 54% of the children were dead before reaching their fifth birthday, largely because of malnutrition.

I subsequently went to the Philippines and encountered more of the same. We decided where mothercraft centers were to be located based on how much malnutrition was present in each village. We focused our efforts on the villages in most need. In a preliminary survey in each village (barrio), children were weighed and their weight for age was compared with a Western reference standard, which was subdivided into first-, second-, and third-degree malnutrition. Third-degree malnutrition, the worst kind, represented children under the sixty-fifth percentile. Keep in mind that a child at the 100th percentile represents only the average for the U.S. Being less than the sixty-fifth percentile means near starvation.

In the urban areas of some of the big cities, as many as 15–20% of the children aged three to six years were judged to be third degree. I can so well remember some of my initial observations of these children. A mother, hardly more than a wisp herself, holding her three-year-old twins with bulging eyes, one at eleven pounds, the other at fourteen pounds, trying to get them to open their mouths to eat some porridge. Older children blind from malnutrition, being led around by their younger siblings to seek a handout. Children without legs or arms hoping to get a morsel of food.

A REVELATION TO DIE FOR

Needless to say, those sights gave us ample motivation to press ahead with our project. As I mentioned, we first had to resolve the problem of AF contamination in peanuts, our preferred protein food.

The first step of investigating AF was to gather some basic information. Who in the Philippines was consuming AF, and who was subject to liver cancer? To answer these questions, I applied for and received an NIH research grant. We also adopted a second strategy by asking another question: How does AF actually affect liver cancer? We wanted to study this question at the molecular level using laboratory rats. I succeeded in getting a second NIH grant for this in-depth biochemical research. These two grants initiated a two-track research investigation, one basic and one applied, which was to continue for the rest of my career. I found studying questions both from the basic and applied perspectives rewarding because it tells us not only the impact of a food or chemical on health, but also why it has that impact. In so doing, we could better understand not only the biochemical foundation of food and health, but also how it might relate to people in everyday life.

We began with a stepwise series of surveys. First, we wanted to know which foods contained the most AF. We learned that peanuts and corn were the foods most contaminated. All twenty-nine jars of peanut butter we had purchased in the local groceries, for example, were contaminated, with levels of AF as much as 300 times the amount judged to be acceptable in U.S. food. Whole peanuts were much less contaminated; none exceeded the AF amounts allowed in U.S. commodities. This disparity between peanut butter and whole peanuts originated at the peanut factory. The best peanuts, which filled "cocktail" jars, were hand-selected from a moving conveyor belt, leaving the worst, moldiest nuts to be delivered to the end of the belt to make peanut butter.

Our second question concerned who was most susceptible to this AF contamination and its cancer-producing effects. We learned that it was children. They were the ones consuming the AF-laced peanut butter. We estimated AF consumption by analyzing the excretion of AF metabolic products in the urine of children living in homes with a partially consumed peanut butter jar.[13] As we gathered this information, an interesting pattern emerged: the two areas of the country with the highest rates of liver cancer, the cities of Manila and Cebu, also were the same areas where the most AF was being consumed. Peanut butter was almost exclusively consumed in the Manila area while corn was consumed in Cebu, the second most populated city in the Philippines. But, as it turned out, there was more to this story. It emerged from my making the acquaintance of a prominent doctor,

Dr. Jose Caedo, who was an advisor to President Marcos. He told me that the liver cancer problem in the Philippines was quite serious. What was so devastating was that the disease was claiming the lives of children before the age of ten. Whereas in the West, this disease mostly strikes people only after forty years of age, Caedo told me that he had personally operated on children younger than four for liver cancer!

That alone was incredible, but what he then told me was even more striking: *the children who got liver cancer were from the best-fed families.* The families with the most money ate what we thought were the healthiest diets, the diets most like our own meaty American diets. *They consumed more protein than anyone else in the country (high-quality animal protein, at that), and yet they were the ones getting liver cancer!*

How could this be? Worldwide, liver cancer rates were highest in countries with the lowest average protein intake. It was therefore widely believed that this cancer was the result of a deficiency in protein. Further, the deficiency problem was a major reason we were working in the Philippines: to increase the consumption of protein by as many malnourished children as possible. But now Dr. Caedo and his colleagues were telling me that the most protein-rich children had the highest rates of liver cancer. This seemed strange to me, at first, but over time my own information increasingly confirmed their observations.

At that time, a research paper from India surfaced in an obscure medical journal.[14] It was an experiment involving liver cancer and protein consumption in two groups of laboratory rats. One group was given AF and then fed diets containing 20% protein. The second group was given the same level of AF and then fed diets containing only 5% protein. Every single rat fed 20% protein got liver cancer or its precursor lesions, but not a single animal fed a 5% protein diet got liver cancer or its precursor lesions. It was not a trivial difference; it was 100% versus 0%. This was very much consistent with my observations for the Philippine children. Those who were most vulnerable to liver cancer were those who consumed diets higher in protein.

No one seemed to accept the report from India. On a flight from Detroit after returning from a presentation at a conference, I traveled with a former but much senior colleague of mine from MIT, Professor Paul Newberne. At the time, Newberne was one of the only people who had given much thought to the role of nutrition in the development of cancer. I told him about my impressions in the Philippines and the paper from India. He summarily dismissed the paper by saying, "They must have gotten the numbers on the animal cages reversed. In no way could a high-protein diet increase the development of cancer."

I realized that I had encountered a provocative idea that stimulated the disbelief, even the ire, of fellow colleagues. Should I take seriously the observation that protein increased cancer development and run the risk of being thought a fool? Or should I turn my back on this story?

In some ways it seemed that this moment in my career had been foreshadowed by events in my personal life. When I was five years old, my aunt who was living with us was dying of cancer. On several occasions my uncle took my brother Jack and me to see his wife in the hospital. Although I was too young to understand everything that was happening, I do remember being struck by the big "C" word: cancer. I would think, "When I get big, I want to find a cure for cancer."

Many years later, just a few years after getting married, at about the time when I was starting my work in the Philippines, my wife's mother was dying of colon cancer at the young age of fifty-one. At that time, I was becoming aware of a possible diet–cancer connection in our early research. Her case was particularly difficult because she did not receive appropriate medical care due to the fact that she did not have health insurance. My wife, Karen, was her only daughter and they had a very close relationship. These difficult experiences were making my career choice easy: I would go wherever our research led me to help get a better understanding of this horrific disease.

Looking back on it, this was the beginning of my career focus on diet and cancer. The moment of deciding to investigate protein and cancer was the turning point. If I wanted to stay with this story, there was only one solution: start doing fundamental laboratory research to see not only if, but also how, consuming more protein leads to more cancer. That's exactly what I did. It took me further than I had ever imagined. The extraordinary findings my colleagues, students, and I generated just might make you think twice about your current diet. But even more than that, the findings led to broader questions, questions that would eventually lead to cracks in the very foundations of nutrition and health.

THE NATURE OF SCIENCE—WHAT YOU NEED TO KNOW TO FOLLOW THE RESEARCH

Proof in science is elusive. Even more than in the "core" sciences of biology, chemistry, and physics, establishing absolute proof in medicine and health is nearly impossible. The primary objective of research investigation is to determine only what is *likely* to be true. This is because research into health is inherently statistical. When you throw a ball in the air, will it come down? Yes, every time. That's physics. If you smoke four packs a day, will you get lung cancer? The answer is maybe. We know that your odds of getting lung cancer are much higher than if you didn't smoke, and we can tell you what those odds (statistics) are, but we can't know with certainty whether you as an individual will get lung cancer.

In nutrition research, untangling the relationship between diet and health is not so straightforward. Humans live all sorts of different ways, have different genetic backgrounds, and eat all sorts of different foods. Experimental limitations such as cost restraints, time constraints, and measurement error are significant obstacles. Perhaps most importantly, food, lifestyle, and health interact through such complex, multifaceted systems that establishing proof for any one factor and any one disease is nearly impossible, even if you had the perfect set of subjects, unlimited time, and unlimited financial resources.

Because of these difficulties, we do research using many different strategies. In some cases, we assess whether a hypothetical cause produces a hypothetical effect by *observing* and measuring the differences that already exist between different groups of people. We might *observe* and compare societies who consume different amounts of fat, then *observe* whether these differences correspond to similar differences in the rates of breast cancer or osteoporosis or some other disease condition. We might *observe* and compare the dietary characteristics of people who already have the disease with a comparable group of people who don't. We might *observe* and compare disease rates in 1950 with disease rates in 1990, then *observe* whether any changes in disease rates correspond to dietary changes.

In addition to *observing* what already exists, we might do an experiment and intentionally *intervene* with a hypothetical treatment to see what happens. We intervene, for example, when testing for the safety and efficacy of drugs. One group of people is given the drug and a second group a placebo (an inactive look-alike substance to please the patient). *Intervening* with diet, however, is far more difficult, especially if people aren't confined to a clinical setting, because then we must rely on everyone to faithfully use the specified diets.

As we do *observational* and *interventional* research, we begin to amass the findings and weigh the evidence for or against a certain hypothesis. When the weight of the evidence favors an idea so strongly that it can no longer be plausibly denied, we advance the idea as a likely truth. It is in this way that I am advancing an argument for a whole foods, plant-based diet (WFPB). As you continue reading, realize that those seeking absolute proof of optimal nutrition in one or two studies will be disappointed and confused. However, I am confident that those seeking the truth regarding diet and health by surveying the weight of the evidence from the variety of available studies will be amazed and enlightened. There are several ideas to keep in mind when determining the weight of the evidence, including the following.

CORRELATION VERSUS CAUSATION

In many studies, you will find that the words *correlation* and *association* are used to describe a relationship between two factors, perhaps even indicating a cause-and-effect relationship. This idea is featured prominently in the China Study. We observed whether there were patterns of associations for different dietary, lifestyle, and disease characteristics within the survey of 65 counties, 130 villages, and 6,500 adults and their families. If protein consumption, for example, is higher among populations that have a *high* incidence of liver cancer, we can say that protein is *positively* correlated or associated with liver cancer incidence; as one goes up, the other goes up. If protein intake is higher among populations that have a *low* incidence of liver cancer, we can say that protein is *inversely* associated with liver cancer incidence. In other words, the two factors go in the opposite direction; as one goes up, the other goes down.

In our hypothetical example, if protein is correlated with liver cancer incidence, this does not prove that protein causes or prevents liver cancer. A classic illustration of this difficulty is that countries with more telephone poles often have a higher incidence of heart disease, and many other diseases. Therefore, telephone poles and heart disease are positively correlated. But this does not prove that telephone poles cause heart disease. In effect, correlation does not equal causation.

This does not mean that correlations are useless. When they are properly interpreted, correlations can be effectively used to study nutrition and health relationships. The China Study, for example, has over 8,000 statistically significant correlations, and this is of immense value. When so many correlations like this are available, researchers can begin to identify patterns of relationships between diet, lifestyle, and disease. These patterns, in turn, are representative of how diet and health processes, which are unusually complex, truly operate. However, if someone wants proof that a single factor causes a single outcome, a correlation is not good enough.

STATISTICAL SIGNIFICANCE

You might think that deciding whether or not two factors are correlated is obvious—either they are or they aren't. But that isn't the case. When you are looking at a large quantity of data, you have to undertake a statistical analysis to determine if two factors are correlated. The answer isn't yes or no. It's a probability, which we call *statistical significance*. Statistical significance is a measure of whether an observed experimental effect is truly reliable or whether it is merely due to the play of chance. If you flip a coin three times and it lands on heads each time, it's probably chance. If you flip it a hundred times and it lands on heads each time, you can be pretty sure the coin has heads on both sides. That's the concept behind *statistical significance*—it's the odds that the correlation (or other finding) is real, that it isn't just random chance.

A finding is said to be statistically significant when there is less than 5% probability that it is due to chance. This means, for example, that there is a 95% chance that we will get the same result if the study is repeated. This 95% cutoff point is arbitrary, but it is the standard, nonetheless. Another arbitrary cutoff point is 99%. In this case, when the result meets this test, it is said to be highly *statistically significant*. In the discussions of diet and disease research in this book, statistical significance pops up from time to time, and it can be used to help judge the reliability, or "weight," of the evidence.

MECHANISMS OF ACTION

Oftentimes correlations are considered more reliable if other research shows that two correlated factors are biologically related. For example, telephone poles and heart disease are positively correlated, but there is no research that shows how telephone poles are biologically related to heart disease. However, there is research that shows the processes by which protein intake and liver cancer might be biologically and causally related (as you will see in chapter three). Knowing the process by which something works in the body means knowing its "mechanism of action." And knowing its mechanism of action strengthens the evidence. Another way of saying this is that the two correlated factors are related in a "biologically plausible" way. If a relationship is biologically plausible, it is considered much more reliable.

META-ANALYSIS

Finally, we should understand the concept of a meta-analysis. A meta-analysis tabulates the combined data from multiple studies and analyzes them as one data set. By accumulating and analyzing a large body of combined data, the result can have considerably more weight. Meta-analysis findings are therefore more substantial than the findings of single research studies, although, as with everything else, there may be exceptions.

After obtaining the results from a variety of studies, we can then begin to use these tools and concepts to assess the weight of the evidence. Through this effort, we can begin to understand what is most likely to be true, and we can behave accordingly. Alternative hypotheses no longer seem plausible, and we can be very confident in the result. Absolute proof, in the technical sense, is unattainable and unimportant. But commonsense proof (99% certainty) is attainable and critical. For example, it was through this process of interpreting research that we formed our beliefs regarding smoking and health. Smoking has never been "100%" proven to cause lung cancer, but the odds that smoking is unrelated to lung cancer are so astronomically low that the matter has long been considered settled.

TURNING OFF
CANCER

Americans dread cancer more than any other disease. Slowly and painfully being consumed by cancer for months, even years, before passing away is a terrifying prospect. This is why cancer is perhaps the most feared of the major diseases.

So when the media reports a newly found chemical carcinogen, the public takes notice and reacts quickly. Some carcinogens cause outright panic. Such was the case a few years ago with Alar, a chemical that was routinely sprayed on apples as a growth regulator. Shortly after a report from the Natural Resources Defense Council titled "Intolerable Risk: Pesticides in Our Children's Food,"[1] the CBS television program *60 Minutes* aired a segment on Alar. In February 1989 a representative of the Council said on *60 Minutes* that the apple industry chemical was "the most potent carcinogen in the food supply."[2,3]

The public reaction was swift. One woman called state police to chase down a school bus to confiscate her child's apple.[4] School systems across the country, in New York, Los Angeles, Atlanta, and Chicago, among others, stopped serving apples and apple products. According to John Rice, former chairman of the U.S. Apple Association, the apple industry took an economic walloping, losing over $250 million.[5] Finally, in response to the public outcry, the production and use of Alar came to a halt in June of 1989.[3]

The Alar story is not uncommon. Over the past several decades, several chemicals have been identified in the popular press as cancer-causing agents. You may have heard of some:

- Aminotriazole (herbicide used on cranberry crops, causing the "cranberry scare" of 1959)

- DDT (widely known after Rachel Carson's book *Silent Spring*)
- Nitrites (a meat preservative and color and flavor enhancer used in hot dogs and bacon)
- Red Dye Number 2
- Artificial sweeteners (including cyclamates and saccharin)
- Dioxin (a contaminant of industrial processes and of Agent Orange, a defoliant used during the Vietnam War)
- Aflatoxin (a fungal toxin found on moldy peanuts and corn)

I know these unsavory chemicals quite well. I was a member of the National Academy of Sciences Expert Panel on Saccharin and Food Safety Policy (1978–79), which was charged with evaluating the potential danger of saccharin at a time when the public was up in arms after the FDA proposed banning the artificial sweetener. I was one of the first scientists to isolate dioxin; I have firsthand knowledge of the MIT lab that did the key work on nitrites; and I spent many years researching and publishing on aflatoxin, one of the most carcinogenic chemicals ever discovered—at least for rats.

But while these chemicals are significantly different in their biochemical properties, they all have a similar story with regard to cancer. In each and every case, research has demonstrated that these chemicals may increase cancer rates in experimental animals. The case of nitrites serves as an excellent example.

THE HOT DOG MISSILE

If you hazard to call yourself "middle-aged" or older, when I say, "Nitrites, hot dogs, and cancer," you might rock back in your chair, nod your head, and say, "Oh yeah, I remember something about that." For the younger folks—well, listen up, because history has a funny way of repeating itself.

The time: the early 1970s. The scene: the Vietnam War was beginning to wind down, Richard Nixon was about to be forever linked to Watergate, the energy crisis was about to create lines at gas stations, and nitrite was becoming a headline word.

> *Sodium Nitrite:* A meat preservative used since the 1920s.[6] It kills bacteria and adds a happy pink color and desirable taste to hot dogs, bacon, and canned meat.

In 1970, the journal *Nature* reported that the nitrite we consume may be reacting in our bodies to form nitrosamines.[7]

Nitrosamines: A scary family of chemicals. No fewer than seventeen nitrosamines are "reasonably anticipated to be human carcinogens" by the U.S. National Toxicology Program.[8]

Hold on a second. Why are these scary nitrosamines "anticipated to be human carcinogens"? The short answer: animal experiments have shown that as chemical exposure increases, incidence of cancer also increases. But that's not adequate. We need a more complete answer.

Let's look at one nitrosamine, NSAR (N-nitrososarcosine). In one study, twenty rats were divided into two groups, each exposed to a different level of NSAR. The high-dose rats were given twice the amount that the low-dose rats received. Of rats given the lower level of NSAR, just over 35% of them died from throat cancer. Of rats given the higher levels, 100% died of cancer during the second year of the experiment.[9–11]

How much NSAR did the rats get? Both groups of rats were given an incredible amount. Let me translate the "low" dose by giving you a little scenario. Let's say you go over to your friend's house to eat every meal. This friend is sick of you and wants to give you throat cancer by exposing you to NSAR. So he gives you the equivalent of the "low" level given to the rats. You go to his house, and your friend offers you a bologna sandwich that has a whole pound of bologna on it! You eat it. He offers you another, and another, and another . . . You'll have to eat 270,000 bologna sandwiches before your friend lets you leave.[9,12] You better like bologna, because your friend is going to have to feed you this way every day for over thirty years! If he does this, you will have had about as much exposure to NSAR (per body weight) as the rats in the "low"-dose group.

Because higher cancer rates were also seen in mice as well as rats, using a variety of methods of exposure, NSAR is "reasonably anticipated" to be a human carcinogen. Although no human studies were used to make this evaluation, it is likely that a chemical such as this, which consistently causes cancer in both mice and rats, can cause cancer in humans at some level. It is impossible to know, however, what this level of exposure might be, especially because the animal dosages are so astronomical. Nonetheless, animal experiments alone are considered enough to conclude that NSAR is "reasonably anticipated" to be a human carcinogen.[9]

So, in 1970, when an article in the prestigious journal *Nature* concluded that nitrites help to form nitrosamines in the body, thereby implying that they help to cause cancer, people became alarmed. Here was the official line: "Reduction of human exposure to nitrites and certain secondary amines, particularly in foods, may result in a decrease in the incidence of human cancer."[7] Suddenly nitrites became a potential killer. Because we humans get exposed to nitrites through consumption of processed meat such as hot dogs and bacon, some products came under fire. Hot dogs were an easy target. Besides containing additives like nitrites, hot dogs can be made out of ground-up lips, snouts, spleens, tongues, throats, and other "variety meats."[13] So as the nitrite/nitrosamine issue heated up, hot dogs weren't looking so hot. Ralph Nader had called hot dogs "among America's deadliest missiles."[14] Some consumer advocacy groups were calling for a nitrite additive ban, and government officials began a serious review of nitrite's potential health problems.[3]

The issue jolted forward again in 1978, when a study at the Massachusetts Institute of Technology (MIT) found that nitrite increased lymphatic cancer in rats. The study, as reported in a 1979 issue of *Science*,[15] found that, on average, rats fed nitrite got lymphatic cancer 10.2% of the time, while animals not fed nitrite got cancer only 5.4% of the time. This finding was enough to create a public uproar. Fierce debate ensued in the government, industry, and research communities. When the dust settled, expert panels made recommendations, industry cut back on nitrite usage, and the issue fell out of the spotlight.

To summarize the story: marginal scientific results can make very big waves in the public when it comes to cancer-causing chemicals. A rise in cancer incidence from 5% to 10% in rats fed large quantities of nitrite caused an explosive controversy. Undoubtedly millions of dollars were spent following the MIT study to investigate and discuss the findings. And NSAR, a nitrosamine possibly formed from nitrite, was "reasonably anticipated to be a human carcinogen" after several animal experiments where exceptionally high levels of chemical were fed to animals for almost half their life span.

BACK TO PROTEIN

The point isn't that nitrite is safe. It is the mere possibility, however unlikely it may be, that it could cause cancer that alarms the public. But what if researchers produced considerably more impressive scientific results that were far more substantial? What if there was a chemical that experimentally turned on cancer in 100% of the test animals and its relative absence limited cancer to 0% of the animals? Furthermore, what if this chemical were capable of acting in this way at routine levels of intake and not the extraordinary levels used in the NSAR experiments? Finding such a chemical would be the holy grail of cancer research. The implications for human health would be enormous. One would assume that this chemical would be of considerably more concern than nitrite and Alar, and even more significant than aflatoxin, a highly ranked carcinogen.

This is exactly what I saw in the Indian research paper[16] when I was in the Philippines. The chemical was protein, fed to rats at levels that are well within the range of normal consumption. Protein! These results were more than startling. In the Indian study, when all the rats had been predisposed to get liver cancer after being given aflatoxin, only the animals fed 20% protein got the cancer while those fed 5% got none.

Scientists, myself included, tend to be a skeptical bunch, especially when confronted with eye-popping results. In fact, it is our responsibility as researchers to question and explore such provocative findings. We might suspect that this finding was unique to rats exposed to aflatoxin and for no other species, including humans. Maybe there were other unknown nutrients that were affecting the data. Maybe my friend, the distinguished MIT professor, was right; maybe the animal identities in the Indian study got mixed up.

The questions begged for answers. To further study this question, I sought and received the two NIH research grants that I mentioned earlier. One was for a human study, the other for an experimental animal study. I did not "cry wolf" in either application by suggesting that protein might promote cancer. I had everything to lose and nothing to gain by acting like a heretic. Besides, I wasn't convinced that protein actually might be harmful. In the experimental animal study, I proposed to investigate the "effect of *various factors* [my italics] on aflatoxin metabolism." The human study mostly focused on aflatoxin's effects on liver cancer in the Philippines, was briefly reviewed in the last chapter, and was concluded after three years. It was later reconsidered in a much more sophisticated study in China (chapter four).

A study of this protein effect on tumor development had to be done extremely well. Anything less would not have convinced anyone, especially my peers, who would review my future request for renewed funding! In hindsight, we must have succeeded. The NIH funding for this study continued for the next twenty-four years and led to additional funding from other research agencies (the American Cancer Society, the American Institute for Cancer Research, and the Cancer Research Foundation of America). On these experimental animal findings alone, this project gave rise to more than 100 scientific papers published in some of the best journals, many public presentations, and several invitations to participate on expert panels.

ANIMAL RIGHTS

The rest of this chapter concerns experimental animal research, all of which has included rodents (rats and mice). I know well that many oppose the use of experimental animals in research. I respect this concern. I respectfully suggest, however, that you consider this: very likely, I would not be advocating a plant-based diet today if it were not for these animal experiments. The findings and the principles derived from these animal studies greatly contributed to my interpretations of my later work, including the China Study, as you will come to see.

One obvious question regarding this issue is whether there was an alternative way to get the same information without using experimental animals. To date, I have found none, even after seeking advice from my animal rights colleagues. These experimental animal studies elaborated some very important principles of cancer causation not obtainable in human-based studies. These principles now have enormous potential to benefit all of our fellow creatures, our environment, and ourselves.

THREE STAGES OF CANCER

Cancer proceeds through three stages: initiation, promotion, and progression. To use a rough analogy, the cancer process is similar to planting a lawn. *Initiation* is when you put the seeds in the soil, *promotion* is when the grass starts to grow, and *progression* is when the grass gets completely out of control, invading the driveway, the shrubbery, and the sidewalk.

So what is the process that successfully "implants" the grass seed in the soil in the first place—that is, initiates cancer-prone cells? Chemicals that do this are called carcinogens. These chemicals are most often the by-products of industrial processes, although small amounts may be formed in nature, as is the case with aflatoxin. These carcinogens genetically transform, or mutate, normal cells into cancer-prone cells. A mutation involves permanent alteration of the genes of the cell, with damage to its DNA.

The entire initiation stage (Chart 3.1) can take place in a very short period of time, even minutes. It is the time required for the chemical carcinogen to be consumed, absorbed into the blood, transported into cells, changed into its active product, bonded to DNA, and passed on to the daughter cells. When the new daughter cells are formed, the process is complete. These daughter cells and all their progeny will forever be genetically

Chart 3.1: Tumor Initiation by Aflatoxin Inside a Liver Cell

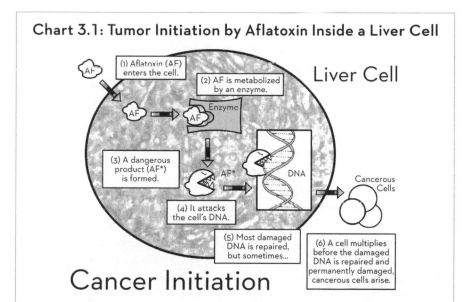

(1) Aflatoxin (AF) enters the cell.

(2) AF is metabolized by an enzyme.

Liver Cell

Enzyme

(3) A dangerous product (AF*) is formed.

DNA

Cancerous Cells

(4) It attacks the cell's DNA.

(5) Most damaged DNA is repaired, but sometimes...

(6) A cell multiplies before the damaged DNA is repaired and permanently damaged, cancerous cells arise.

Cancer Initiation

After entering our cells (Step 1) most carcinogens do not, themselves, initiate the cancer process. They first must be converted to products that are more reactive (Steps 2 & 3), with the help of critically important enzymes. These carcinogen products then bind tightly to the cell's DNA to form carcinogen-DNA complexes, or adducts (Step 4).

Unless repaired or removed, carcinogen-DNA adducts have the potential to create chaos with the genetic workings of the cell. But nature is smart. These adducts can be repaired, and most adducts are repaired fairly quickly (Step 5). However, if they remain in place while cells are dividing to form new "daughter" cells, genetic damage occurs and this new genetic defect (or mutation) is passed on to all new cells formed thereafter (Step 6).[17]

damaged, giving rise to the potential for cancer. Except in rare instances, completion of the initiation phase is considered irreversible.

At this point in our lawn analogy, the grass seeds have been put in the soil and are ready to germinate. Initiation is complete. The second growth stage is called promotion. Like seeds ready to sprout blades of grass and turn into a green lawn, our newly formed cancer-prone cells are ready to grow and multiply until they become a visibly detectable cancer. This stage occurs over a far longer period of time than initiation, often many years for humans. It is when the newly initiated cluster multiplies and grows into larger and larger masses and a clinically visible tumor is formed.

But just like seeds in the soil, the initial cancer cells will not grow and multiply unless the right conditions are met. The seeds in the soil, for example, need a healthy amount of water, sunlight, and other nutrients before they make a full lawn. If any of these factors are denied or are missing, the seeds will not grow. If any of these factors are missing after growth starts, the new seedlings will become dormant, while awaiting further supply of the missing factors. This is one of the most profound features of promotion. *Promotion is reversible, depending on whether the early cancer growth is given the right conditions in which to grow.* This is where certain dietary factors become so important. These dietary factors, called promoters, feed cancer growth. Other dietary factors, called anti-promoters, slow cancer growth. Cancer growth flourishes when there are more promoters than anti-promoters; when anti-promoters prevail, cancer growth slows or stops. It is a push-pull process. The profound importance of this reversibility cannot be overemphasized.

The third phase, progression, begins when a bunch of advanced cancer cells progress in their growth until they have done their final damage. It is like the fully grown lawn invading everything around it: the garden, driveway, and sidewalk. Similarly, a developing cancer tumor may wander away from its initial site in the body and invade neighboring or distant tissues. When the cancer takes on these deadly properties, it is considered malignant. When it actually breaks away from its initial home and wanders, it is metastasizing. This final stage of cancer results in death.

At the start of our research, the stages of cancer formation were known only in vague outline. But we knew enough about these stages of cancer to be able to structure our research more intelligently. We had no shortage of questions. Could we confirm the findings from India that a low-protein diet represses tumor formation? More importantly, why does protein affect the cancer process? What are the mechanisms; that is, how does protein work? With plenty of questions to be answered, we went about our experimental studies meticulously and in depth to obtain results that would withstand the harshest of scrutiny.

PROTEIN AND INITIATION

How does protein intake affect cancer initiation? Our first test was to see whether protein intake affected the enzyme principally responsible for aflatoxin metabolism, the mixed function oxidase (MFO). This enzyme is very complex because it also metabolizes pharmaceuticals and other chemicals, friend or foe, to the body. Paradoxically, this enzyme both detoxifies and activates aflatoxin. It is an extraordinary transformation substance.

THE ENZYME "FACTORY"

(1) Aflatoxin (AF) enters the cell.

(2) AF is metabolizes by an enzyme.

AF

AF → AF Enzyme

In a simplistic way, the MFO enzyme system can be thought of as a factory within the industrious workings of the cell. Various chemical "raw materials" are fed into the factory, where all the complex reactions are performed. The raw materials may be disassembled or assembled. After a transforming process, the raw material chemicals are ready to be shipped out of the factory as mostly normal, safe products. But there also may be by-products of these complex processes that are exceptionally dangerous. Think of the smokestack at a real-life factory. If someone told you to stick your face down a smokestack and breathe deeply for a couple hours, you'd refuse. Within the cell, the dangerous by-products, if not held in check, are the highly reactive aflatoxin metabolites that go on to attack the cell's DNA and damage its genetic blueprint.

At the time we started our research, we hypothesized that the protein we consume alters tumor growth by changing how aflatoxin is detoxified by the enzymes present in the liver.

We initially determined whether the amount of protein that we eat could change this enzyme activity. After a series of experiments (Chart 3.2[18]), the answer was clear. Enzyme activity could be easily modified simply by changing the level of protein intake.[18–21]

Decreasing protein intake like that done in the original research in India (20% to 5%) not only greatly decreased enzyme activity, but did so very quickly.[22] What does this mean? Decreasing enzyme activity via low-protein diets implied that less aflatoxin was being transformed into the dangerous aflatoxin metabolite that had the potential to bind and to mutate the DNA.

We decided to test this implication: Did a low-protein diet actually decrease the binding of aflatoxin product to DNA, resulting in fewer adducts? An undergraduate student in my lab, Rachel Preston, did the experiment (Chart 3.3) and showed that the lower the protein intake, the lower the amount of aflatoxin-DNA adducts.[23]

Chart 3.2: Effect of Dietary Protein on Enzyme Activity

Chart 3.3: Decrease in Carcinogen Binding to Nucleus Components Caused by Low-Protein Feeding

We now had impressive evidence that low protein intake could markedly decrease enzyme activity and prevent dangerous carcinogen binding to DNA. These were very impressive findings, to be sure. It might even be enough information to "explain" how consuming less protein leads to less cancer. But we wanted to know more and be doubly assured of this effect, so we continued to look for other explanations. As time passed, we were to learn something really quite remarkable. Almost every time we searched for a way, or mechanism, by which protein works to produce its effects, we found one! For example, we came to discover that low-protein diets, or their equivalents, reduce tumors by the following mechanisms:

- less aflatoxin entered the cell[24-26]
- cells multiplied more slowly[18]
- multiple changes occurred within the enzyme complex to reduce its activity[27]
- the quantity of critical components of the relevant enzymes was reduced[28, 29]
- less aflatoxin-DNA adducts were formed[23, 30]

The fact that we found more than one way (mechanism) that low-protein diets work was eye-opening. It added a great deal of weight to the results of the Indian researchers. It also suggested that biological effects, although often described as operating through single reactions, more likely operate through a large number of varied simultaneous reactions, very likely acting in a highly integrated and concerted manner. Could this mean that the body had lots of backup systems in case one was bypassed in some way? As research unfolded in the subsequent years, the truth of this thesis became increasingly evident.

From our extensive research, one idea seemed to be clear: lower protein intake dramatically decreased tumor initiation. This finding, even though well substantiated, would be enormously provocative for many people—so much so that few if any professionals in this area of science want to talk about it or even acknowledge its existence. Such an observation—that increased consumption of protein was capable of initiating the first stage of cancer—questioned our worship of this nutrient, so it had to be wrong!

PROTEIN AND PROMOTION

To go back to the lawn analogy, sowing the grass seeds in the soil was the initiation process. We found, conclusively, through a number of experiments, that a low-protein diet could decrease, at the time of planting, the number of seeds in our "cancerous" lawn. That was an incredible finding, but we needed to do more. We wondered: What happens during the promotion stage of cancer, the all-important reversible stage? Would the benefits of low protein intake achieved during initiation continue through promotion?

Practically speaking, it was difficult to study this stage of cancer because of time and money. It is an expensive study that allows rats to live until they develop full tumors. Each such experiment would take more than two years (the normal lifetime of rats) and would have cost well over $100,000 (even more money today). To answer the many questions that we had, we could not proceed by studying full tumor development; I would still be in the lab, thirty-five years later!

This is when we learned of some exciting work just published by others[31] that showed how to measure tiny clusters of cancer-like cells that appear right after initiation is complete. These little microscopic cell clusters were called foci.

Foci are precursor clusters of cells that grow into tumors. Although most foci do not become full-blown tumor cells, they are predictive of tumor development.

By watching foci develop and measuring how many there are and how big they become,[32] we could learn indirectly how tumors also develop and what effect protein might have. By studying the effects of protein on the promotion of foci instead of tumors, we could avoid spending a lifetime and a few million dollars working in the lab.

What we found was truly remarkable. *Foci development was almost entirely dependent on how much protein was consumed, regardless of how much aflatoxin was consumed!*

This was documented in many interesting ways, first done by my graduate students Scott Appleton[33] and George Dunaif[34] (a typical comparison is shown in Chart 3.4). After initiation with aflatoxin, foci grew (were promoted) far more with the 20% protein diet than with the 5% protein diet.[33,34]

Chart 3.4: Dietary Protein and Foci Formation

Chart 3.5: Carcinogen Dose Versus Protein Intake

Up to this point, all of the animals were exposed to the same amount of aflatoxin. But what if the initial aflatoxin exposure is varied? Would protein still have an effect? We investigated this question by giving two groups of rats either a high-aflatoxin dose or a low-aflatoxin dose, along with a standard baseline diet. Because of this, the two groups of rats were starting the cancer process with different amounts of initiated, cancerous "seeds." Then, during the promotion phase, we fed a low-protein diet to the high-aflatoxin-dose groups and a high-protein diet to the low-aflatoxin-dose group. We wondered whether the animals that start with lots of cancerous seeds are able to overcome their predicament by eating a low-protein diet.

Again, the results were remarkable (Chart 3.5). Animals starting with the most cancer initiation (high-aflatoxin dose) developed *substantially less foci* when fed the 5% protein diet. In contrast, animals initiated with a low-aflatoxin dose actually produced *substantially more foci* when subsequently fed the 20% protein diet.

A principle was being established. Foci development, initially determined by the amount of the carcinogen exposure, is actually controlled far more by dietary protein consumed during promotion. Protein during promotion trumps the carcinogen, regardless of initial exposure.

With this background information, we designed a much more substantial experiment. Here is a step-by-step sequence of experiments, carried out by my graduate student Linda Youngman.[35] All animals were dosed with the same amount of carcinogen, then alternately fed either 5% or 20% dietary protein during the twelve-week promotion stage. We divided this twelve-week promotion stage into four periods of three weeks each. Period 1 represents weeks one to three, period 2 represents weeks four to six, and so on.

When animals were fed the 20% protein diet during periods 1 and 2 (20-20), foci continued to enlarge, as expected. But when animals were switched to the low-protein diet at the beginning of period 3 (20-20-5), there was a sharp decrease in foci development. And, when animals were subsequently switched back to the 20% protein diet during period 4 (20-20-5-20), foci development was turned on once again.

In another experiment, in animals fed 20% dietary protein during period 1 but switched to 5% dietary protein during period 2 (20-5), foci development was sharply decreased. But when these animals were returned to 20% dietary protein during period 3 (20-5-20), we again saw the dramatic power of dietary protein to promote foci development.

These several experiments, taken together, were quite profound. Foci growth could be reversed, up and down, by switching the amount of protein being consumed, and at all stages of foci development.

These experiments also demonstrated that the body could "remember" early carcinogen insults,[35,36] even though they might then lie dormant with low protein intake. That is, exposure to aflatoxin left a genetic "imprint" that remained dormant with 5% dietary protein until nine weeks later, when this imprint reawakened to form foci with 20% dietary protein. In simple terms, the body holds a grudge. It suggests that if we are exposed in the past to a carcinogen that initiates a bit of cancer that remains dormant, this cancer can still be "reawakened" by bad nutrition at a later point in time.

These studies showed that cancer development is modified by relatively modest changes in protein consumption. But how much protein is too much or too little? Using rats, we investigated a range of 4–24% dietary protein (Chart 3.6[37]). Foci did not develop with up to about 10% dietary protein. Beyond 10%, foci development increased dramatically with increases in dietary protein. The results were later repeated a second time in my laboratory by a visiting professor from Japan, Fumiyiki Horio.[38]

The most significant finding of this experiment was this: foci developed only when the animals met or exceeded the amount of dietary protein (12%) needed to satisfy their body growth rate.[39] That is, when the animals met and surpassed their requirement for protein, disease onset began.

This finding may have considerable relevance for humans even though these were rat studies. I say this because the protein required for growth in young rats and humans as well as the protein required to maintain health for adult rats and humans is remarkably similar.[40,41]

According to the recommended daily allowance (RDA) for protein consumption, we humans should be getting about 10% of our energy from

Chart 3.6: Foci Promotion by Dietary Protein

protein. This is considerably more than the actual amount required (about 5–6%). But because requirements may vary from individual to individual, 10% dietary protein is recommended to ensure adequate intake for virtually all people (note the difference between "requirement" and "recommendation"). What do most of us routinely consume? Remarkably, it is considerably more than the recommended 10%. The average American consumes 15–16% protein, while the government recommends levels as high as 17–21%. Does this place us at risk for getting cancer? These animal studies suggest that it does so—not necessarily due only to the specific effects of protein, but also to the displacement of those foods that oppose this protein effect.

Ten percent dietary protein is equivalent to eating about 50–60 grams of protein per day, depending on body weight and total calorie intake. The national average of 15–16% is about 70–100 grams of protein per day, with men at the upper part of the range and women at the lower end. In food terms, there are about twelve grams of protein in 100 calories of spinach (fifteen ounces) and five grams of protein in 100 calories of raw chickpeas (just over two tablespoons). There are about thirteen grams of protein in 100 calories of porterhouse steak (just over one and a half ounces). (Later in this chapter, we will show the consequences of our choosing how much and what kind of protein to consume.)

Yet another research question of ours was whether protein consumption could modify the all-important relationship between aflatoxin dose and foci formation. A chemical is usually not considered a carcinogen unless higher doses yield higher incidences of cancer. For example, as the aflatoxin dose becomes greater, foci and tumor growth should be correspondingly greater. If an increasing response is not observed for a suspect chemical carcinogen, serious doubt arises whether it really is carcinogenic.

To investigate this dose-response question, ten groups of rats were administered increasing doses of aflatoxin, then fed either regular levels (20%) or low levels (5–10%) of protein during the promotion period (Chart 3.7[34]).

Chart 3.7: Aflatoxin Dose—Foci Response

Legend:
- 20% Protein
- 5% Protein

Y-axis: Foci Response
X-axis: 200, 235, 275, 300, 350
Aflatoxin Dose (mcg/kg body weight/day)

In the animals fed the 20% level of protein, foci increased in number and size, as expected, when the aflatoxin dose was increased. The dose-response relationship was strong and clear. However, in the animals fed 5% protein, *the dose-response curve completely disappeared.* There was no foci response, even when animals were given the maximum tolerated aflatoxin dose. This was yet another result demonstrating that a low-protein diet could override the cancer-causing effect of a very powerful carcinogen, aflatoxin.

Is it possible that chemical carcinogens, in general, do not cause cancer unless the nutritional conditions are "right"? Is it possible that, for much of our lives, we are being exposed to small amounts of cancer-causing chemicals, but cancer does not occur unless we consume foods that promote and nurture tumor development? Can we control cancer through nutrition?

NOT ALL PROTEINS ARE ALIKE

If you have followed the story so far, you have seen how provocative these findings are. Controlling cancer through nutrition was, and still is, a radical idea. But as if this weren't enough, one more issue would yield explosive information: Did it make any difference what type of protein was used in these experiments? For all of these experiments, we were using casein, which makes up 80–85% of cow's milk protein. So the next logical question was whether plant protein, tested in the same way, has the same effect on cancer promotion as casein. The answer is an astonishing "NO." *In these experiments, plant protein did not promote cancer growth, even at the higher levels of intake.* An undergraduate premedical student doing an honors degree with me, David Schulsinger, did the study (Chart 3.8[42]). *Gluten, the protein of wheat, did not produce the same result as casein, even when fed at the same 20% level.*

Chart 3.8: Protein Type and Foci Response

We also examined whether soy protein had the same effect as casein on foci development. Rats fed 20% soy protein diets did not form early foci, just like the 20% wheat protein diets. Suddenly protein, milk protein in this case, wasn't looking so good. We had discovered that low protein intake reduces cancer initiation and works in multiple synchronous ways. As if that weren't enough, we were finding that high protein intake, in excess of the amount needed for growth, promotes cancer after initiation. Like flipping a light switch on and off, we could control cancer promotion merely by changing levels of protein, regardless of initial carcinogen exposure. But the cancer-promoting factor in this case was cow's milk protein. It was difficult enough for my colleagues to accept the idea that protein might help cancer grow, but cow's milk protein? Was I crazy?

ADDITIONAL QUESTIONS

For those readers who want to know somewhat more, I've included a few questions in Appendix A.

THE GRAND FINALE

Thus far we had relied on experiments where we measured only the early indicators of tumor development, the early cancer-like foci. Now, it was time to do the big study, the one where we would measure complete tumor formation. We organized a very large study of several hundred rats and examined tumor formation over their lifetimes using several different approaches.[36,43]

The effects of protein feeding on tumor development were nothing less than spectacular. Rats generally live for about two years; thus the study was 100 weeks in length. All animals that were administered aflatoxin and fed the regular 20% levels of casein either were dead or near death from liver tumors at 100 weeks.[36,43] All animals administered the same level of aflatoxin but fed the low 5% protein diet were alive and active, with sleek hair coats, at 100 weeks. This was a virtual 100 to 0 score, something almost never seen in research and almost identical to the original research in India.[16]

In this same experiment,[36] we switched the diets of some rats at either forty or sixty weeks, to again investigate the reversibility of cancer promotion. Animals switched from a high-protein to a low-protein diet had significantly less tumor growth (35–40% less!) than animals fed a high-protein diet. Animals switched from a low-protein diet to a high-protein diet halfway through their lifetime started growing tumors again. These findings involving

Chart 3.9a: Tumor Development at 100 Weeks

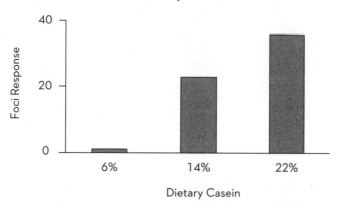

Chart 3.9b: Early Foci, "Lifetime"

full-blown tumors confirmed our earlier findings using foci—namely, nutritional manipulation can turn cancer "on" and "off."

We also measured early cancer growth, or foci, in these "lifetime" studies to see if their response to dietary protein was similar to that of subsequent cancer growth. The correspondence between foci growth and tumor growth could not have been more impressive (Chart 3.9A).[36, 43] The development of foci was impressively predictive of later cancer growth.

How much more did we need to find out? I would never have dreamed that our results up to this point would be so incredibly consistent, biologically plausible, and statistically significant. We had fully confirmed the original work from India and had done it in exceptional depth.

Let there be no doubt: cow's milk protein is an exceptionally potent cancer promoter in rats dosed with aflatoxin. The fact that this promotion effect occurs at dietary protein levels (10–20%) commonly used both in rodents and humans makes it especially tantalizing—and provocative.

OTHER CANCERS, OTHER CARCINOGENS

Okay, so here's the central question: How does this research apply to human health and human liver cancer in particular? One way to investigate this question is to research other species, other carcinogens, and other organs. If casein's effect on cancer is consistent across these categories, it becomes more likely that humans better take note. So our research became broader in scope, to see whether our discoveries would hold up.

While our rat studies were under way, studies were published[44,45] claiming that chronic infection with hepatitis B virus (HBV) was the major risk factor for human liver cancer. It was thought that people who remained chronically infected with HBV had twenty to forty times the risk of getting liver cancer.

Over the years, considerable research had been done on how this virus causes liver cancer.[46] In effect, a piece of the virus gene inserts itself into the genetic material of the mouse liver where it initiates liver cancer. When this process, called *transfection*, is done experimentally, the animals are considered *transgenic*.

Virtually all of the research done in other laboratories on HBV transgenic mice—and there was a lot of it—was done primarily to understand the molecular mechanism by which HBV worked. No attention was given to nutrition and its effect on tumor development. I watched with some amusement for several years how one community of researchers argued for aflatoxin as the key cause of human liver cancer and another community argued for HBV. No one in either community dared to suggest that nutrition had anything to do with this disease.

We wanted to know about the effect of casein on HBV-induced liver cancer in mice. This was a big step. It went beyond aflatoxin as a carcinogen and rats as a species. A brilliant young graduate student from China in my group, Jifan Hu, initiated studies to answer this question and was later joined by Dr. Zhiqiang Cheng. We needed a colony of these transgenic mice. There were two such "breeds" of mice, one living in La Jolla, California, the other in Rockville, Maryland. Each strain had a different piece of HBV gene stuck in the genes of their livers, and each was therefore highly prone to liver cancer. I contacted the responsible researchers and inquired about their helping us to establish our own mouse colony. Both research groups asked what we wanted to do and both were inclined to think that studying the protein effect was foolish. I also sought a research grant to study this question and it was rejected. The reviewers did not take kindly to the idea of a nutritional effect on a virus-induced cancer, especially of a dietary protein effect. I was beginning to wonder: Was I now being too provocative in questioning the mythical health value of protein? The reviews of the grant proposal certainly indicated this possibility.

We eventually obtained funding, did the study on both strains of mice, *and got essentially the same result as we did with the rats*.[47,48] You can see the results for yourself. The adjoining picture (Chart 3.10[47]) shows what a cross section of the mouse livers looks like under a microscope. The dark-colored material is indicative of cancer development (ignore the "hole"; that's only a cross section of a vein). There is intense early cancer formation in the 22% casein animals (D), much less in the 14% casein animals (C), and none in the 6% casein animals (B); the remaining picture (A) shows a liver having no virus gene (the control).

The adjoining graph (Chart 3.11[47]) shows the expression (activity) of two HBV genes that cause cancer inserted in the mouse liver. Both the picture and the graph show the same thing: the 22% casein diet turned on expression of the viral gene to cause cancer, whereas the 6% casein diet showed almost no such activity.

By this time, we had more than enough information to conclude that casein, that sacred protein of cow's milk, dramatically promotes liver cancer in:

- rats dosed with aflatoxin
- mice infected with HBV

Not only were these effects substantial, but we also discovered a network of complementary mechanisms that created the effects.

Next question: Can we generalize these findings to other cancers and to other carcinogens? At the University of Illinois Medical Center in Chicago, another research group was working with mammary (breast) cancer in rats.[49–51] This research showed that increasing the amounts of casein in

Chart 3.10: Dietary Protein Effect on Genetically Based (HBV) Liver Cancer (MICE)

Non-transgenic Mice (Control) with 22% Casein Diet
A

Transgenic Mice with 6% Casein Diet
B

Transgenic Mice with 14% Casein Diet
C

Transgenic Mice with 22% Casein Diet
D

Chart 3.11: Dietary Protein Effect on Gene Expression (MICE)

rats' diets promoted the development of mammary (breast) cancer. They found that higher casein intake:

- promotes breast cancer in rats dosed with two experimental carcinogens: 7,12-dimethybenz(a)anthracene (DBMA) and N-nitroso-methylurea (NMU)
- operates through a network of reactions that combine to increase cancer
- operates through the same female hormone system that operates in humans

LARGER IMPLICATIONS

An impressively consistent pattern was beginning to emerge. For two different organs, four different carcinogens, and two different species, casein promotes cancer growth while using a highly integrated system of mechanisms. It is a powerful, convincing, and consistent effect. For example, casein affects the way that cells interact with carcinogens, DNA reacts with carcinogens, and cancerous cells grow. The depth and consistency of these findings strongly suggest that they are relevant for humans, for four reasons. First, rats and humans have an almost identical need for protein. Second, protein operates in humans virtually the same way it does in rats. Third, the level of protein intake causing tumor growth is the same level that humans consume. And fourth, in both rodents and humans the initiation stage is far less important than the promotion stage of cancer. This is because we are very likely "dosed" with a certain (albeit very small) amount of carcinogens in our everyday lives, but whether they lead to fully developed tumors depends on their promotion, or lack thereof.

Even though I became convinced that increasing dietary casein promotes cancer, I still had to be wary of generalizing too much. This was an exceptionally provocative finding that drew fierce skepticism and even wanton hostility. But these findings nonetheless were a hint of things to come. I wanted to broaden my evidence still more. Perhaps these findings were a seed that might expose a far greater truth. What effect did other nutrients have on cancer, and how did they interact with different carcinogens and different organs? Might the effects of other nutrients, carcinogens, or organs cancel each other, or might there be consistency of effect for nutrients within certain types of food? Would promotion continue to be reversible? If so, cancer might be readily controlled, even reversed, simply by decreasing the intakes of the promoting nutrients and/or increasing the intakes of the anti-promoting nutrients.

We initiated more studies using several different nutrients, including fish protein, dietary fats, and the antioxidants known as carotenoids. A couple of excellent graduate students of mine, Tom O'Connor and Youping He, measured the ability of these nutrients to affect liver and pancreatic cancer. *The results of these, and many other studies, showed nutrition to be far more important in controlling cancer promotion than the dose of the initiating carcinogen.* The idea that nutrients primarily affect tumor development during promotion was beginning to appear to be a general property of nutrition and cancer relationships. The *Journal of the National Cancer Institute*, which is the official publication of the U.S. National Cancer Institute, took note of these studies and featured some of our findings on its cover.[52]

Furthermore, a pattern was beginning to emerge: *nutrients from animal-based foods increased tumor development while nutrients from plant-based foods decreased tumor development.* In our large lifetime study of rats with aflatoxin-induced tumors, the pattern was consistent. In mice with hepatitis B virus–altered genes, the pattern was consistent. In studies done by another research group, with breast cancer and different carcinogens, the pattern was consistent. In studies of pancreatic cancer and other nutrients, the pattern was consistent.[52,53] In studies on carotenoid antioxidants and cancer initiation, the pattern was consistent.[54,55] From the first stage of cancer initiation to the second stage of cancer promotion, the pattern was consistent. From one mechanism to another, the pattern was consistent.

Since the publication of these research findings in top-flight, peer-reviewed scientific journals during the 1970s, 1980s, and 1990s, then publication of a summary of this evidence in the first edition of this book, I have witnessed the public's reaction to this information. There is no doubt that many people—including well over a million readers—have taken note.

Although reactions have varied widely, as expected, it is clear that these reactions have been intensely personal.

Some, when reading this chapter, have said, "That's it," and committed themselves to dietary change forevermore. The thought that their most revered nutrient, when consumed in excess, enhanced development of their most feared disease, was enough to alter their eating, no further explanation needed. Others, deeply embedded in cultural dietary practices, also have said, "That's it!"—but their reactions were to read no further, then go on a tirade questioning why this research was ever done in the first place. Either way, this evidence has touched intensely held beliefs.

Still, then as now, I could not ignore the possibility that this evidence, still narrow in its scope but stunningly impressive and consistent, might be of great significance to human health. But I needed to be cautious, especially because this evidence had been mostly gathered in experimental animal studies. Although there are strong arguments that these provocative findings are *qualitatively* relevant to human health, we cannot know the *quantitative* relevance. In other words, are these principles regarding animal protein and cancer critically important for all humans in all situations, or are they merely marginally important for a minority of people in fairly unique situations? Are these principles involved in one thousand human cancers every year, one million human cancers every year, or more? We needed direct evidence from human research. Ideally, this evidence would be gathered with rigorous methodology and would investigate dietary patterns comprehensively, using large numbers of people who had similar lifestyles and genetic backgrounds, yet had widely varying occurrence of disease.

Having the opportunity to do such a study is rare, at best, but by incredibly good luck we were given exactly the opportunity we needed. In 1980 I had the good fortune of welcoming in my laboratory a most personable and professional scientist from mainland China, Dr. Junshi Chen. With this remarkable man, opportunities arose to search for some larger truths. We were given the chance to do a human study that would take all of these principles we had begun to uncover in the lab to the next level. It was time to study the role of nutrition, lifestyle, and disease in the most comprehensive manner ever undertaken in the history of medicine. We were on to the China Study.

LESSONS FROM
CHINA

A SNAPSHOT IN TIME

Have you ever had the sensation of wanting to permanently capture a moment? Such moments can grip you in a way you will never forget. For some people, those moments center on family, close friends, or related activities; for others, those moments may center on nature, spirituality, or religion. For most of us, I suspect, it can be a little of each. They become the personal moments, both happy and sad, that define our memories. It's these moments in which everything just "comes together." They are the snapshots of time that define much of our life experience.

The value of a snapshot of time is not lost on researchers, either. We construct experiments, hoping to preserve and analyze the specific details of a certain moment for years to come. I was fortunate enough to be privy to such an opportunity in the early 1980s, after a distinguished senior scientist from China, Dr. Junshi Chen, came to Cornell to work in my lab. He was deputy director of China's premier health research laboratory and one of the first handful of Chinese scholars to visit the U.S. following the establishment of relations between our two countries.

THE CANCER ATLAS

In the early 1970s, the premier of China, Zhou Enlai, was dying of cancer. In the grips of this terminal disease, Premier Chou initiated a nationwide survey to collect information about a disease that was not well understood. It was to be a monumental survey of death rates for twelve different kinds of cancer for more than 2,400 Chinese counties and 880 million (96%) of their citizens. The survey was remarkable in many ways. It involved 650,000 workers, the most ambitious biomedical research project ever undertaken. The end result of the survey was a beautiful, color-coded atlas showing where certain types of cancer were high and where they were almost nonexistent.[1]

Chart 4.1: Sample Cancer Atlas in China

This atlas made it clear that in China cancer was geographically localized. Some cancers were much more common in some places than in others. Earlier studies had set the stage for this idea, showing that cancer incidence also varies widely between different countries.[2-4] But these China data were more remarkable because the geographic variations in cancer rates were much greater (Chart 4.2). They also occurred in a country where 87% of the population is the same ethnic group, the Han people.

Why was there such a massive variation in cancer rates among different counties when genetic backgrounds were similar from place to place? Might it be possible that cancer is largely due to environmental/lifestyle factors, and not genetics? A few prominent scientists had already reached that conclusion. The authors of a major review on diet and cancer, prepared for

Chart 4.2: Range of Cancer Rates in Chinese Counties

Cancer Site	Males	Females
All Cancers	35–721	35–491
Nasopharynx	0–75	0–26
Esophagus	1–435	0–286
Stomach	6–386	2–141
Liver	7–248	3–67
Colorectal	2–67	2–61
Lung	3–59	0–26
Breast	—	0–20

*Age-adjusted death rates, representing # cases/100,000 people/year

the U.S. Congress in 1981, estimated that genetics only determines about *2–3% of total cancer risk.*[4]

The data behind the China cancer atlas were profound. Cancer rates in the counties with the highest rates of some cancers were more than 100 times greater than in counties with the lowest rates of these cancers. These are truly remarkable figures. By way of comparison, we in the U.S. see, at most, two to three times the cancer rates from one part of the country to another.

In fact, very small and relatively unimportant differences in cancer rates make big news, big money, and big politics. There has been a long-standing story in my state of New York about the increased rates of breast cancer in Long Island. Large amounts of money (about $30 million[5]) and years and years of work have been spent examining the issue. What sorts of rates were causing such a furor? Two counties in Long Island had rates of breast cancer only 10–20% higher than the state average. This difference was enough to make front-page news, scare people, and move politicians to action. Contrast this with the findings in China where some parts of the country had cancer rates 100 times (10,000%) higher than others.

Because China is relatively homogenous genetically, it was clear that these differences had to be explained by environmental causes. This raised a number of critical questions:

- Why was cancer so high in some rural Chinese counties and not in others?
- Why were these differences so incredibly large?
- Why was overall cancer, in the aggregate, less common in China than in the U.S.?

The more Dr. Chen and I talked, the more we wished that we had a snapshot in time of the dietary and environmental conditions in rural China. If only we could look into these people's lives, note what they eat, how they live, what is in their blood and their urine, and how they die. If only we could construct a picture of their experience with unprecedented clarity and detail so that we could study it for years to come. If we could do that, we might be able to offer some answers to our "why" questions.

Occasionally science, politics, and financing come together in a way that allows a truly extraordinary study to take place. This happened for us, and we got the opportunity to do everything we wanted, and more. We were able to create the most comprehensive snapshot of diet, lifestyle, and disease ever taken.

PULLING IT TOGETHER

We assembled a world-class scientific team. There was Dr. Chen, who was the deputy director of the most significant government diet and health research laboratory in all of China. We enlisted Dr. Junyao Li, one of the authors of the *Cancer Atlas Survey* and a key scientist in China's Academy of Medical Sciences in the Ministry of Health. The third member was Richard Peto of Oxford University. Considered one of the premier epidemiologists in the world, Peto has since been knighted and has received several awards for cancer research. I rounded out the team as the Project Director.

Everything was coming together. It was to be the first major research project between China and the United States. We cleared the necessary funding hurdles, weathering both CIA intrusiveness and Chinese government reticence. We were on our way.

We decided to make the study as comprehensive as possible. From the *Cancer Atlas*, we had access to disease mortality rates for more than four dozen different kinds of disease, including individual cancers, heart diseases, and infectious diseases.[6] We gathered data on 367 variables and then compared each variable with every other variable. We went into sixty-five counties across China and administered questionnaires and blood tests on 6,500 adults. We took urine samples, directly measured everything families ate over a three-day period, and analyzed food samples from marketplaces around the country.

The sixty-five counties selected for the study were located in rural to semi-rural parts of China. This was intentionally done because we wanted to study people who mostly lived and ate food in the same area for most of their lives. This was a successful strategy, as we were to learn that an average of 90–94% of the adult subjects in each county still lived in the same county where they were born.

When we were done, we had *more than 8,000 statistically significant associations* between lifestyle, diet, and disease variables. We had a study that was unmatched in terms of comprehensiveness, quality, and uniqueness. We had what the *New York Times* termed "the Grand Prix of epidemiology." In short, we had created that revealing snapshot of time that we had originally envisioned.

This was the perfect opportunity to test the principles that we discovered in the animal experiments. Were the findings in the lab going to be consistent with the human experience in the real world? Were our discoveries about the effects of dietary protein on aflatoxin-induced liver cancer in rats going to apply to other types of cancer and other types of diseases in humans?

FOR MORE INFORMATION

We take great pride in the comprehensiveness and quality of the China Study. To see why, read Appendix B on page 373. You'll find a more complete discussion of the basic design and characteristics of the study.

THE CHINESE DIETARY EXPERIENCE

Critical to the importance of the China project was the type of diet consumed in rural China. It was a rare opportunity to study health-related effects of a mostly plant-based diet.

In America, an average of 15–16% of our total calories comes from protein and upwards of 81% of this amount comes from animal-based foods.[7] But in rural China only 9–10% of total calories comes from protein and only 10% of this protein comes from animal-based foods.[8] This means that there are major nutritional differences in the Chinese and American diets, as shown in Chart 4.3.

The findings shown in Chart 4.3 are standardized for a body weight of sixty-five kilograms (143 pounds). This is the standard way that Chinese authorities record such information and it allows us to easily compare different populations. (For an American adult male of seventy-seven kilograms, calorie intake will be about 2,400 calories per day. For an average rural Chinese adult male of seventy-seven kilograms, calorie intake will be about 3,000 calories per day.)

Chart 4.3: Chinese and American Dietary Intakes

Nutrient	China	United States
Calories (kcal/day)[9]	2,641	1,989
Total fat (% of calories)	14.5	34–38
Dietary fiber (g/day)	33	12
Total protein (g/day)	64	91
Animal protein (% of calories)	0.8	10–11
Total iron (mg/day)	34	18

In every category seen above, there are massive dietary differences between the Chinese and American experiences: much more overall calories, less fat, less protein, much less animal foods, more fiber, and much more iron are consumed in China. These dietary differences are supremely important.

While the eating pattern in China is far different from that of the United States, there is still a lot of variation within China. Experimental variation (i.e., a range of values) is essential when we investigate diet and health associations. Fortunately, in the China Study considerable variation existed for most of the measured factors. There was exceptional variation in disease rates (Chart 4.2) and more than adequate variation for clinical measurements and food intakes. For example, blood cholesterol ranged—as county averages—from highest to lowest almost twofold, blood beta-carotene about ninefold, blood lipids about threefold, fat intake about sixfold, and fiber intake about fivefold. This was crucial, as we primarily were concerned with comparing each county in China with every other county.

Ours was the first large study that investigated this particular range of dietary experience and its health consequences. In effect, we were comparing, within the Chinese range, diets rich in plant-based foods to diets very rich in plant-based foods. In almost all other studies, all of which are Western, scientists are comparing diets rich in animal-based foods to diets very rich in animal-based foods. The difference between rural Chinese diets and "Western" diets, and the ensuing disease patterns, is enormous. It was this distinction, as much as any other, that made this study so important.

The media called the China Study a "landmark study." An article in the *Saturday Evening Post* said the project "should shake up medical and nutrition researchers everywhere."[10] Some in the medical establishment said another study like this could never be done. What I knew was that our study offered an opportunity to investigate many of the most contentious ideas that I was forming about food and health.

Now, I want to show you what we learned from this study and how twenty more years of research, thought, and experience have changed not only the way I think about the connection between nutrition and health, but the way my family and I eat as well.

DISEASES OF POVERTY AND AFFLUENCE

It doesn't take a scientist to figure out that the possibility of death has been holding pretty steady at 100% for quite some time. There's only one thing that we have to do in life, and that is to die. I have often met people who use this fact to justify their ambivalence toward health information. But I take a different view. I have never pursued health hoping for immortality. Good health is about being able to fully enjoy the time we do have. It is about being as functional as possible throughout our entire lives and avoiding disabling, painful, and lengthy battles with disease. There are many better ways to die, and to live.

Because the China *Cancer Atlas* had mortality rates for more than four dozen different kinds of disease, we had a rare opportunity to study the many ways that people die. We wondered: Do certain diseases tend to cluster in certain areas of the country? For example, did colon cancer occur in the same regions as diabetes? If this proved to be the case, we could assume that diabetes and colon cancer (or other diseases that clustered) shared common causes. These causes could include a variety of possibilities, ranging from the geographic and environmental to the biological. However, because all diseases are biological processes (gone awry), we can assume that whatever "causes" are observed, they will eventually operate through biological events.

When these diseases were cross-listed in a way that allowed every disease rate to be compared with every other disease rate,[11] two groups of diseases emerged: those typically found in more economically developed areas (diseases of affluence) and those typically found in rural agricultural areas (diseases of poverty)[12] (Chart 4.4).

The diseases shown in Chart 4.4 tend to be associated with diseases in their own list but not in the opposite list. A region in rural China that has a high rate of pneumonia, for example, will not have a high rate of breast cancer, but will have a high rate of a parasitic disease. The disease that kills most Westerners, coronary heart disease, is more common in areas where breast cancer also is more common. Coronary heart disease, by the way, is relatively uncommon in many developing societies of the world. This is not because people die at a younger age, thus avoiding these Western diseases.

Chart 4.4: Disease Groupings Observed in Rural China

Disease of Affluence (Nutritional extravagance)	Cancer (colon, lung, breast, leukemia, childhood brain, stomach, liver), diabetes, coronary heart disease
Disease of Poverty (Nutritional inadequacy and poor sanitation)	Pneumonia, intestinal obstruction, peptic ulcer, digestive disease, pulmonary tuberculosis, parasitic disease, rheumatic heart disease, metabolic and endocrine disease other than diabetes, diseases of pregnancy, and many others

These comparisons are age-standardized rates, meaning that people of the same age are being compared.

Disease associations of this kind have been known for quite some time. What the China Study added, however, was an unsurpassed amount of data on death rates for many different diseases and a unique range of dietary experience. As expected, certain diseases do cluster together in the same geographic areas, implying that they have shared causes.

These two disease groups have usually been referred to as diseases of affluence and diseases of poverty. As a developing population accumulates wealth, people change their eating habits, lifestyles, and sanitation systems. As wealth accumulates, more and more people die from "rich" diseases of affluence than "poor" diseases of poverty. Because these diseases of affluence are so tightly linked to eating habits, diseases of affluence might be better named "diseases of nutritional extravagance." The vast majority of people in the United States and other Western countries die from diseases of affluence. For this reason, these diseases are often referred to as Western diseases. Some rural counties had few diseases of affluence while other counties had far more. The core question of the China Study was this: Is it because of differences in dietary habits?

STATISTICAL SIGNIFICANCE

As I go through this chapter, I will indicate the statistical significance of various observations with Roman numeral superscripts. Roman numeral one (I) means 95+% probability; numeral two (II) means 99+% probability; and numeral three (III) means 99.9+% probability. No Roman numeral means that the association is something less than 95% probability.[13] These probabilities also can be described as the chance or odds that an observation is real. A 95% probability means a 19 in 20 chance that the observation is real; a 99% probability means a 99 in 100 chance that the observation is real; and a 99.9% probability means a 999 in 1,000 chance that the observation is real.

BLOOD CHOLESTEROL AND DISEASE

We compared the prevalence of Western diseases with diet and lifestyle variables[14] and, to our surprise, one of the strongest predictors of Western diseases was blood cholesterol.[III]

IN YOUR FOOD—IN YOUR BLOOD

There are two main categories of cholesterol. *Dietary cholesterol* is present in the food we eat. It is a component of food, much like sugar, fat, protein, vitamins, and minerals. This cholesterol is found only in animal-based food and is the "cholesterol" we find on food labels. How much dietary cholesterol you consume is *not* something your doctor can know when he or she checks your blood cholesterol levels. The doctor can't measure dietary cholesterol any more than he or she can measure how many hot dogs and chicken breasts you've been eating. Instead, the doctor measures the amount of cholesterol present in your blood; this cholesterol is mostly made in the liver. Blood cholesterol and dietary cholesterol, although chemically identical, are determined by different factors. A similar situation occurs with fat. Dietary fat is the stuff you eat: the grease on your French fries, for example. Body fat, on the other hand, is the stuff made by your body and is very different from the fat that you spread on your toast in the morning (butter or margarine). Dietary fats and cholesterol don't necessarily turn into body fat and blood cholesterol. The way the body makes body fat and blood cholesterol is extremely complex, involving hundreds of different chemical reactions and dozens of nutrients. Because of this complexity, the health effects of eating dietary fat and cholesterol may be very different from the health effects of having high blood cholesterol (what your doctor measures) or having too much body fat.

As blood cholesterol levels in rural China rose in certain counties, the incidence of Western diseases also increased. What made this so surprising was that Chinese levels were far lower than we had expected. The average level of blood cholesterol was only 127 mg/dL, which is almost 100 points less than the American average (215 mg/dL)![15] Some counties had average levels as low as 94 mg/dL. For two groups of about twenty-five women in the inner part of China, average blood cholesterol was at the amazingly low level of 80 mg/dL.

If you know your own cholesterol levels, you'll appreciate how low these values really are. In the U.S., our range is around 170–290 mg/dL. Our low values are near the high values for rural China. Indeed, in the U.S., there was a myth that there might be health problems if cholesterol levels were below 150 mg/dL. If we followed that line of thinking, about 85% of the rural Chinese would appear to be in trouble. But the truth is quite different. *Lower blood cholesterol levels are linked to lower rates of heart disease, cancer, and other Western diseases, even at levels far below those considered "safe" in the West.*

I was perplexed and doubtful that these levels could be right because the existing literature, to my knowledge at that time, had never shown total cholesterol to be much below about 140–150 mg/dL. Was it possible that our methodology was unreliable? We therefore compared these findings with two additional assay methods and explored whether some of the cholesterol in the samples may have escaped analysis because it had separated out from the solution. But the low cholesterol levels we found in rural China were not the result of a methodological issue. They really were that low, prompting the realization that we had to tweak our knowledge about blood cholesterol, and especially its relationship to disease.

At the outset of the China Study, no one could or would have predicted that there would be a relationship between cholesterol and any of the disease rates. What a surprise we got! As blood cholesterol levels decreased from 170 mg/dL to 90 mg/dL, cancers of the liver,[II] rectum,[I] colon,[II] male lung,[I] female lung, breast, childhood leukemia, adult leukemia,[I] childhood brain, adult brain,[I] stomach, and esophagus (throat) decreased. As you can see, this is a sizable list. Most Americans know that if you have high cholesterol, you should worry about your heart, but they don't know that you might want to worry about cancer as well.

There are several types of blood cholesterol, including LDL and HDL cholesterol. LDL is the "bad" kind and HDL is the "good" kind. In the China Study, higher levels of the bad LDL cholesterol also were associated with Western diseases.

Keep in mind that by Western standards, these diseases were relatively rare in China and blood cholesterol levels were quite low. Our findings made a convincing case that many Chinese had an advantage at the lower cholesterol levels, even below 170 mg/dL. Now imagine a country where the inhabitants had blood cholesterol levels far higher than the Chinese average. You might expect that these relatively rare diseases, such as heart disease and some cancers, would be prevalent, perhaps even the leading killers!

Of course, this is exactly the case in Western societies. To give a couple of examples at the time of our study, the death rate from coronary heart disease was *seventeen times higher* among American men than rural Chinese men.[16] The American death rate from breast cancer was *five times higher* than the rural Chinese rate.

Even more remarkable were the extraordinarily low rates of coronary heart disease in the southwestern Chinese provinces of Sichuan and Guizhou. During a three-year observation period (1973–1975), not one single person died of coronary heart disease before the age of sixty-four, among 246,000 men in a Guizhou county and 181,000 women in a Sichuan county![17]

After these low cholesterol data were made public, I learned from three very prominent heart disease researchers and physicians, Drs. Bill Castelli, Bill Roberts, and Caldwell Esselstyn, Jr., that in their long careers they had never seen a heart disease fatality among their patients who had blood cholesterol levels below 150 mg/dL. Dr. Castelli was the long-time director of the famous Framingham Heart Study of NIH; Dr. Esselstyn was a renowned surgeon at the Cleveland Clinic who did a remarkable study on reversing heart disease (chapter five); and Dr. Roberts has long been editor of the prestigious medical journal *Cardiology*.

BLOOD CHOLESTEROL AND DIET

Blood cholesterol is clearly an important indicator of disease risk. The big question is: How will food affect blood cholesterol? In brief, animal-based foods were correlated with increasing blood cholesterol (Chart 4.5). With almost no exceptions, nutrients from plant-based foods were associated with *decreasing* levels of blood cholesterol.

Several studies have now shown, in both experimental animals and in humans, that consuming animal-based protein increases blood cholesterol levels.[18–21] Saturated fat and dietary cholesterol also associate with blood cholesterol, although these nutrients are not as effective as animal protein.[18–21] In contrast, plant-based foods contain no cholesterol and, in varied ways, help to decrease the amount of cholesterol made by the body. All of this was consistent with the findings from the China Study.

Chart 4.5: Foods Associated with Blood Cholesterol

As intakes of meat,[I] milk, eggs, fish,[I-II] fat,[I] and animal protein go up . . .	Blood Cholesterol goes up.
As intakes of plant-based foods and nutrients (including plant protein,[I] dietary fiber,[II] cellulose,[II] hemicellulose,[I] soluble carbohydrate,[II] B-vitamins of plants [carotenes, B_2, B_3],[I] legumes, light-colored vegetables, fruit, carrots, potatoes, and several cereal grains) go up . . .	Blood Cholesterol goes down.

These disease associations with blood cholesterol were remarkable, because blood cholesterol and animal-based food consumption both were so low by American standards. In rural China, individuals' animal protein intake averages only 7.1 g/day whereas an equivalent American's averages a whopping 70 g/day. To put this into perspective, seven grams of animal protein is found in about three chicken nuggets from McDonald's. We expected that when animal protein consumption and blood cholesterol levels were as low as they are in rural China, there would be no further association with the Western diseases. But we were wrong. Even this low range of animal-based food in rural China appeared to be associated with Western diseases, as indicated by the highly significant association of blood cholesterol with Western diseases (in the aggregate) and the association of blood cholesterol with animal protein.

The same effects were observed for each type of blood cholesterol. Animal protein consumption by men was associated with increasing levels of "bad" blood cholesterol[III] whereas plant protein consumption was associated with decreasing levels of this same cholesterol.[II]

Walk into almost any doctor's office and ask which dietary factors affect blood cholesterol levels, and he or she will likely mention saturated fat and dietary cholesterol. In more recent decades, some might also mention the cholesterol-lowering effect of soy or high-fiber bran products, but few will say that animal protein has anything to do with blood cholesterol levels.

It has always been this way. While on sabbatical at the University of Oxford, I attended lectures given to medical students on the dietary causes of heart disease by one of their prominent professors of medicine. He went on and on about the adverse effects of saturated fat and cholesterol intakes on coronary heart disease as if these were the only dietary factors that were important. He was unwilling to concede that animal protein consumption had anything to do with blood cholesterol levels, even though the evidence at that time made it abundantly clear that animal protein was more strongly correlated with blood cholesterol levels than saturated fat and dietary cholesterol.[18] Like too many others, his blind faith in the dietary status quo and in the importance of animal protein left him unwilling to be open-minded. As these findings poured in, I was beginning to discover that being open-minded was not a luxury, but a necessity.

FAT AND BREAST CANCER

If there were some sort of nutrition parade, and each nutrient had a float, by far the biggest would belong to fat. So many people, from researchers to educators, from government policy makers to industry representatives, have investigated or made pronouncements on fat for so long. People from a huge number of different communities have been constructing this behemoth for over half a century.

As this strange parade got started on Main Street, USA, the attention of everyone sitting on the sidewalks would inevitably be drawn to the fat float, where bystanders would be invited to have a taste. Most people might see the fat float and say, "I should stay away from that," but then climb on and eat a hefty piece of it. Others might climb on but remain on the unsaturated half of the float, saying that these fats are healthy because only saturated fats are bad. Many scientists would point fingers at the fat float and claim that the heart disease and cancer clowns are hiding inside. Meanwhile, some self-proclaimed diet gurus, like the late Dr. Robert Atkins and many of his low-carb pals, might set up shop on the float and start selling books. At the end of the day the average person who gorged on the float would be left scratching his head and feeling queasy, wondering what he should have done and why.

There's good reason for the average consumer to be confused. The unanswered questions on fat remain unanswered, as they have for the past forty years. How much fat can we have in our diets? What kind of fat? Is polyunsaturated fat better than saturated fat? Is monounsaturated fat better than either? What about those special fats like omega-3, omega-6, trans fats, and DHA? Should we avoid coconut fat? What about fish oil? Is there something special about flaxseed oil? What's a high-fat diet anyway? A low-fat diet?

This can be confusing, even for trained scientists. The details that underlie these questions, *when considered in isolation*, are very misleading. As you shall see, considering how networks of chemicals behave instead of isolated single chemicals is far more meaningful.

In some ways, however, it is this foolish mania regarding isolated aspects of fat consumption that teaches us the best lessons. Therefore, let's look a little more closely at this story of fat as it has emerged during the past forty years. It illustrates why the public is so confused both about fat and about diet in general.

On average, we consume 35–40% of our total calories as fat.[22] We have been consuming high-fat diets like this since the late nineteenth century, at the onset of our industrial revolution. Because we had more money, we began consuming more meat and dairy, which are relatively high in fat. We were demonstrating our affluence by consuming such foods.

Then came the mid- to late twentieth century when scientists began to question the advisability of consuming diets so high in fat. National and international dietary recommendations[23–26] emerged to suggest that we should decrease our fat intake to or below 30% of calories. That lasted for a couple decades, but now, the fears surrounding high-fat diets are abating. Some authors of popular books even advocate increased fat intake! Some experienced researchers have suggested that it is not necessary to go below 30% fat, as long as we consume the right kind of fat.

The level of 30% fat has become a benchmark, even though there is no evidence to suggest that this is a vital threshold. Let's get some perspective on this figure by considering the fat contents of a few foods, as seen in Chart 4.6.

Chart 4.6: Fat Content of Sample Foods

Food	Percent of calories derived from fat
Butter	100%
McDonald's Double Cheeseburger	67%
Whole Cow's Milk	64%
Ham	61%
Hot Dog	54%
Soybeans	42%
"Low-Fat" (or 2%) Milk	35%
Chicken	26%
Spinach	14%
Wheaties Breakfast Cereal	8%
Skim Milk	5%
Peas	5%
Carrots	4%
Green Beans	3.5%
Whole Baked Potatoes	1%

With a few exceptions, animal-based foods contain considerably more fat than plant-based foods.[27] This is well illustrated by comparing the amount of fat in the diets of different countries. Fat and animal protein intake are more than 90% correlated.[28] This means that fat intake increases in parallel with animal protein intake, which further means that dietary fat is an indicator of how much animal-based food is in the diet. It is almost a perfect match.

FAT AND A FOCUS ON CANCER

The 1982 National Academy of Sciences (NAS) report on Diet, Nutrition, and Cancer, of which I was a co-author, was the first expert panel report that deliberated on the association of dietary fat with cancer. This report was the first to recommend a maximum fat intake of 30% of calories for cancer prevention. Previously, the U.S. Senate Select Committee on Nutrition chaired by Senator George McGovern[29] held widely publicized hearings on diet and heart disease and recommended a maximum intake of 30% dietary fat. Although the McGovern report generated a public discourse on diet and disease, it was the 1982 NAS report that gave momentum to this debate. Its focus on cancer, as opposed to heart disease, increased public interest and concern. It spurred additional research activity and public awareness of the importance of diet in disease prevention.

Many of the reports at the time[23,30,31] were centered on the question of how much dietary fat was appropriate for good health. The unique attention given to fat was motivated by international studies showing that the amount of dietary fat consumed was closely associated with the incidence of breast cancer, large bowel cancer, and heart disease. These were the diseases that kill the majority of people in Western countries before their time. Clearly, this correlation was destined to attract great public attention. The China Study was begun in the midst of this environment.

The best known study,[32] in my view, was that of the late Ken Carroll, professor at the University of Western Ontario in Canada. His findings showed a very impressive relationship between dietary fat and breast cancer (Chart 4.7).

This finding, which corresponded to the earlier reports of others,[3,33] became especially intriguing when compared with migrant studies.[34,35] These studies showed that people who migrated from one area to another and who started eating the typical diet of their new residency assumed the disease risk of the area to which they moved. This strongly implied that diet and lifestyle were the principal causes of these diseases. It also suggested that genes are not necessarily that important. As noted earlier, a very prominent report by Sir Richard Doll and Sir Richard Peto of the University of Oxford (U.K.), submitted to the U.S. Congress, summarized many of these studies and concluded that only 2–3% of all cancers could be attributed to genes.[4]

Do the data from these international and migrant studies mean that we can lower our rate of breast cancer to almost zero if we make perfect lifestyle choices? The information certainly suggests that this could be the case. Concerning the evidence in Chart 4.7, the solution seems obvious: if we eat less fat, then we'll lower our breast cancer risk. Most scientists made this conclusion and some surmised that dietary fat caused breast cancer. But that interpretation was too simple. Other charts prepared by Professor Carroll were largely, almost totally, ignored (Charts 4.8 and 4.9). They show that breast cancer was associated with animal fat intake but not with plant fat.

In rural China, dietary fat intake (at the time of the survey in 1983) was very different from the United States in two ways. First, fat was only 14.5% of calorie intake in China, compared with about 36% in the U.S. Second, the amount of fat in the diets of rural China depended almost entirely on the amount of animal-based food in the diet, just like the findings in Chart 4.7. The correlation between dietary fat and animal protein in rural China was very high, at 70–84%,[36] similar to the 93% seen when comparing different countries.[28]

This is important because in China and the international studies, fat consumption was only an indication of *animal-based food* consumption. Thus, the association between fat and breast cancer might really be telling us that as consumption of animal-based foods goes up, so does breast cancer. This is not the case in the U.S., where we selectively add or remove fat

Chart 4.7: Total Fat Intake and Breast Cancer

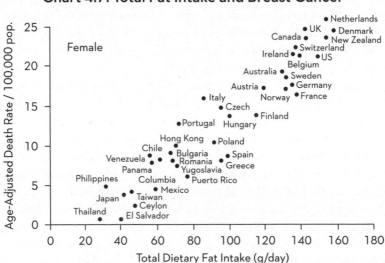

from our foods and our diets. We get as much or more fat from plant-based food (potato chips, French fries) as we get from processed animal-based foods (skim milk, lean cuts of meat). China does not tinker with fat in their food supply as we do here.

At this very low range of dietary fat in China, from 6–24%, I initially thought that dietary fat would not be linked with diseases like heart disease or the various cancers, as it is in the West. Some people in the U.S.—like many of my colleagues in science and medicine—call a 30% fat diet a "low-fat" diet. Therefore, a low-fat diet containing only 25–30% fat was thought to be low enough to obtain the maximum amount of health benefits. This implied that going lower provided no further benefit. Surprise!

Findings from rural China showed that reducing dietary fat from a "high" of 24% to a low of 6% was associated with lower breast cancer risk. However, lower dietary fat in rural China meant less consumption not only of fat but, more importantly, of animal-based food.

This connection of breast cancer with dietary fat, and thus with animal-based foods, brought into consideration other factors that also place a woman at risk for breast cancer:

- Early age of menarche (age of first menstruation)
- High blood cholesterol
- Late menopause
- High exposure to female hormones

Chart 4.8: Animal Fat Intake and Breast Cancer

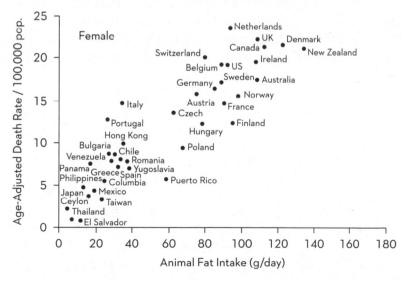

Chart 4.9: Plant Fat Intake and Breast Cancer

What does the China Study show regarding these risk factors? Higher dietary fat (and the animal protein that its presence indicates) is associated with higher blood cholesterol,[I] and both of these factors, along with higher female hormone levels, are associated, in turn, with more breast cancer[I] and earlier age of menarche.[I]

The much later age of menarche in rural China is remarkable. Twenty-five women in each of the 130 villages in the survey were asked when they had their first menstrual period. The range of village averages was fifteen to nineteen years, with an average of seventeen years. The U.S. average is roughly eleven years!

Many studies have shown that earlier menarche leads to higher risk for breast cancer.[37] Menarche is triggered by the growth rate of the girl; the faster the growth, the earlier the age of onset. It also is well established that rapid growth of young girls often leads to greater adult body height and more body weight and body fatness, each of which is associated with higher breast cancer risk. Early age of menarche, both in Chinese and in Western women, also leads to higher levels of blood hormones such as estrogen. These hormone levels remain high throughout the reproductive years if consumption of a diet rich in animal-based food is maintained. Under these conditions, age of menopause is deferred by three to four years,[I] thus extending the reproductive life from beginning to end by about nine to ten years and greatly increasing lifetime exposure to female hormones. Other studies have shown that an increase in years of reproductive life is associated with increased breast cancer risk.[38,39]

This network of relationships becomes still more impressive. Higher fat consumption is associated with higher blood levels of estrogen during the critical ages of thirty-five to forty-four years[III] and higher blood levels of the female hormone prolactin during the later ages of fifty-five to sixty-four years.[III] These hormones are highly correlated with animal protein intake,[III] milk,[III] and meat.[II] Unfortunately, we could not demonstrate whether these hormone levels were directly related to breast cancer risk in China because the rate of disease is so low.[40]

Nonetheless, when hormone levels among Chinese women were compared with those of British women,[41] Chinese estrogen levels were only about one-half those of the British women, who have an equivalent hormone profile to that of American women. Because the length of the reproductive life of a Chinese woman is only about 75% of that of the British (or American) woman, this means that with lower estrogen levels, the Chinese woman only experiences about 35–40% of the lifetime estrogen exposure of British (and American) women. This corresponds to Chinese breast cancer rates that are only one-fifth of those of Western women.

The strong association of a high-animal protein, high-fat diet with reproductive hormones and early age of menarche, both of which raise the risk of breast cancer, is an important observation. It makes clear that we should not have our children consume diets high in animal-based foods. If you are a woman, would you ever have imagined that eating diets higher in animal-based foods would expand your reproductive life by about nine to ten years? As an aside, an interesting implication of this observation, as noted by *Ms.* magazine founder Gloria Steinem, is that eating the right foods could reduce teenage pregnancy by delaying the age of menarche.

Beyond the hormone findings, is there a way to show that animal-based food intake relates to overall cancer rates? This is somewhat difficult, but one of the factors we measured was how much cancer there was in each family. Animal protein intake was convincingly associated in the China Study with the prevalence of cancer in families.[III] This association is an impressive and significant observation, considering much of the population's unusually low intake of animal protein.

Diet and disease factors such as animal protein consumption or breast cancer incidence lead to changes in the concentrations of certain chemicals in our blood. These chemicals are called biomarkers. As an example, blood cholesterol is a biomarker for heart disease. We measured six blood biomarkers that are associated with animal protein intake.[42] Do they confirm the finding that animal protein intake is associated with cancer in families? Absolutely. Every single animal protein–related blood biomarker is significantly associated with the amount of cancer in a family.[II–III]

In this case, multiple observations, tightly networked into a web, show that animal-based foods are strongly linked to breast cancer. What makes this conclusion especially compelling are two kinds of evidence. First, the individual parts of this web were consistently correlated and, in most cases, were statistically significant. Second, this effect occurred *at unusually low intakes of animal-based foods.*

Our investigation of breast cancer (detailed further in chapter eight) is a perfect example of what makes the China Study so convincing. Rather than a single, simple association of fat and breast cancer,[1] we were able to construct a much more expansive web of information about how diet affects breast cancer risk. We were able to examine in multiple ways the role of diet and cholesterol, age of menarche, and female hormone levels, all of which are known risk factors for breast cancer. When each new finding pointed in the same direction, we were able to see a picture that was convincing, consistent, and biologically plausible.

THE IMPORTANCE OF FIBER

The late professor Denis Burkitt, of Trinity College, Dublin, was unusually articulate. His commonsense, scientific credibility and sense of humor made quite an impression on me when I first met him at a Cornell seminar. The subject of his work was dietary fiber. He had traveled 10,000 miles in a jeep over rugged countryside to study the dietary habits of Africans.

He asserted that even though fiber was not digested, it was vital for good health. Fiber was able to pull water from the body into the intestines to keep things moving along. These undigested fibers, like stick-um paper, also gather up nasty chemicals that find their way into our intestines and that might be carcinogenic. If we don't consume enough fiber, we are susceptible to constipation-based diseases. According to Burkitt, these include large bowel cancer, diverticulosis, hemorrhoids, and varicose veins.

In 1993, Dr. Burkitt was awarded the prestigious Bower Award, the richest award in the world next to the Nobel Prize. He invited me to speak at his award ceremony at the Franklin Institute in Philadelphia, only two months before his unfortunate passing. He offered his opinion that our China Study was the most significant work on diet and health in the world at that time.

Dietary fiber is exclusively found in plant-based foods. This material, which gives rigidity to the cell walls of plants, comes in thousands of different chemical variations. It is mostly made of highly complex carbohydrate molecules. We digest very little or no fiber. Nonetheless, fiber, having few or no calories itself, helps dilute the caloric density of our diets, creates a sense of fullness, and helps to shut down appetite, among other things. In doing so, it satisfies our hunger and minimizes the overconsumption of calories.

Average fiber intake (Chart 4.10) is about three times higher in China than in the U.S.[43] These differences are exceptional, especially considering the fact that many county averages were even much higher.

But according to some "experts" in the U.S., there is a dark side to dietary fiber. They contend that if fiber intake is too high our bodies are not able to absorb as much iron and related minerals, which are essential for health. The fiber may bind with these nutrients and carry them through our system before we are able to digest them. They say that the maximum level of fiber intake should be around thirty to thirty-five grams per day, which is only about the average intake of the rural Chinese.

Chart 4.10: Average Intakes of Dietary Fiber, GM/Day

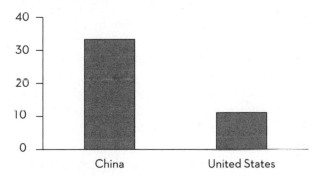

We studied this iron/fiber issue very carefully in the China Study. As it turns out, fiber is not the enemy of iron absorption as so many experts claim it to be. We measured how much iron the Chinese were consuming and how much was in their bodies. Iron was measured in six different ways (four blood biomarkers and two estimates of iron intake), and when we compared these measurements with fiber intake, *there was no evidence showing that increasing fiber intake impaired iron absorption in the body.* In fact, we found the opposite effect. A good indicator of how much iron is in the blood, hemoglobin, actually increased with greater intakes of dietary fiber.[I] As it turns out, high-fiber foods, like wheat and corn (but not the polished rice consumed in China), also happen to be high in iron, meaning that the higher the consumption of fiber, the higher the consumption of iron.[III] Iron intake in rural China (34 mg/day) was surprisingly high when compared to the average American intake (18 mg/day) and it was far more associated with plant-based foods than with animal-based foods.[44]

The China findings on dietary fiber and iron, like so many other observations in this study, did not support the common view of Western scientists. People who consume more plant-based foods, thus more dietary fiber, also consume more iron,[III] all of which results in statistically significant higher levels of hemoglobin. Unfortunately, a bit of confusion has arisen over the fact that some people in rural China, including women and children, have low iron levels. This is especially true in areas where parasitic diseases are more common. In areas of rural China where parasitic diseases were more common, iron status was lower.[I] This has given some the opportunity to claim that these people need more meat, but the evidence indicates that the problem would be much better corrected by reducing parasitism in these areas.

Much of the initial interest in dietary fiber arose with Burkitt's travels in Africa and his claim that large bowel cancer is lower among populations who consume high-fiber diets. Burkitt made this claim popular but the story is at least 200 years old. In England during the late eighteenth and early nineteenth centuries, it was claimed by some of the leading physicians that constipation, which was associated with less bulky diets (i.e., low-fiber diets), was associated with a higher risk of cancer (usually breast and "intestinal" cancers).

At the beginning of the China Study, this belief that fiber might prevent large bowel cancer was the prevailing view, although the 1982 National Academy of Sciences Committee on Diet, Nutrition and Cancer "found no conclusive evidence to indicate that dietary fiber . . . exerts a protective effect against colorectal cancer in humans." The report went on to conclude, "If there is such an effect, specific components of fiber, rather than total dietary fiber, are more likely to be responsible."[23] In hindsight, our discussion of this issue was inadequate. The question, the review of the research literature, and the interpretation of the evidence were too focused on looking for a specific type of fiber as the responsible cause. Finding none, the fiber hypothesis was dismissed.

It was a mistake. The China Study provided evidence that there is a link with certain cancers. The results showed that high-fiber intake was consistently associated with lower rates of cancers of the rectum and colon. High-fiber intakes also were associated with lower levels of blood cholesterol.[I,II] Of course, high-fiber consumption reflected high plant-based food consumption; foods such as beans, leafy vegetables, and whole grains are all high in fiber.

ANTIOXIDANTS, A BEAUTIFUL COLLECTION

One of the more obvious characteristics of plants is their wide range of bright colors. If you admire how food is presented, it's hard to beat a plate of fruits and vegetables. The reds, greens, yellows, purples, and oranges of plant foods are tempting and very healthy. This link between nicely colored vegetables and their exceptional health benefits has often been noted. It turns out that there is a beautiful, scientifically sound story behind this color/health link.

The colors of fruits and vegetables are derived from a variety of chemicals called antioxidants. These chemicals are almost exclusively found in plants. They are only present in animal-based foods to the extent that animals eat them and store a small amount in their own tissues.

Living plants illustrate nature's beauty, both in color and in chemistry. They take the energy of the sun and transform it into life through the process of photosynthesis. In this process, the sun's energy is first turned into simple sugars, and then into more complex carbohydrates, fats, and proteins.

This complex process amounts to some pretty high-powered activity within the plant, all of which is driven by the exchange of electrons between molecules. Electrons are the medium of energy transfer. The site at which photosynthesis takes place is a bit like a nuclear reactor. The electrons zooming around in the plant that are changing the sunlight into chemical energy must be managed very carefully. If they stray from their rightful places in the process, they may create free radicals, which can wreak havoc in the plant. It would be like the core of a nuclear reactor leaking radioactive materials (free radicals) that can be very dangerous to the surrounding area.

So how does the plant manage these complex reactions and protect against errant electrons and free radicals? It puts up a shield around potentially dangerous reactions that sponges up these highly reactive substances. The shield is made up of antioxidants that intercept and scavenge electrons that might otherwise stray from their course.

Antioxidants are usually colored because the same chemical property that sponges up excess electrons also creates visible colors. Some of these antioxidants are called carotenoids, of which there are hundreds. They vary in color from the yellow color of beta-carotene (squash), to the red color of lycopene (tomatoes), to the orange color of the odd-sounding cryptoxanthins (oranges). Other antioxidants may be colorless and these include chemicals such as ascorbic acid (vitamin C) and vitamin E, which act as antioxidants in other parts of plants that need to be protected from the hazards of wayward electrons.

What makes this remarkable process relevant for us animals, however, is that we produce low levels of free radicals throughout our lifetime. Simply being exposed to the sun's rays, to certain industrial pollutants, and to improperly balanced nutrient intakes creates a background of unwanted free radical damage. Free radicals are nasty. They can cause our tissues to become rigid and limited in their function. It is a bit like old age, when our bodies become creaky and stiff. To a great extent, this is what aging is. This uncontrolled free radical damage also is part of the processes that give rise to cataracts, to hardening of the arteries, to cancer, to emphysema, to arthritis, and many other ailments that become more common with age.

But here's the kicker: we do not naturally build shields to protect ourselves against free radicals. As we are not plants, we do not carry out photosynthesis and therefore do not produce any of our own antioxidants. Fortunately the antioxidants in plants work in our bodies the same way they work in plants. It is a wonderful harmony. The plants make the antioxidant shields, and at the same time make them look incredibly appealing with beautiful, appetizing colors. Then we animals, in turn, are attracted to the plants and eat them and borrow their antioxidant shields for our own health. Whether you believe in God, evolution, or just coincidence, you must admit that this is a beautiful, almost spiritual, example of nature's wisdom.

In the China Study, we assessed antioxidant status by recording the intakes of vitamin C and beta-carotene and measuring the blood levels of vitamin C, vitamin E, and carotenoids. Among these antioxidant biomarkers, vitamin C provided the most impressive evidence.

The most significant vitamin C association with cancer was its relationship with the number of cancer-prone families in each area.[45] When levels of vitamin C in the blood were low, these families were *more likely* to have a high incidence of cancer.[III] Low vitamin C was prominently associated with higher risk for esophageal cancer,[III] leukemia, and cancers of the nasopharynx, breast, stomach, liver, rectum, colon, and lung. It was esophageal cancer that first attracted *NOVA* television program producers to report on cancer mortality in China. It was this television program that spurred our own survey to see what was behind this story. Vitamin C primarily comes from fruit, and eating fruit was also inversely associated with esophageal cancer.[II,46] Cancer rates were five to eight times higher for areas where fruit intake was lowest. The same vitamin C effect existing for these cancers also existed for coronary heart disease, hypertensive heart disease, and stroke.[II] Vitamin C intake from fruits clearly showed a powerful protective effect against a variety of diseases.

The other measures of antioxidants, blood levels of alpha- and beta-carotene (a vitamin precursor), and alpha and gamma tocopherol (vitamin

E) are poor indicators of the effects of antioxidants. These antioxidants are transported in the blood by lipoprotein, which is the carrier of "bad" cholesterol. So anytime we measured these antioxidants, we were simultaneously measuring unhealthy biomarkers. This was an experimental compromise that diminished our ability to detect the beneficial effects of the carotenoids and the tocopherols, even when these benefits are known to exist.[47] We did, however, see a correlation between stomach cancer and beta-carotene in which stomach cancer was higher when the blood levels of beta-carotene were lower.[48]

Can we say that vitamin C, beta-carotene, and dietary fiber are solely responsible for preventing these cancers? In other words, can a pill containing vitamin C and beta-carotene or a fiber supplement create these health effects? No. The triumph of health lies not in the individual nutrients, but in the whole foods that contain those nutrients: plant-based foods. In a bowl of spinach salad, for example, we have fiber, antioxidants, and countless other nutrients that are orchestrating a wondrous symphony of health *as they work in concert* within our bodies. The message could not be simpler: eat as many whole fruits, vegetables, and whole grains as you can, and you will probably derive all of the benefits noted above as well as many others.

I have been making this point about the health value of whole, plant-based foods ever since vitamin supplements were introduced on a large scale in the marketplace. And I have watched in dismay how the industry and the media convinced so many Americans that these products represent the same good nutrition as do whole, plant-based foods. As we shall see in later chapters, the promised health benefits of taking single-nutrient supplements are proving to be highly questionable. The "take-home message": if you want vitamin C or beta-carotene, don't reach for the pill bottle—reach for the fruit or leafy green vegetables.

THE ATKINS CRISIS

In case you haven't noticed, there is an elephant in the room, and it goes by the name "low-carb diet." At the time of the first edition of this book, it had become very popular. Almost all diet books on store shelves were variations of this one theme: eat as much protein, meat, and fat as you want, but stay away from those "fatty" carbs.

Today the low-carb phenomenon remains alive and well, although punctuated by my authoring a very small book in 2013 called *The Low-Carb Fraud*.[49] (The book was originally intended only as a chapter in *Whole*,[50] also published in 2013, before our publisher decided that it deserved to be a stand-alone book. Tom also addressed these popular diets in *The China Study Solution*. All three titles include longer discussions of the material summarized here.) In fact, there seems to have been an increasing number of books in the last couple of decades that advocate a diet very low in total carbohydrates. Though their titles vary—*The Zone Diet* by Barry Sears, *The South Beach Diet* by Arthur Agatston, *Wheat Belly* by William Davis, *Good Calories, Bad Calories* and *Why We Get Fat* by Gary Taubes, *Grain Brain* by David Perlmutter, *The Paleo Diet* by Loren Cordain, *The Big Fat Surprise* by Liz Teicholz, *The New Atkins for a New You* by Eric Westman, and many, many more—they have only minor, mostly cosmetic differences in message. They all promote an Atkins-type diet that is very low in carbohydrates.

Aren't some of these authors talking about refined carbohydrates like sugar and white flour, not carbohydrates in general, you might ask? If this were the case—if they were to limit their remarks to the adverse health effects of refined carbohydrates—we could share some common ground. However, most of these authors hardly make this distinction, if at all. One of the more recent of these authors, David Perlmutter, sums it up by clearly stating that he is "not referring to the refined white flours, pastas, and rice" but "to all the grains that so many of us have embraced as being healthful—whole wheat, whole germ, multigrain, seven-grain, live grain, stone-ground, and so on."[51]

The authors of these books advocate keeping dietary carbohydrates as low as 15–20% of total calories. By definition, this means that they are advocating very high-fat, very high-protein diets; the only way to make up the other 80–85% of calories is through fat and protein. Fifty percent of the calories in the standard American diet already comes from fat and protein, and these books' agenda is to raise that number even further. Most of these authors only pay lip service to vegetables (even less, if any, to fruit or whole grains), creating menus loaded with fat and protein of animal origin.

As you have seen already in this book, my research findings and my point of view show that eating this way is perhaps the single greatest threat to American health we currently face. So what is the story, anyway?

One of the fundamental arguments at the beginning of most low-carbohydrate, high-protein diet books is that America has been wallowing in low-fat mania at the advice of experts for the past twenty years, yet people are fatter than ever. This argument has an intuitive appeal, but there is one inconvenient fact about this period of time that these books consistently ignore: according to a report[52] summarizing government food statistics, "Americans consumed thirteen *pounds* [my emphasis] more [added] fats and oils per person in 1997 than in 1970, up from 52.6 to 65.6 pounds." It is true that we have had a trend to consuming fewer of our total calories as fat, when considered as a percentage, but that's only because we have outpaced our gorging on fat by gorging on sugary junk food. Simply by looking at the numbers, anybody can see that America has not adopted the "low-fat" experiment—not by any stretch of the imagination.

In fact, the claim that the low-fat "brainwashing" experiment has been tried and failed is often the first of many statements of fact in current diet books that can be described either as severe ignorance or opportunistic deceit. It is difficult to know where to begin to refute the maze of misinformation and false promises commonly made by authors completely untrained in nutrition, authors who have never conducted any peer-reviewed, professionally based experimental research. And yet these books are immensely popular. Why? Because people do lose weight, at least in the short term.

In one published study[53] funded by the Atkins Center for Complementary Medicine, researchers put fifty-one obese people on the Atkins Diet.[54] The forty-one subjects who maintained the diet over the course of six months lost an average of twenty pounds. In addition, average blood cholesterol levels decreased slightly,[53] which was perhaps even more important. Because of these two results, this study was presented in the media as real, scientific proof that the Atkins Diet works and is safe. Unfortunately, the media didn't go much deeper than that.

The first sign that all is not rosy is that these obese subjects were severely restricting their calorie intake during the study. The average American consumes about 2,250 calories per day.[55] When the study participants were on the diet, they consumed an average of 1,450 calories per day. That's 35% fewer calories! I don't care if you eat worms and cardboard; if you eat 35% fewer calories, you will lose weight and your cholesterol levels will improve[56] in the short run, but that is not to say that worms and cardboard form a healthy diet. One may argue that those 1,450 calories are so satisfying that people feel full on this diet, but if you compare calorie input and calorie expenditure, it's a matter of simple math that a person cannot sustain this amount of calorie restriction over a period of years or decades without either becoming an invalid or melting away into nothing. People are notoriously unsuccessful at significantly restricting their energy intake over any long period of time, and that is why there has yet to be a long-term study that shows success with the "low-carb" diets. This, however, is only the beginning of the problems.

In this same study, funded by the Atkins group, researchers report, "At some point during the twenty-four weeks, twenty-eight subjects (68%) reported constipation, twenty-six (63%) reported bad breath, twenty-one (51%) reported headache, four (10%) noted hair loss, and one woman (1%) reported increase menstrual bleeding."[53] They also refer to other research, saying, "Adverse effects of this diet in children have included calcium oxa-late and urate kidney stones . . . vomiting, amenorrhea [when a woman misses her period], hypercholesterolemia [high cholesterol] and . . . vitamin deficiencies."[53] Additionally, they found that the dieters had a stunning 53% increase in the amount of calcium they excreted in their urine,[53] which may spell disaster for their bone health. The weight loss, some of which is sim-ply initial fluid loss,[57] may come with a very high price.

A different review of low-carbohydrate diets published by researchers in Australia concludes, "Complications such as heart arrhythmias, cardiac contractile function impairment, sudden death, osteoporosis, kidney dam-age, increased cancer risk, impairment of physical activity and lipid abnor-malities can all be linked to long-term restriction of carbohydrates in the diet."[57] According to a 2002 report, a teenage girl died suddenly after being on a high-protein diet.[58,59]

In short, most people will be unable to maintain this diet for the rest of their lives, and even if anybody manages to do so, they may be asking for seri-ous health problems down the road. In fact, I know of little if any evidence on diet and human disease that is more convincing than the findings that show that a low-carb diet is dangerous for human health. I have heard one doctor call high-protein, high-fat, low-carbohydrate diets "make-yourself-sick" diets, and I think that's an appropriate moniker. You can also lose weight by undergoing chemotherapy or starting a heroin addiction, but I wouldn't recommend those, either.

So far, no study has directly and correctly compared a low-carb diet with a whole foods, plant-based diet. One study with the potential to shed some light on the differences in health benefits between high-carb and low-carb diets compared the very high-protein Paleo diet with the stan-dard American diet (already high in fat and protein).[60] The Paleo subjects lost ground, health-wise; they showed increased blood total cholesterol ($p < 0.05$), LDL cholesterol ($p < 0.01$), and triglycerides ($p < 0.05$), and decreased HDL cholesterol ($p < 0.05$). Similarly, a 2013 meta-analysis of seventeen well-performed studies (totaling 272,216 subjects) concluded that there was a *31% increase in total deaths* for those using diets lower in carbohydrates.[61]

It is quite remarkable that these adverse effects of the Paleo variation of the low-carb diet are statistically significant when the sensitivity for detecting such effects was so limited—the diets being compared were both composed of high amounts of protein. It stands to reason that were the Paleo or other low-carb diets directly compared with the WFPB diet, the adverse effects likely would be much more substantial, as there is extensive evidence from many other studies showing that people who eat a diet low in carbohydrates and high in animal fat and protein for a lifetime incur more, not less, breast cancer,[62] colon cancer,[63] and heart disease[64] and many other ailments typically observed in Western societies. Together, these findings suggest to me that there never will be evidence showing that the low-carb diet can reverse diseases, as there is for the WFPB diet.

One final thought: the diet is not all that Atkins recommends. Indeed, most diet books are merely one part of huge food and health empires. In the case of Dr. Atkins' diet, he states that many of his patients require nutrient supplements, some of which are used to combat "common dieters' problems."[65] In one passage, after making unsubstantiated claims about the efficacy of antioxidant supplements that contradicted subsequent studies,[66] he wrote, "Add to the [antioxidants] the vita-nutrients known to be useful for each of the myriad medical problems my patients face, and you'll see why many of them take over thirty vitamin pills a day."[67] *Thirty pills a day?*

There are snake oil salesmen, who have no professional research, professional training, or professional publications in the field of nutrition; and there are scientists, who have formal training, have conducted research, and have reported on their findings in professional forums. Perhaps it is a testament to the power of modern marketing savvy that an obese man with heart disease and high blood pressure[68] became one of the richest snake oil salesmen ever to live, selling a diet that promises to help you lose weight, to keep your heart healthy, and to normalize your blood pressure.

THE TRUTH ABOUT CARBOHYDRATES

An unfortunate outcome of the popularity of diet books in recent decades is that people are more confused than ever about the health value of carbohydrates. As you will see in this book, there is a mountain of scientific evidence to show that the healthiest diet you can possibly consume is a *high-carbohydrate* diet. It has been shown to reverse heart disease, reverse diabetes, prevent a plethora of chronic diseases, and yes, it has been shown many times to cause significant weight loss. But it's not quite as simple as that.

Unless isolated, refined, and put into a sugar bowl or a flour bin, most of the carbohydrates we consume are from fruits, vegetables, and grains. These natural carbohydrates are composed of long chains of simpler carbohydrate molecules and are digested (broken down) in a controlled, regulated manner to yield the simpler molecules (e.g., sucrose, as in table sugar) for subsequent metabolism. Complex carbohydrates include the many forms of dietary fiber, almost all of which remain undigested while still providing substantial health benefits. The carbohydrates present in whole foods also are packaged with generous amounts of vitamins, minerals, and accessible forms of energy. Fruits, vegetables, and whole grains are the healthiest foods you can consume, and they are primarily made of carbohydrates.

On the opposite end of the carbohydrate spectrum are the simple carbohydrates, which generally are highly processed, or refined, and stripped of their fiber, vitamins, and minerals. They are typically found in foods like white bread, processed snack items including crackers and chips made with white flour, sweets including pastries and candy bars, and sugar-laden soft drinks. These highly refined carbohydrates originate from grains or sugar plants, like sugar cane or the sugar beet. They are readily broken down during digestion to the simplest carbohydrate molecular units, which are absorbed into the body to give blood sugar, or glucose.

Unfortunately, most Americans consume voluminous amounts of simple, refined carbohydrates and paltry amounts of complex carbohydrates. For example, in 1996, 42% of Americans ate cakes, cookies, pastries, or pies on any given day, while only 10% ate dark green vegetables.[52] In another ominous sign, only three vegetables accounted for half of the total vegetable servings in 1996[52]: potatoes, which were mostly consumed as fries and chips; head lettuce, one of the least nutrient-dense vegetables you can consume; and canned tomatoes, which generally accompany pizza and pasta consumption. We said in the first edition that the average American consumed *thirty-two teaspoons of added sugars per day in 1996*,[52] but it is now clear, in retrospect, that this is a difficult estimate to establish. The most reliable present estimate seems to be 19 teaspoons a day as of 2007–2008, having declined from 25 teaspoons a day in 1999–2000, primarily because of a drop in soda consumption.[69] This newer, somewhat lower estimate may also reflect a decision by the USDA in 2000 to distinguish between *added refined sugar* and *natural sugar*. Natural sugar, because it is accompanied by vitamins, minerals, and dietary fiber in whole plants, is thought to be much less of a problem—unless it contributes to a burden of excessive added sugar in one's diet.

Our intemperate consumption of refined carbohydrates is why carbohydrates as a whole have gotten such a bad rap; the vast majority of carbohydrates consumed in America are found in junk food or grains so refined that, to convince consumers they carry any claim to healthfulness at all, they must be supplemented with vitamins and minerals, consumption of which is not as effective as in their natural form in whole foods. On this point, the popular diet authors and I agree. For example, you could eat a low-fat, high-carbohydrate diet by exclusively eating the following foods: pasta made from refined flour, baked potato chips, soda, sugary cereals, and low-fat candy bars. Eating this way is a *bad* idea. You will not derive the health benefits of a plant-based diet eating these foods, because they are not in whole food form. In experimental research, the health benefits of a high-carbohydrate diet come from eating the complex carbohydrates found in whole grains, fruits, and vegetables. Eat an apple, a zucchini, or a plate of brown rice topped with beans and other vegetables instead.

THE CHINA STUDY WEIGHS IN

With regard to weight loss, there are some surprising findings from the China Study that shed light on the weight loss debate. When we started the China Study, I thought that China had the opposite problem from that of the U.S. I had heard that China could not feed itself, that it was prone to famines, and that there was not enough food for people to attain their full adult height—that, very simply, there were not enough calories to go around. Although China has, during the last fifty to sixty years, had its share of nutritional problems, we were to learn that these earlier views on China's calorie intake were dead wrong.

We wanted to compare the calorie consumption in China and America, but there was a catch. Chinese are more physically active than Americans, especially in rural areas, where manual labor is the norm. To compare an extremely active laborer with an average American would be misleading. It would be like comparing the amount of energy consumed by a manual laborer at hard work with the amount of energy consumed by an accountant. The vast difference in calorie intake sure to exist between these individuals would tell us nothing of value and only confirm that the manual laborer is more active.

To overcome this problem, we ranked the Chinese into five groups according to their levels of physical activity. After figuring out the calorie intakes of the *least active* Chinese, the equivalent of office workers, we then compared their calorie intake with the *average* American. What we found was astonishing.

Average calorie intake, per kilogram of body weight, was 30% *higher* among the least active Chinese than among average Americans. Yet, body weight was 20% *lower* (Chart 4.11). How can it be that even the least active Chinese consume more calories yet have no overweight problems? What is their secret?

There are two possible explanations for this apparent paradox. First, even the Chinese office workers are more physically active than average Americans. Many office workers in rural China, during the time of our survey, were

Chart 4.11: Calorie Consumption (kcal/kg) and Body Weight

Calorie Intake (kcal/kg)

China   U.S.

Average Body Mass Index

China   U.S.

traveling on bicycles almost every place they went. Thus, they would need to consume more calories in order to perform their daily chores and be healthy. Even so, we cannot tell how much of the extra calorie consumption was due to physical activity and how much to something else, perhaps their food.

We do know, however, that some people use the calories they consume differently from other people. We often say that "they have a higher rate of metabolism" or "it's in their genes." You know these people. They are the ones who seem to eat all they want and still not gain weight. Then there are most of us, who need to watch our calorie intake—or so we think. This is the simplistic interpretation.

I have a more comprehensive interpretation that is based on our own considerable research and on the studies of others. It goes like this. Provided that we aren't restricting our calorie intake, those of us who consume a high-fat, high-protein diet simply retain more calories than we need. We store these calories as body fat, perhaps weave it into our muscle fibers (we call it "marbling" in beef animals), and perhaps store it in the more obvious places, like our butt, our midsection, or around our face and upper thighs.

Here's the clincher: only a small amount of calories needs to be retained by our body to cause significant change in body weight. For example, if we retain only an extra fifty calories per day, this can lead to an extra ten pounds per year. You may not think that this is a lot, but over a period of five years, that's an extra fifty pounds.

Some people would hear this and might be inclined to just eat fifty fewer calories per day. This, theoretically, could make a difference, but it is entirely impractical. It is impossible to keep track of daily calorie intake with such precision. Think about eating a meal at a restaurant. Do you know how many calories each meal has? What about the casserole you might fix? What about the steak you might buy? Do you know the number of calories they contain? Of course not.

The truth is this: despite any short-term caloric restriction regimes we may follow, our body, through many mechanisms, will ultimately choose how many calories to take in and what to do with them. Our attempts to limit calorie intake are short-lived and imprecise, whether we do it by limiting carbohydrates or fat.

The body employs a delicate balancing act and some very intricate mechanisms in deciding how to use the calories being consumed. When we treat our body well by eating the right foods, it knows how to partition the calories away from body fat and into the more desirable functions like keeping the body warm, running the body metabolism, supporting and encouraging physical activity, or just disposing of any excess. The body is using multiple intricate mechanisms to decide how calories get used, stored, or "burned off."

Consuming diets *high* in protein and fat transfers calories away from their conversion into body heat to their storage form—as body fat (unless severe calorie restriction is causing weight loss). In contrast, diets low in protein and fat cause calories to be "lost" as body heat. In research, we say that storing more calories as fat and losing less as heat means being more efficient. I bet that you would rather be a little more inefficient and convert it into body heat rather than body fat, right? Well, simply consuming a diet lower in fat and protein can do this.

This is what our China Study data show. Chinese consume more calories both because they are more physically active and because their consumption of low-fat, low-protein diets shifts conversion of these calories away from body fat to body heat. This is true even for the least physically active Chinese. Remember, it takes very little, only fifty calories a day, to change our storage of body fat and thus change our body weight.[70]

We saw the same phenomenon in our experimental animals fed the low-protein diets. They routinely consumed slightly more calories, gained less weight, disposed of the extra calories as body heat,[71] and voluntarily exercised more,[72] while still having far less cancer than animals on standard diets. We found that calories were "burned" at a faster rate and transformed into body heat as more oxygen was consumed.[71]

Understanding that diet can cause small shifts in calorie metabolism that lead to big shifts in body weight is an important and useful concept. It means that there is an orderly process of controlling body weight over time that does work, as opposed to the disorderly process of crash diets that don't work. It also accounts for the frequent observations (discussed in chapter six) that people who consume low-protein, low-fat diets composed of whole plant foods have far less difficulty with weight problems, even if they consume the same, or even slightly more, total calories.

DIET AND BODY SIZE

We now know that eating a low-fat, low-protein diet high in complex carbohydrates from fruits and vegetables will help you lose weight. But what if you want to become bigger? A desire to be as big as possible is pervasive in most cultures. During Europe's colonial period in Asia and Africa, Europeans even considered smaller people to be less civilized. Body size seems to be a mark of prowess, manliness, and dominance.

Most people think they can be bigger and stronger by eating protein-rich animal-based foods. This belief stems from the idea that consuming protein (a.k.a. meat) is needed for physical power. This has been a common notion the world over for a long time. The Chinese have even officially recommended a higher-protein diet in order to encourage bigger athletes and to better compete in the Olympics. Animal-based foods have more protein, and this protein is considered to be of "higher quality." Animal protein enjoys the same reputation in a rapidly modernizing China as everywhere else.

There is, however, a problem with the idea that consuming animal-based foods is a good way of becoming bigger. The people who eat the most animal protein have the most heart disease, cancer, and diabetes. In the China Study, for example, animal protein consumption was associated with taller and heavier[I] people, but was also associated with higher levels of total and bad cholesterol.[II] Furthermore, body weight, associated with animal protein intake,[I] was associated with more cancer[II–III] and more coronary heart disease.[II] It seems that being bigger, and presumably better, comes with very high costs. But might it be possible for us to achieve our full growth potential, while simultaneously minimizing disease risks?

Childhood growth rates were not measured in the China Study but adult height and weight were. This information proved surprising. Consuming more protein was associated with greater body size ([III] for men and [II] for women).[73] However, this effect was primarily attributed to plant protein, because it makes up 90% of the total Chinese protein intake. Animal protein consumption was indeed associated with greater body weight,[I] and consumption of protein-rich milk seemed to be effective as well.[II] But the good news is this: *greater plant protein intake was closely linked to greater height*[II] *and body weight*.[II] Body growth is linked to protein in general and both animal and plant proteins are effective!

This means that individuals can achieve their genetic potential for growth and body size by consuming a plant-based diet. So why is it that people in developing nations, who consume few or no animal-based foods, are consistently smaller than Western people? This is because plant-based diets in poor areas of the world usually have insufficient variety, inadequate quantity and quality, and are associated with poor public health conditions where childhood diseases are prevalent. Under these conditions, growth is stunted and people do not reach their genetic potential for adult body size. In the China Study, low adult height and weight were strongly associated with areas having high mortality rates for pulmonary tuberculosis,[III] parasitic diseases,[III] pneumonia ([III] for height), "intestinal obstruction,"[III] and digestive diseases.[III]

These findings support the idea that body stature can be achieved by consuming a low-fat, plant-based diet, provided that public health conditions effectively control the diseases of poverty. Under these conditions, the diseases of affluence (heart disease, cancers, diabetes, etc.) can be simultaneously minimized.

The same low-animal protein, low-fat diet that helps prevent obesity also allows people to reach their full growth potential while working other wonders as well. It better regulates blood cholesterol and reduces heart disease and a variety of cancers.

What are the odds that all of these associations (and many others) favoring a plant-based diet are due to pure chance? It is extremely unlikely, to say the least. Such consistency of evidence across a broad range of associations is rare in scientific research. It points to a new worldview, a new paradigm. It defies the status quo, promises new health benefits, and demands our attention.

CIRCLING BACK

In the beginning of my career, I concentrated on the biochemical processes of liver cancer. Chapter three delineates the decades-long laboratory work we did with experimental animals, work that passed the requirements to be called "good science." The finding: casein, and very likely all animal proteins, may be the most relevant cancer-causing substance that we consume. Adjusting the amount of dietary casein has the power to turn on and turn off cancer growth, and to override the cancer-producing effects of aflatoxin, a very potent Class IA carcinogen, but even though these findings were substantially confirmed, they still applied to experimental animals.

It was therefore with great anticipation that I looked to the China Study for evidence on the causes of liver cancer in humans.[74]

Liver cancer rates are very high in rural China, exceptionally high in some areas. Why was this? The primary culprit seemed to be chronic infection with hepatitis B virus (HBV). On average, about 12–13% of our study subjects were chronically infected with the virus. In some areas, one-half of the people were chronically infected! To put this into perspective, only 0.2–0.3% of Americans are chronically infected with this virus.

But there's more. In addition to the virus being a cause of liver cancer in China, it seems that diet also plays a key role. How do we know? The blood cholesterol levels provided the main clue. Liver cancer is strongly associated with increasing blood cholesterol,[III] and we already know that animal-based foods are responsible for increases in cholesterol.

So, where does HBV fit in? The experimental mice studies gave a good signal. In mice, HBV initiated the liver cancer, but the cancer grew in response to the feeding of higher levels of casein. In addition, blood cholesterol also increased. These observations fit perfectly with our human findings. Individuals who are chronically infected with HBV and who consume animal-based foods have high blood cholesterol and a high rate of liver cancer. The virus provides the gun, and bad nutrition pulls the trigger.

A very exciting story was taking shape, at least to my way of thinking. It was a story full of meaning and suggestive of important principles that might apply to other diet and cancer associations. It also was a story that had not been told to the public, and yet it was capable of saving lives. Eventually, it was a story that was leading to the idea that our most powerful weapon against cancer is the food we eat every day.

So there we had it. The years of animal experiments illuminated profound biochemical principles and processes that greatly helped to explain the effect of nutrition on liver cancer. But now we could see that these processes were relevant for humans as well. People chronically infected with hepatitis B virus also had an increased risk of liver cancer. But our findings suggested those who were infected with the virus and who were simultaneously eating more animal-based foods had higher cholesterol levels and more liver cancer than those infected with the virus and not consuming animal-based foods. The experimental animal studies and the human studies made a perfect fit.

PULLING IT TOGETHER

Almost all of us in the United States will die of diseases of affluence. In our China Study, we saw that nutrition has a very strong effect on these diseases. Plant-based foods are linked to lower blood cholesterol; animal-based foods are linked to higher blood cholesterol. Animal-based foods are linked to higher breast cancer rates; plant-based foods are linked to lower rates. Fiber and antioxidants from plants are linked to a lower risk of cancers of the digestive tract. Plant-based diets and active lifestyles result in a healthy weight, yet permit people to become big and strong. Our study was comprehensive in design and comprehensive in its findings. From the labs of Virginia Tech and Cornell University to the far reaches of China, it seemed that science was painting a clear, consistent picture: we can minimize our risk of contracting deadly diseases just by eating the right food.

When we first started this project, we encountered significant resistance from some people. One of my colleagues at Cornell, who had been involved in the early planning of the China Study, got quite heated in one of our meetings. I had put forth the idea of investigating how lots of dietary factors, some known but many unknown, work together to cause disease. Thus we had to measure lots of factors, regardless of whether or not they were justified by prior research. If that was what we intended to do, he said he wanted nothing to do with such a "shotgun" approach.

This colleague was expressing a view that was more in line with mainstream scientific thought than with my evolving perception of nutrition, and indeed, of science research. He and like-minded colleagues think that science is best done when investigating single—mostly known—factors in isolation. An array of largely unspecified factors doesn't show anything, they say. It's okay to measure the specific effect of, say, selenium on breast cancer, but it's not okay to measure multiple nutritional conditions in the same study, in the hope of identifying important dietary patterns.

I prefer the broader picture, for we are investigating the incredible complexities and subtleties of nature itself. I wanted to investigate how dietary patterns related to disease, now the most important point of this book. *Everything in food works together to create health or disease.* The more we think that a single chemical characterizes a whole food, the more we stray into idiocy. As we shall see in Part IV of this book, this way of thinking has generated a lot of poor science.

So I say we need more, not less, of the "shotgun approach." We need more thought about overall dietary patterns and whole foods. Does this mean that I think the shotgun approach is the only way to do research? Of course not. Do I think that the China Study findings constitute absolute scientific proof? Of course not. Does it provide enough information to inform some practical decision-making? Absolutely.

An impressive and informative web of information was emerging from this study. But does every potential strand (or association) in this mammoth study fit perfectly into this web of information? No. Although most statistically significant strands readily fit into the web, there were a few surprises. Most, but not all, have since been explained.

Some associations observed in the China Study, at first glance, were at odds with what might have been expected from Western experience.

I've had to use care in separating unusual findings that could be due to chance and experimental insufficiency from those that truly offered new insights into our old ways of thinking. As I mentioned earlier, the range of blood cholesterol levels in rural China was a surprise. At the time when the China Study was begun, a blood cholesterol range of 200–300 milligrams per deciliter (mg/dL) was considered normal, and lower levels were suspect. In fact, some in the scientific and medical communities considered cholesterol levels lower than 150 mg/dL to be dangerous. In fact, my own cholesterol was 260 mg/dL in the late 1970s, not unlike other members of my immediate family. The doctor told me it was "fine, just average."

But when we measured the blood cholesterol levels in China, we were shocked. They ranged from 70–170 mg/dL! Their high was our low, and their low was off the chart you might find in your doctor's office! It became obvious that our idea of "normal" values (or ranges) only applies to Western subjects consuming the Western diet. It so happens, for example, that our "normal" cholesterol levels present a significant risk for heart disease. Sadly, it's also "normal" to have heart disease in America. Over the years, standards have been established that are consistent with what we see in the West. We too often have come to the view that U.S. values are "normal" because we have a tendency to believe that the Western experience is likely to be right.

At the end of the day, the strength and consistency of the majority of the evidence is enough to draw valid conclusions. Namely, whole, plant-based foods are beneficial, and animal-based foods are not. Few other dietary choices, if any, can offer the incredible benefits of looking good, growing tall, and avoiding the vast majority of premature diseases in our culture.

The China Study was an important milestone in my thinking. Standing alone, it does not *prove* that diet *causes* disease. Absolute proof in science is nearly unattainable. Instead, a theory is proposed and debated until the weight of the evidence is so overwhelming that everyone commonly accepts that the theory is most likely true. In the case of diet and disease, the China Study adds a lot of weight to the evidence. Its experimental features (multiple diet, disease, and lifestyle characteristics; an unusual range of dietary experience; a good means of measuring data quality) provided an unparalleled opportunity to expand our thinking about diet and disease in ways that previously were not available. The study was like a flashlight that illuminated a path I had never fully seen before.

The results of the China Study, in combination with evidence I discerned from the work of others, convinced me to turn my dietary lifestyle around. I stopped eating meat twenty-five years ago, and I stopped eating almost all animal-based foods, including dairy, within the past sixteen to eighteen years, except on very rare occasions. My cholesterol has dropped, even as I've aged; I am more physically fit now than when I was twenty-five; and I am forty-five pounds lighter now than I was when I was thirty years old. I am now at an ideal weight for my height. My entire family, including our children, their spouses, and our grandchildren, has also adopted this way of eating, thanks in large part to my wife, Karen, who has managed to create an entire new dietary lifestyle that is attractive, tasty, and healthy. All of us are about as close to a WFPB diet as you will find. And let me assure you that it seems to be working very well. Our transitions were originally made for health reasons, as a result of my research findings, but have come with an increasing sensitivity to ethical and environmental reasons for eating a plant-based diet. From a boyhood of drinking at least two quarts of milk a day to an early professional career of scoffing at vegetarians, I have taken an unusual turn in my life, and my family has followed suit.

However, I must stress that it was not *only* the China Study that changed my thinking. Since publication of the first edition, some self-anointed "scientists" have spoken of the conclusions of this book as if they were drawn solely from our findings in rural China. Nonsense! This chapter alone addresses our findings from rural China; the rest of this book draws on the findings from my own laboratory and on the findings from many, many other research groups. It is the *breadth* of this evidence—from basic to applied research, from far-ranging experimental study designs, from information on how public policy frames the difficulties of science reporting—that adds *weight* of evidence that informs my interpretation of our findings in China.

The most oft-quoted complaint of these critics is that I have inferred causation from correlation alone, a false allegation. I know this principle well, as I discussed in chapter two. This criticism also assumes that scientific hypotheses should always focus on very reductionist cause–effect relationships, wherein one specific entity causes one specific effect or outcome, involving specific mechanisms presumably acting independently. But this is not how nutrition, or our bodies, work. Nutritional effects involve countless nutritional "causes" acting in concert through countless mechanisms (a wholistic phenomenon extensively explained in my more recent book, *Whole*[75]).

Virtually all of the evidence on how diet and nutrition works to produce health or disease is reductionist evidence because reductionism is the normal strategy for doing this research. We mostly study hypotheses in isolation, nutrients out of their natural context, mechanisms as if they are singular events (see chapter three), and specific diseases as if they bore little or no relationship to other health outcomes. These reductionist details are important when used to construct the fabric of the whole. However, they are the source of great confusion when interpreted outside of the whole of which they are a part.

Over the years, I have gone well beyond our own research findings to see what other researchers have found regarding diet and health. As our research findings expanded from the specific to the general, the picture has continued to enlarge, as the work of other scientists has allowed us to seek and more accurately see the larger context. As you shall see, the picture of health that has emerged is nothing short of astonishing.

PART II

DISEASES OF AFFLUENCE

Here in America, we are affluent, and we die certain deaths because of it. We eat like feasting kings and queens every day of the week, and it kills us. You probably know people who suffer from heart disease, cancer, stroke, Alzheimer's, obesity, or diabetes. There's a good chance that you yourself suffer from one of these problems, or that one of these diseases runs in your family. As we have seen, these diseases are relatively unknown in traditional cultures that subsist mostly on whole plant foods, as in rural China. But these ailments arrive when a traditional culture starts accumulating wealth and starts eating more and more meat, dairy, and refined plant products (like crackers, cookies, and soda).

In public lectures, I start my presentation by telling the audience my personal story, just as I have done in this book. Invariably, I get a question at the end of the lecture from someone who wants to know more about diet and a specific disease of affluence. Chances are that you yourself also have a question about a specific disease. Chances are, too, that this specific disease is a disease of affluence, because that's what we die of here in America.

You might be surprised to know that the disease that interests you has much in common with other diseases of affluence, especially when it comes to nutrition. There is no such thing as a special diet for cancer and a different, equally special diet for heart disease. The evidence now amassed from researchers around the world shows that the same diet that is good for the prevention of cancer is also good for the prevention of heart disease, as well as obesity, diabetes, cataracts, macular degeneration, Alzheimer's, cognitive dysfunction, multiple sclerosis, osteoporosis, and other diseases. Furthermore, this diet seems to benefit everyone, regardless of his or her genes or personal dispositions. People constantly come up to tell me after my lectures of the ailments, some quite rare, that resolved for them when they adopted this diet.

All of these diseases, and others, spring forth from the same influence: an unhealthy, largely toxic diet and lifestyle that has an excess of sickness-promoting factors and a deficiency of health-promoting factors. In other words, the Western diet. Conversely, there is one diet to counteract all of these diseases: a whole foods, plant-based (WFPB) diet.

The following chapters are organized by disease, or disease grouping. Each contains evidence showing how food relates to that disease. As you read each chapter, you will begin to see the breadth and depth of the astonishing scientific argument favoring a WFPB diet. For me, the consistency of evidence regarding such a disparate group of diseases has been the most convincing aspect of this argument. When a WFPB diet is demonstrably beneficial for such a wide variety of diseases, is it possible that humans were meant to consume any other diet? I say no, and I think you'll agree.

America and most other Western nations have gotten it wrong when it comes to diet and health, and we have paid a grave price. We are sick, overweight, and confused. As I have moved on from the laboratory studies and the China Study and encountered the information discussed in Part II, I have become overwhelmed. I have come to realize that some of our most revered conventions are wrong and real health has been grossly obscured. Most unfortunately, the unsuspecting public has paid the ultimate price. In large measure, this book is my effort to right these wrongs. As you will come to see in the following chapters, from heart disease to cancer, and from obesity to blindness, there is a better path to optimal health.

As a doctor, Tom has seen the ravages of these diseases. They are the harbingers of personal tragedy that so many of us have experienced. Beyond the personal costs, they fuel the medical care expenditures that threaten our economy. These diseases also fuel the frustration of those medical professionals who got in the business to help people. It can be frustrating to work so hard to help people and yet, over and over, see their health steadily decline.

All of these problems beg for a new type of solution that addresses the root cause of our illnesses. As you will see in the pages ahead, the solution could not be more plain.

BROKEN HEARTS

Put your hand on your chest and feel your heart beat. Now put your hand where you can feel your pulse. That pulse is the signature of your being. Your heart, creating that pulse, is working for you every minute of the day, every day of the year, and every year of your entire life. If you live an average lifetime, your heart will beat about 3 billion times.[1]

Now take a moment to realize that during the time it took you to read that paragraph, an artery in the heart of roughly one more American clogged up, cutting off blood flow downstream and starting a rapid process of tissue and cell death. This process is better known, of course, as a heart attack. By the time you finish reading this page, four Americans will have had a heart attack, and another four will have fallen prey to stroke or heart failure.[2] Over the next twenty-four hours, 3,000 Americans will have heart attacks,[2] roughly the same number of people who perished in the terrorist attacks of September 11, 2001.

The heart is the centerpiece of life and, more often than not in America, it is the centerpiece of death. Malfunction of the heart and/or circulatory system will kill 40% of Americans,[3] more than those killed by any other injury or ailment, including cancer. Heart disease has been our number one cause of death for almost 100 years.[4] This disease does not recognize gender or race boundaries; all are affected. If you were to ask most women what disease poses the greatest risk to them, heart disease or breast cancer, many women would undoubtedly say breast cancer. But they would be wrong. Women's death rate from heart disease is *eight times higher* than their death rate from breast cancer.[5,6]

If there is an "American" game, it is baseball; an "American" dessert, apple pie. If there is an "American" disease, it is heart disease.

EVERYONE'S DOING IT

In 1950, Judy Holliday could be seen on the big screen, Ben Hogan dominated the world of golf, the musical *South Pacific* won big at the Tony Awards, and on June 25, North Korea invaded South Korea. The American administration was taken aback but responded quickly. Within days, President Truman sent in troops on the ground and bombers overhead to push back the North Korean army. Three years later, in July of 1953, a formal cease-fire agreement had been signed and the Korean War was over. During this period of time, over 30,000 American soldiers were killed in battle.

At the end of the war, a landmark scientific study was reported in the *Journal of the American Medical Association*. Military medical investigators had examined the hearts of 300 male soldiers killed in action in Korea. The soldiers, at an average age of twenty-two years, had never been diagnosed with heart problems. In dissecting these hearts, researchers found startling evidence of disease in an exceptional number of cases. *Fully 77.3% of the hearts they examined had "gross evidence" of heart disease.*[7] (In this instance, "gross" means large.)

That number, 77.3%, is startling. Coming at a time when our number one killer was still shrouded in mystery, the research clearly demonstrated that heart disease develops over an entire lifetime. Furthermore, almost everyone was susceptible! These soldiers were not couch-potato slouches; they were in top condition in the prime of their physical lives. Since that time, several other studies have confirmed that heart disease is pervasive in young Americans.[8]

THE HEART ATTACK

But what is heart disease? One of the key components is plaque. Plaque is a greasy layer of proteins, fats (including cholesterol), immune system cells, and other components that accumulate on the inner walls of the coronary arteries. I have heard one surgeon say that if you wipe your finger on a plaque-covered artery, it has the same feel as wiping your finger across a warm cheesecake. If you have plaque building up in your coronary arteries, you have some degree of heart disease. Of the autopsied soldiers in Korea, one out of twenty diseased men had so much plaque that 90% of an artery was blocked.[7] That's like putting a kink in a garden hose and watering a desperately dry garden with the resulting trickle of water!

Why hadn't these soldiers had a heart attack already? After all, only 10% of the artery was open. How could that be enough? It turns out that if the plaque on the inner wall of the artery accumulates slowly, over several years, blood flow has time to adjust. Think of blood flowing through your artery as a raging river. If you put a few stones on the sides of a river every day over a period of years, like plaque accumulating on the walls of the artery, the water will find another way to get to where it wants to be. Maybe the river will form several smaller streams over the stones. Perhaps the river will go under the stones, forming tiny tunnels, or maybe the water will flow through small side streams, taking a new route altogether. These new tiny passageways around or through the stones are called "collaterals." The same thing happens in the heart. If plaque accumulates over a period of several years, there will be enough collateral development that blood can still travel throughout the heart. However, too much plaque buildup can cause severe blood restriction, and debilitating chest pain, or angina, can result. But this buildup only rarely leads to heart attacks.[9,10]

So what leads to heart attacks? It turns out that it's the less severe accumulations of plaque, blocking under 50% of the artery, that often cause heart attacks.[11] These accumulations each have a layer of cells, called the cap, which separates the core of the plaque from the blood flowing by. In the dangerous plaques, the cap is weak and thin (undoubtedly related to a diet that produces a tissue environment with excessive amounts of reactive oxygen species and inadequate amounts of antioxidants, meaning a diet having excess amounts of animal-based foods and inadequate amounts of plant-based foods).[12] Consequently, as blood rushes by, it can erode the cap until it ruptures. When the cap ruptures, the core contents of the plaque mix with the blood. The blood then begins clotting around the site of rupture. The clot grows and can quickly block the entire artery. When the artery becomes blocked over such a short period of time, there is little chance for collateral blood flow to develop. When this happens, blood flow downstream of the rupture is severely reduced and the heart muscles don't get the oxygen they require. At this point, as heart muscle cells start to die, heart-pumping mechanisms begin to fail, and the person may feel a crushing pain in the chest, or a searing pain down into an arm and up into the neck and jaw. In short, the victim starts to die. This is the process behind most of the 1.1 million heart attacks that occur in America every year. One out of three people who have a heart attack will die from it.[9,10]

We now know that the small to medium accumulation of plaque, the plaque that blocks less than 50% of the artery, is the most deadly.[11,13] So how can we predict the timing of heart attacks? Unfortunately, with existing technologies, we can't. We can't know which plaque will rupture, when, or how severe it might be. What we do know, however, is our relative risk for having a heart attack. What once was a mysterious death, which claimed people in their most productive years, has been "demystified" by science. Historically, no study has been more influential than that of the Framingham Heart Study.

FRAMINGHAM

After World War II, the National Heart Institute[14] was created with a modest budget[4] and a difficult mission. Scientists knew that the greasy plaques that lined the arteries of diseased hearts were composed of cholesterol, phospholipids, and fatty acids,[15] but they didn't know why these lesions developed, how they developed, or exactly how they led to heart attacks. In the search for answers, the Institute decided to follow a population over several years, to keep detailed medical records of everybody in the population, and to see who got heart disease and who didn't. The scientists headed to Framingham, Massachusetts.

Located just outside of Boston, Framingham is steeped in American history. European settlers first inhabited the land in the seventeenth century. Over the years the town has had supporting roles in the Revolutionary War, the Salem Witch Trials, and the abolition movement. More recently, in 1948, the town assumed its most famous role. Over 5,000 residents of Framingham, both male and female, agreed to be poked and prodded by scientists over the years so that we might learn something about heart disease.

And learn something we did. By watching who got heart disease and who didn't, and comparing their medical records, the Framingham Heart Study developed the concept of risk factors such as cholesterol, blood pressure, physical activity, cigarette smoking, and obesity. Because of the Framingham Study, we now know that these risk factors play a prominent role in causing heart disease. For years doctors have used a Framingham prediction model to tell who is at high risk for heart disease and who is not. Over 1,000 scientific papers have been published from this study, and it continues to this day, having now studied four generations of Framingham residents.

The shining jewel of the Framingham Study is its findings on blood cholesterol. In 1961, they convincingly showed a strong correlation between high blood cholesterol and heart disease. Researchers noted that men with cholesterol levels "over 244 mg/dL (milligrams per deciliter) have more than three times the incidence of coronary heart disease as do those with cholesterol levels less than 210 mg/dL."[16] The contentious question of whether blood cholesterol levels could predict heart disease was, to a considerable extent, laid to rest. Cholesterol levels do make a difference. In this same paper, high blood pressure was also demonstrated to be an important risk factor for heart disease.

The importance given to risk factors signaled a conceptual revolution. When this study was started, most doctors believed that heart disease was an inevitable "wearing down" of the body, and we could do little about it. Our hearts were like car engines; as we got older, the parts didn't work as well and sometimes gave out. By demonstrating that we could anticipate the disease in advance by measuring risk factors, the idea of preventing heart disease suddenly had validity. Researchers wrote, "It appears that a preventive program is clearly necessary."[16] Simply lower the risk factors, such as blood cholesterol and blood pressure, and you lower the risk of heart disease.

In modern-day America cholesterol and blood pressure are household terms. We spend over $30 billion a year on drugs to control these risk factors and other aspects of cardiovascular disease.[2] Almost everyone now knows that he or she can work to prevent a heart attack by keeping his or her risk factors at the right levels. This awareness is only about fifty years old and due in large measure to the scientists and subjects of the Framingham Heart Study.

OUTSIDE OUR BORDERS

Framingham is the most well-known heart study ever done, but it is merely one part of an enormous body of research conducted in this country over the past sixty years. Early research led to the alarming conclusion that we have some of the highest rates of heart disease in the world. One study published in 1959 compared the coronary heart disease death rates in twenty different countries (Chart 5.1).[17]

These studies were examining Westernized societies. If we look at more traditional societies, we tend to see even more striking disparities in the incidence of heart disease. The Papua New Guinea Highlanders, for example, pop up in research quite a bit because heart disease is rare in their society.[18] Remember, for example, how low the rate of heart disease was in rural China. American men died from heart disease at a rate almost seventeen times higher than their Chinese counterparts.[19]

Why were we succumbing to heart disease in the sixties and seventies, when much of the world was relatively unaffected?

Quite simply, it was a case of death by food. The cultures that have lower heart disease rates eat less saturated fat and animal protein and more

Chart 5.1: Heart Disease Death Rates for Men Aged 55 to 59 Across 20 Countries, Circa 1955[17]

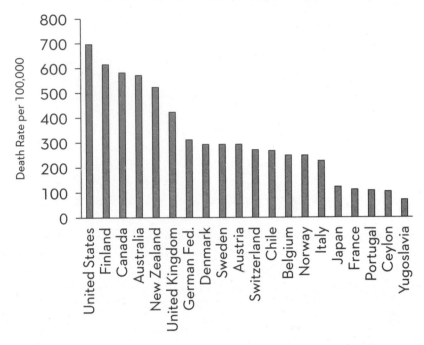

whole grains, fruits, and vegetables. In other words, they subsist mostly on plant foods while we subsist mostly on animal foods.

But might it be that the genetics of one group might just make them more susceptible to heart disease? We know that this is not the case, because within a group with the same genetic heritage, a similar relationship between diet and disease is seen. For example, Japanese men who live in Hawaii or California have a much higher blood cholesterol level and incidence of coronary heart disease than Japanese men living in Japan.[20,21] The cause is clearly environmental, as most of these people have the same genetic heritage. Smoking habits are not the cause because men in Japan, who were more likely to smoke, still had less coronary heart disease than the Japanese Americans.[20] The researchers pointed to diet, writing that blood cholesterol increased "with dietary intake of saturated fat, animal protein and dietary cholesterol." On the flip side, blood cholesterol "was negatively associated with complex carbohydrate intake."[21] In simple terms, animal foods were linked to higher blood cholesterol; plant foods were linked to lower blood cholesterol.

This research clearly implicated diet as one possible cause of heart disease. Furthermore, the early results were painting a consistent picture: the more saturated fat and cholesterol (as indicators of animal food consumption) people eat, the higher their risk for getting heart disease. And as other cultures have come to eat more like us, they also have seen their rates of heart disease skyrocket. In more recent times, several countries now report higher death rates from heart disease than America.

RESEARCH AHEAD OF ITS TIME

So now we know what heart disease is and what factors determine our risk for it, but what do we do once the disease is upon us? When the Framingham Heart Study was just beginning, some doctors were already trying to figure out how to treat heart disease, rather than just prevent it. In many ways, these investigators were ahead of their time because their interventions, which were the most innovative, successful treatment programs at the time, utilized the least advanced technology available: the knife and fork. These doctors noticed the ongoing research at the time and made some commonsense connections. They recognized that[22]:

- excess fat and cholesterol consumption caused atherosclerosis (the hardening of the arteries and the accumulation of plaque) in experimental animals
- eating cholesterol-laden food caused a rise in cholesterol in the blood
- high blood cholesterol might predict and/or cause heart disease
- most of the world's population didn't have heart disease, and these heart disease–free cultures had radically different dietary patterns, consuming less fat and cholesterol

So they decided to try to alter heart disease in their patients by having them eat less fat and cholesterol. One of the most progressive doctors was Dr. Lester Morrison of Los Angeles. He started a study in 1946 (two years before the Framingham Study) to "determine the relationship of dietary fat intake to the incidence of atherosclerosis."[23] In his study he instructed fifty heart attack survivors to maintain their normal diet and fifty different heart attack survivors to consume an experimental diet.

In the experimental diet group he reduced the consumption of fat and cholesterol. One of his published sample menus allowed the patient to have only a small amount of meat two times a day: two ounces of "cold roast lamb, lean, with mint jelly" for lunch, and another two ounces of "lean meats" for dinner.[23] Even if you loved cold roast lamb with mint jelly, you weren't allowed to eat much of it. In fact, the list of prohibited foods in the experimental diet was fairly long and included cream soups, pork, fat meats, animal fats, whole milk, cream, butter, egg yolks, and breads and desserts made with butter, whole eggs, and whole milk.[23]

Did this progressive diet accomplish anything? After eight years, only twelve of fifty people eating their normal American diet were alive (24%). In the diet group, twenty-eight people were still alive (56%), almost two and one-half times the amount of survivors in the control group. After twelve years, every single patient in the control group was dead. In the diet group, however, nineteen people were still alive, a survival rate of 38%.[23] While it was unfortunate that so many people in the dietary group still died, it was clear that they were staving off their disease by eating moderately less animal foods and moderately more plant foods (see Chart 5.2).

Chart 5.2: Survival Rate of Dr. Morrison's Patients

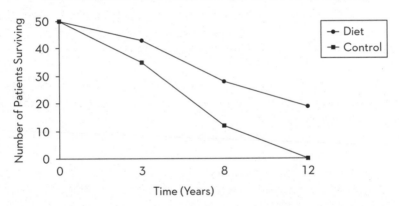

In 1946, when this study began, most scientists believed that heart disease was an inevitable part of aging, and nothing much could be done about it. While Morrison didn't cure heart disease, he proved that something as simple as diet could significantly alter its course, even when the disease is so advanced that it has already caused a heart attack.

Another research group proved much the same thing at about that time. A group of doctors in Northern California took a larger group of patients with advanced heart disease and put them on a low-fat, low-cholesterol diet. These doctors found that the patients who ate the low-fat, low-cholesterol diet died at a rate *four times lower* than patients who didn't follow the diet.[24]

It was now clear that there was hope. Heart disease wasn't the inevitable result of old age, and even when a person had advanced disease, a low-fat, low-cholesterol diet could significantly prolong his or her life. This was a remarkable advance in our understanding of the number one killer in

America. Furthermore, this new understanding made diet and other environmental factors the centerpieces of heart disease. Any discussion of diet, however, was narrowly focused on fat and cholesterol. These two isolated food components became the bad guys.

We now know that the attention paid to fat and cholesterol was misguided. The possibility that no one wanted to consider was that fat and cholesterol were merely indicators of animal food intake. For example, look at the relationship between animal protein consumption and heart disease death in men aged fifty-five to fifty-nine across twenty different countries in Chart 5.3.[17]

This study suggests that the more animal protein you eat, the more heart disease you have. In addition, dozens of experimental studies show that feeding rats, rabbits, and pigs animal protein (e.g., casein) dramatically raises cholesterol levels, whereas plant protein (e.g., soy protein) dramatically lowers cholesterol levels.[25] Studies in humans not only mirror these findings, but also show that eating plant protein has even greater power to lower cholesterol levels than reducing fat or cholesterol intake.[26]

While some of these studies implicating animal protein were conducted in the past thirty years, others were published well over sixty years ago when the health world was first beginning to discuss diet and heart disease. In 1941, it was shown that animal protein (casein) induced a fivefold greater severity of atherosclerosis than plant protein (soy) in rabbits.[27] Even earlier experimental research investigating the possible dietary origin of heart disease *over a century ago* also implicated animal protein. Back then, those who hypothesized a dietary cause largely fell into two schools of thought, one focused on dietary fat and cholesterol, the other focused on protein, especially animal protein.[28] Although dietary fat was found to induce formation of early atherosclerosis in experimental rabbits, animal-based protein (such as casein) proved even more effective. As early as 1909, Dr. Alexander Ignatowski attributed the formation of atherosclerosis to animal protein.[29] Reviews of this early literature[30] report that animal protein was substantially more effective than cholesterol in inducing the formation of early heart disease.

Yet somehow animal protein has remained in the shadows while saturated fat and cholesterol have taken the brunt of the criticism. These three nutrients (fat, animal protein, and cholesterol) characterize animal-based food in general. So isn't it perfectly reasonable to wonder whether animal-based food, and not just these isolated nutrients, causes heart disease? (If only this early research on the importance of animal-based protein in heart disease been taken seriously over the past century, progress in understanding the dietary cause of heart disease would have been far greater, with much less confusion and dispute!)

Chart 5.3: Heart Disease Death Rates for Men Aged 55 to 59 Years and Animal Protein Consumption Across 20 Countries[17]

Of course, no one pointed a finger at animal-based foods in general. It would have led immediately to professional isolation and ridicule (for reasons discussed in Part IV). These were contentious times in the nutritional world. A conceptual revolution was taking place, and a lot of people didn't like it. Even talking about diet was too much for many scientists. Preventing heart disease by diet was a threatening idea because it implied that something about the good old meaty American diet was so bad for us that it was destroying our hearts. The status quo boys didn't like it.

One status quo scientist had a good time making fun of people who appeared to have a low risk of heart disease. In 1960, he wrote the following piece of "humor" to mock the then-recent findings[31]:

Thumbnail Sketch of the Man Least Likely to Have Coronary Heart Disease:

An effeminate municipal worker or embalmer, completely lacking in physical and mental alertness and without drive, ambition or competitive spirit who has never attempted to meet a deadline of any kind. A man with poor appetite, subsisting on fruit and vegetables laced with corn and whale oils, detesting tobacco, spurning ownership of radio, TV or motor car, with full head of hair and scrawny and un-athletic in appearance, yet constantly straining his puny muscles by exercise; low in income, B.P. (blood pressure), blood sugar, uric acid and cholesterol, who has been taking nicotinic acid, pyridoxine and long term anticoagulant therapy ever since his prophylactic castration.

The author of this passage might just as well have said, "Only REAL men have heart disease." Also notice how a diet of fruits and vegetables is described as "poor" even though the author suggests that this diet is eaten by those people who are least likely to have heart disease. The unfortunate association of meat with physical ability, general manliness, sexual identity, and economic wealth all cloud how the status quo scientists viewed food, regardless of the health evidence. This view had been passed down from the early protein pioneers described in chapter two.

Perhaps this author should have met a friend of mine, Chris Campbell (no relation). Chris is a two-time NCAA Division I wrestling champion, three-time U.S. Senior wrestling champion, two-time Olympic wrestler, and Cornell Law School graduate. At the age of thirty-seven he became the oldest American ever to win an Olympic medal in wrestling, weighing in at 198 pounds. Chris Campbell is a vegetarian. Many more athletes have begun eschewing animal foods, including several professional football players and UFC fighters. I think they might disagree with the characterization that they might be "effeminate municipal workers or embalmers."

The battle between the status quo and the dietary prevention camp was intense. I remember attending a lecture at Cornell University during the late 1950s when a famous researcher, Ancel Keys, came to talk about preventing heart disease by diet. Some scientists in the audience just shook their heads in disbelief, saying diet can't possibly affect heart disease. In those first decades of heart disease research, a heated, personal battle flared, and open-mindedness was the first casualty.

RECENT HISTORY

Today, this epic battle between defenders of the status quo and advocates of diet is as strong as ever. Since the first edition of this book, a highly energized discussion has erupted on the internet and in the media in which popular opinion suggests that blood cholesterol is a cause of heart disease, and others (mostly those who deny that animal-based foods—the dietary source of cholesterol—might be a health problem, and mostly in discussion groups on the internet) argue that it is not. (Neither is technically correct. Blood cholesterol is only a marker or estimator of disease risk, and is most useful when discussing populations of people. For individuals, it is only a crude estimate of disease risk.)

Although we are still engaging in the same arguments, there have been significant changes in the landscape of heart disease. How far have we come, and how have we proceeded to fight this disease? Mostly, the status quo has been protected. Despite the potential of diet and disease prevention, most of the attention given to heart disease has been on mechanical and chemical intervention for those people who have advanced disease. Diet has been pushed aside. Surgery, drugs, electronic devices, and new diagnostic tools have stolen the spotlight.

We now have coronary bypass surgery, where a healthy artery is "pasted" over a diseased artery, thereby bypassing the most dangerous plaque on the artery. The ultimate surgery, of course, is the heart transplant, which even utilizes an artificial heart on occasion. We also have a procedure that doesn't require cracking the chest plate open, called coronary angioplasty, where a small balloon is inflated in a narrowed, diseased artery, squishing the plaque back against the wall, and opening up the passage for increased blood flow. We have defibrillators to revive hearts, pacemakers, and precise imaging techniques so that we can observe individual arteries without having to expose the heart.

The past sixty years have truly been a celebration of chemicals and technology (as opposed to diet and prevention). In summarizing the initial widespread research on heart disease, one doctor highlighted the mechanical:

> It was hoped that the strength of science and engineering developed after World War II could be applied to this battle [against heart disease] . . . The enormous advances in mechanical engineering and electronics that had been stimulated by the war seemed to lend themselves particularly well to the study of the cardiovascular system.[4]

Some great advances have been made, to be sure, which is thought to account for the fact that our death rate from heart disease is a full 58% lower than what it was in 1950.[2] A 58% reduction in the death rate seems a great victory for chemicals and technology. One of the greatest strides has come from better emergency room treatment of heart attack victims. In 1970, if you were older than sixty-five years, had a heart attack, and were lucky enough to make it to the hospital alive, you had a 38% chance of dying. Today, if you make it to the hospital alive, you only have a 15% chance of dying. The hospital's emergency response is much better, and consequently huge numbers of lives are being spared, at least for that moment.[2]

In addition, the number of people smoking has steadily been decreasing,[32,33] which in turn lowers our death rate from heart disease. Between hospital advances, mechanical devices, drug discoveries, lower smoking rates, and more surgical options, there clearly seems to be much to cheer about. We've made progress, so it seems.

Or have we?

After all, heart disease is still our number one cause of death. Every twenty-four hours, almost 2,000 Americans will die from this disease.[2] For all the advances, there are a huge number of people still succumbing to broken hearts.

In fact, the incidence rate (not death rate) for heart disease[34] is about the same as it was in the early 1970s.[2] In other words, while we don't die as much from heart disease, we still get it as often as we used to. In fact, very recent research finds that patients presenting with heart attacks are younger than ever before.[35] It seems that we simply have gotten slightly better at postponing death from heart disease, but *we have done nothing to stop the rate at which our hearts become diseased.*

SURGERY: THE PHANTOM SAVIOR

The mechanical interventions that we use in this country are much less effective than most people realize. Bypass surgery is popular. As many as 380,000 bypass operations were performed in 1990,[36] meaning that about 1 out of 750 Americans underwent this extreme surgery. During the operation, the patient's chest is split open, blood flow is rerouted by a series of clamps, pumps, and machines, and a leg vein or chest artery is cut out and sewn over a diseased part of the heart, thereby allowing blood to bypass the most clogged arteries.

The costs are enormous. More than one of every fifty elective patients will die because of complications[37] during the procedure,[38] which a recent estimate, based on a 2011 report by the American Heart Association,[39] listed at between $70,000 and $200,000 (up from the $46,000 cited in this book's first edition). Other side effects include heart attack, respiratory complications, bleeding complications, infection, high blood pressure, and stroke. When the vessels around the heart are clamped shut during the operation, plaque breaks off of the inner walls. Blood then carries this debris to the brain, where it causes numerous "mini" strokes. Researchers have compared the intellectual capabilities of patients before and after the operation, and found that a stunning 79% of patients "showed impairment in some aspect of cognitive function" seven days after the operation.[40]

Why do we put ourselves through this? The most pronounced benefit of this procedure is relief of angina, or chest pain. About 70–80% of patients who undergo bypass surgery remain free of this crippling chest pain for one year.[41] *But this benefit doesn't last.* Within three years of the operation, up to one-third of patients will suffer from chest pain again.[42] Within ten years half of the bypass patients will have died, had a heart attack, or had their chest pain return.[43] Long-term studies indicate that only certain subsets of heart disease patients live longer because of their bypass operation.[13] Furthermore, these studies demonstrate that *those patients who undergo bypass operation do not have fewer heart attacks than those who do not have surgery.*[13]

Remember which plaque buildups cause heart attacks? The deadly buildups are the smaller, less stable plaques that tend to rupture. The bypass operation, however, is targeted to the largest, most visible plaques, which may be responsible for chest pain, but not for heart attacks.

Angioplasty is a similar story. The procedure is expensive and carries significant risks. After identifying blockages in a coronary artery, a balloon is inserted into the artery and inflated. It pushes the plaque back against the vessel, thereby allowing more blood to flow. This balloon procedure is often accompanied with stent placement. A small wire-mesh coil is placed into the narrowed section of the artery and expanded to prop it open for a longer period of time. This has become a popular procedure, as it relieves chest pain. In the decade prior to 2013, an estimated 7 million Americans have had a stent placed, at a cost of over $110 billion.[44] Unfortunately, even with the newer drug-eluting stents that are designed to keep the artery open even longer, as many as 5–10% of all stents will "clog" up, requiring as many as 200,000 procedures annually to go back in and open up blood flow again.[45] Worse, there is little or no evidence that these stents extend life when they are used in stable disease[46] (versus in-progress heart attacks, when they can be lifesaving); not surprisingly, a number of lawsuits have been filed for their overuse.[47]

So, upon closer examination, our seemingly beneficent mechanical advances in the field of heart disease are severely disappointing. When used for stable disease, *bypass surgery, angioplasty, and stents do not address the cause of heart disease, prevent heart attacks, or extend the lives of any but the sickest heart disease patients.*

What's going on here? Despite the positive public relations surrounding the past sixty years of heart disease research, we must ask ourselves: Are we winning this war? Maybe we should ask ourselves what we might do differently. For example, whatever happened to the dietary lessons learned fifty years ago? Whatever happened to the dietary treatments discovered by Dr. Lester Morrison, as discussed earlier?

Those discoveries largely faded away. I only learned about this 1940s and 1950s research in recent years. I am bewildered because the professionals I heard during my graduate student days in the late 1950s and early 1960s vigorously denied that any such work was being done or even being contemplated. In the meanwhile, America's eating habits have only gotten worse. According to the U.S. Department of Agriculture, we consume significantly more meat and added fat than we did thirty years ago.[48] Clearly we are not moving in the right direction.

As this information has resurfaced in the past two decades, the fight against the status quo has been heating up again. A few rare doctors are proving that there is a better way to defeat heart disease. They are demonstrating revolutionary success, using the most simple of all treatments: food.

DR. CALDWELL B. ESSELSTYN, JR.

If you were to guess the location of the best cardiac care center in the country, maybe the world, what city would you name? New York? Los Angeles? Chicago? A city in Florida, perhaps, near elderly people? As it turns out, the best medical center for cardiac care is located in Cleveland, Ohio, according to *US News and World Report*. Patients fly in to the Cleveland Clinic from all over the world for the most advanced heart treatment available, administered by prestigious doctors.

One of the doctors at the Clinic, Dr. Caldwell B. Esselstyn, Jr., has quite a resume. As a student at Yale University, Dr. Esselstyn rowed in the 1956 Olympics, winning a gold medal. After being trained at the Cleveland Clinic, he went on to earn the Bronze Star as an army surgeon in the Vietnam War. He then became a highly successful doctor at one of the top medical institutions in the world, the Cleveland Clinic, where he was president of the staff, member of the Board of Governors, chairman of the Breast Cancer Task Force, and head of the Section of Thyroid and Parathyroid Surgery. Having published over 100 scientific papers, Dr. Esselstyn was named one of the best doctors in America in 1994–1995.[49] From knowing this man personally, I get the feeling that he has excelled at virtually everything he has done in his life. He reached the pinnacle of success in his professional and personal life, and did it with grace and humility.

The quality I find most appealing about Dr. Esselstyn, however, is not his resume or awards; it is his principled search for the truth. Dr. Esselstyn has had the courage to take on the establishment. For the Second National Conference on Lipids in the Elimination and Prevention of Coronary Artery Disease (which he organized and in which he kindly asked me to participate), Dr. Esselstyn wrote:

> *Eleven years into my career as a surgeon, I became disillusioned with the treatment paradigm of U.S. medicine in cancer and heart*

*disease. Little had changed in 100 years in the management of
cancer, and in neither heart disease nor cancer was there a serious
effort at prevention. I found the epidemiology of these diseases
provocative, however: Three-quarters of the humans on this planet
had no heart disease, a fact strongly associated with diet.[50]*

Dr. Esselstyn started to reexamine the standard medical practice.
"Aware that medical, angiographic and surgical interventions were treating only the symptoms of heart disease and believing that a fundamentally different approach to treatment was necessary," Dr. Esselstyn decided to test the effects of a whole foods, plant-based (WFPB) diet on people with established coronary disease.[51] By using a minimal amount of cholesterol-lowering medication and a very low-fat, plant-based diet, he has gotten the most spectacular results ever recorded in the treatment of heart disease.[51,52]

In 1985, Dr. Esselstyn began his study with the primary goal of reducing his patients' blood cholesterol to below 150 mg/dL. He asked each patient to record everything he or she ate in a food diary. Every two weeks, for the next five years, Dr. Esselstyn met with his patients to discuss the process, administer blood tests, and record blood pressure and weight. He followed up this daytime meeting with an evening telephone call to report the results of the blood tests and further discuss how the diet was working. In addition, all of his patients met together a few times a year to talk about the program, socialize, and exchange helpful information. In other words, Dr. Esselstyn was diligent, involved, supportive, and compassionately stern on a personal level with his patients.

The diet they, including Dr. Esselstyn and his wife, Ann, followed was free of all added fat and almost all animal products. Dr. Esselstyn and his colleagues report, "[Participants] were to avoid oils, meat, fish, fowl and dairy products, except for skim milk and nonfat yogurt."[51] About five years into the program, Dr. Esselstyn recommended to his patients that they stop consuming any skim milk and yogurt, as well.

Five of his patients dropped out of the study within the first two years; that left eighteen. These eighteen patients originally had come to Dr. Esselstyn with severe disease. *Within the eight years leading up to the study, these eighteen people had suffered through forty-nine coronary events,* including angina, bypass surgery, heart attacks, strokes, and angioplasty. These were not healthy hearts. One might imagine that they were motivated to join the study by the panic created when premature death is near.[51,52]

These eighteen patients achieved remarkable success. At the start of the study, the patients' average cholesterol level was 246 mg/dL. *During the course of the study, the average cholesterol was 132 mg/dL, well below the 150 mg/dL target.*[52] Their levels of "bad" LDL cholesterol dropped just as dramatically.[51] In the end, though, the most impressive result was not the blood cholesterol levels, but how many coronary events occurred since the start of the study.

In the following eleven years, there was exactly ONE coronary event among the eighteen patients who followed the diet. That one event was from a patient who strayed from the diet for two years. After straying, the patient consequently experienced clinical chest pain (angina) and then resumed a healthy whole food, plant-based diet. The patient eliminated his angina, and has not experienced any further events.[52]

Not only has the disease in these patients been stopped, it has even been reversed. *Seventy percent of his patients have seen an opening of their clogged arteries.*[52] Eleven of his patients had agreed to angiography, a procedure in which specific arteries in the heart can be "x-rayed." Of these eleven, the blockages in the arteries were, on average, reduced in size by 7% over the first five years of his study. This may sound like a small change but it should be noted that the volume of blood delivered is at least 30% greater when the diameter is increased by 7%.[53] More importantly, this is the difference between the presence of pain (from angina) and absence of pain, indeed between life and death. Authors of the five-year report note, "This is the longest study of minimal fat nutrition used in combination with cholesterol-lowering drugs conducted to date, and our finding of a mean decrease of arterial stenosis [blockage] of 7.0% is greater than any reports in previous research."[51]

One physician took special note of Dr. Esselstyn's study. He was only forty-four years of age and seemingly healthy when he found himself with a heart problem, culminating in a heart attack. Because of the nature of his heart disease, there was nothing that conventional medicine could safely offer him. He visited Dr. Esselstyn, decided to commit to the dietary program, and *after thirty-two months, without any cholesterol-lowering medication, he reversed his heart disease and lowered his blood cholesterol to 89 mg/dL.* What follows is the dramatic image of this patient's diseased artery before and after Dr. Esselstyn's dietary advice (Chart 5.4).[8] The light part of the picture is blood flowing through an artery. The picture on the left (A) has a section marked by a parenthesis where severe coronary disease had reduced the amount of blood flow. After adopting a WFPB diet, that same artery opened up, reversing the ravages of heart disease and allowing a much more normal blood flow, as shown in the picture on the right (B).

Is it possible that Dr. Esselstyn just got a lucky group of patients? The answer is no. Patients this sick with heart disease don't spontaneously heal

Chart 5.4: Coronary Artery Before and After Consuming Plant-Based Diet

themselves. Another way to check the likelihood of this degree of success is to look at the five patients that dropped out of the dietary program and resumed their standard care. *As of 1995, these five people had fallen prey to ten new coronary events.*[51] Meanwhile, as of 2003, seventeen years into the study, all but one patient following the diet were still alive, headed into their seventies and eighties.[54] By 2011, 25 years later, only five of the original eighteen patients in that study had passed—and none from coronary heart disease.[55]

Can any sane person dispute these findings? It seems impossible. If you remember nothing else about this chapter, remember the forty-nine to zero score; forty-nine coronary events prior to a WFPB diet, and zero events for those patients who adhered to a WFPB diet.

As if this study were not convincing enough, consider Dr. Esselstyn's latest contribution, the findings of which were published in July 2014.[56] After counseling patients with evidence of heart disease for about seven years, he decided to follow up to determine how they had fared. Of the original 198 patients, he learned that 177 (89.3%) had, since their one and only five-hour counseling session, complied with the advice provided to them. That advice included information on how to adhere to a WFPB diet, while leaving their drug use protocol as advised by their primary care doctors. Their average age when they attended the counseling session was 62.9 years, and a mean of 3.7 years had passed since.

Major cardiac events attributed to progression of disease for this compliant group was <1% (one stroke among 177 patients). Among the 21 patients who did not adhere to a WFPB diet, 62% suffered such events. This finding (<1% vs. 62%) is truly remarkable, substantially exceeding the findings of any other "nutritional" intervention. (Previous research, it should be noted, has indicated that a 20–25% disease recurrence for nonadherents might be more traditional.)

Dr. Esselstyn has done what "Big Science" has been trying to do, without success, for over sixty-five years: *he defeated heart disease.*

DR. DEAN ORNISH

In the past twenty-five years another giant in this field, Dr. Dean Ornish, has been instrumental in bringing diet to the forefront of medical thought. A graduate of Harvard Medical School, he has been featured prominently in popular media, succeeded in having his heart disease treatment plan covered by a number of insurance carriers, and written several best-selling books. If you have heard of the diet/heart disease connection, chances are that it may well be because of Dr. Ornish's work.

His best-known research is the Lifestyle Heart Trial, in which he treated twenty-eight heart disease patients with lifestyle changes alone.[57] He put these patients on an experimental treatment plan and twenty additional patients on the standard treatment plan. He followed both groups carefully and measured several health indicators, including artery blockages, cholesterol levels, and weight.

Dr. Ornish's treatment plan was very different from the standards of high-tech modern medicine. He put the twenty-eight patients in a hotel for the first week of treatment and told them what they had to do to take control of their health. He asked them to eat a low-fat, plant-based diet for at least a year. Only about 10% of their calories were to come from fat. They could eat as much food as they wanted, as long as it was on the acceptable food list, which included fruits, vegetables, and grains. As researchers noted, "No animal products were allowed except egg white and one cup per day of non-fat milk or yogurt."[57] In addition to diet, the group was to practice various forms of stress management, including meditation, breathing exercises, and relaxation exercises for at least one hour per day. The patients were also asked to exercise three hours per week at levels customized to the severity of their disease. To help the patients make these lifestyle changes, the group met twice a week for four hours at a time for mutual support. Dr. Ornish and his research group did not use any drugs, surgery, or technology to treat these patients.[57]

The experimental patients adhered to pretty much everything that the researchers asked of them and were rewarded with improved health and vitality. On average, their total cholesterol dropped from 227 mg/dL to 172 mg/dL, and their "bad" LDL cholesterol dropped from 152 mg/ dL to 95 mg/dL. And after one year, the frequency, duration, and severity of their chest pains plummeted. Further, it was clear that the closer the patients adhered to the lifestyle recommendations, the more their hearts healed. The patients who had the best adherence over the course of the year saw the blockages in their arteries diminish by over 4%. Four percent may seem like a small number, but remember that heart disease builds up over a life-time, so a 4% change in only a year is a fantastic result. *In all, 82% of the patients in the experimental group had regression in their heart disease over the course of a year*.

The control group did not fare so well, despite the fact that they received the usual care. Their chest pain became worse in terms of frequency, dura-tion, and severity. For example, although the experimental group experi-enced a 91% reduction in the frequency of chest pain, the control group experienced a 165% rise in the frequency of chest pain. Their cholesterol levels were significantly worse than those of the experimental patients, and the blockages in their arteries also became worse. The patients in the group who were the least attentive to diet and lifestyle changes had blockages that increased in size by 8% over the course of the year.[57]

Between Dr. Ornish, Dr. Esselstyn, and others before them, like Dr. Morrison, I believe that we have found the strategic link in our heart dis-ease battle plan. Their dietary treatments not only relieve the symptoms of chest pain, but they also treat the cause of heart disease and can eliminate future coronary events. There are no surgical or chemical heart disease treatments, at the Cleveland Clinic or anywhere else, that can compare to these impressive results.

THE FUTURE

The future is filled with hope. We now know enough to nearly eliminate our most common type of heart disease. We know not only how to prevent the disease, but how to successfully treat it. We do not need to crack open our breast plates to reroute our arteries, and we do not need a lifetime of powerful drugs in our blood. By eating the right food, we can keep our hearts healthy.

The next step is to implement this dietary approach on a large scale, which is exactly what Dr. Dean Ornish has done. Dr. Ornish began the Multicenter Lifestyle Demonstration Project, in which teams of health professionals at eight diverse sites were trained to treat heart disease patients with Dr. Ornish's lifestyle intervention program. Patients eligible to participate were those who had documented heart disease severe enough to warrant surgery. Instead of surgery, they enrolled in a one-year lifestyle program. This program was started in 1993, and by 1998 forty insurance programs were covering the costs for selected patients.[38]

As of 1998, almost 200 people had taken part in the Lifestyle Project, and the results were phenomenal. After one year of treatment, 65% of patients had eliminated their chest pain. The effect was long lasting, as well. After three years, over 60% of the patients continued reporting no chest pain.[38] As of 2011, nearly 4,000 patients have benefitted from Dr. Ornish's Program for Reversing Heart Disease.

The health benefits are equaled by the economic benefits. At the writing of the first edition of this book, over one million heart disease surgeries were being undertaken every year.[38] In 2002, physician services and hospital care for heart disease patients cost $78.1 billion (that does not include drug costs, home health care, or nursing home care).[2] In the 1990s, the angioplasty procedure alone cost $31,000, and bypass surgery cost $46,000; the cost has only risen since.[38] In marked contrast, the year-long lifestyle intervention program only cost $7,000. By comparing the patients who underwent the lifestyle program with those patients who underwent the traditional route of surgery, Dr. Ornish and his colleagues demonstrated that the lifestyle intervention program cut costs by an average of $30,000 per patient[38]—a success recognized by Medicare, which, as of January 2011, is now covering medical costs for patients who adopt Dr. Ornish's program.

As of the writing of this second edition, however, a few updates to the state of heart disease treatment are in order. Although the total number of heart disease surgeries appears to be either the same,[58] or slightly smaller,[59] the types of surgeries being performed have changed. Between 2001–2002 and 2007–2008,[59] more invasive bypass operations declined by 38%, while angioplasty and stent placement operations remained approximately the same. Although there has been considerable discussion about which type of heart surgery best suits the cardiac patient[60]—amid huge amounts of money being spent to compare surgical interventions—there has been virtually no serious discussion in the cardiology community about the possible use of dietary intervention to treat heart disease patients. This is a glaring omission, and—considering the side effects and costs of stent and bypass operations—it is an undeniable tragedy perpetrated on the American public. Annually, thousands of Americans suffer adverse outcomes, including death, during these procedures. A stent operation costs from $11,000 to over $41,000,[61] and a bypass costs $117,000, not including doctor fees (according to the American Heart Association).[62]

Compare all of this to the cost of Esselstyn's dietary advice, which may require as few as five hours of time and yield superior results: only $900 per session-person.[63]

When viewed nationwide, the costs continue to mount. The *Telegraph* reports that, according to IMS Health, the cost of "cholesterol treating medicines—including statins" was estimated at $35 billion for 2010.[64] And there's more: according to the American Heart Association, the total cost of treating heart disease is projected to rise from $273 billion (in 2011) to $818 billion in 2030 (although much of this is due to an increasing number of people moving into ages where heart disease is more common).[65] If the heart disease treatment community were a nation, this figure would make it the twenty-seventh richest among the world's almost 200 countries.[66] This American Heart Association report, it should be noted, offers no new insight on how this rapidly growing business might be reversed through dietary lifestyle—except to advocate almost mundane population-based prevention programs like "reducing dietary fat intakes and improving lipid levels" or "personalized approaches to prevention that include assessments of genetic variants, biomarkers and imaging modalities."[67] And there is little or no evidence that these approaches have, or can, do anything to cause meaningful change.

Clearly, much work remains to be done. The health care establishment is structured to profit from chemical and surgical intervention. Diet still takes the backseat to drugs and surgery, if it is mentioned to patients at all. One criticism that is constantly leveled at the dietary argument is that patients will not make such fundamental changes. One doctor charges that Dr. Esselstyn's patients change their eating habits simply because of Esselstyn's "zealous belief."[68] This criticism is not only wrong and insulting to patients and Dr. Esselstyn; it is also self-fulfilling. If doctors do not believe that patients will change their diets, they will neglect to talk about diet, or will do it in an off-handed, disparaging way. There is no greater disrespect a doctor can show patients than that of withholding potentially lifesaving information based on the assumption that patients do not want to change their lifestyle.

Well-meaning institutions are not exempt from such closed-mindedness. The American Heart Association recommends a diet for heart disease that favors moderation. The National Cholesterol Education Program does the same thing. These organizations pitch moderate diets with trivial changes as being healthy lifestyle "goals." If you are at high risk for heart disease, or if you already have the disease, they recommend that you adopt a diet containing 30% of total calories as fat (7% of total calories as saturated fat) and less than 200 mg/day of dietary cholesterol.[69,70] According to them, we should also keep our total blood cholesterol level under the "desirable" level of 200 mg/dL.[70]

These venerable organizations are not giving the American public the most up-to-date scientific information. While we are told that a total blood cholesterol level of 200 mg/dL is "desirable," *we know that 35% of heart attacks strike Americans who have cholesterol levels between 150 and 200 mg/dL*[71] (a truly safe cholesterol level is under 150 mg/dL). We also know that the most aggressive reversal of heart disease ever demonstrated occurred when fat was about 10% of total calorie intake. Studies have clearly demonstrated that many patients who follow the more moderate government-recommended diets *see a progression of heart disease.*[72] The innocent victims are health-conscious Americans who follow these recommendations, keeping their total cholesterol around 180 or 190 mg/dL, only to be rewarded with a heart attack leading to a premature death.

To top it off, the National Cholesterol Education Program dangerously writes, "Lifestyle changes are the most cost-effective means to reduce risk for CHD [coronary heart disease]. Even so, to achieve maximal benefit, many persons will require LDL [cholesterol]-lowering drugs."[70] No wonder America's health is failing. The dietary recommendations for the most diseased hearts among us, given by supposedly reputable institutions, are severely watered down and followed by the caveat that we'll probably need a lifetime of drugs anyway.

Our leading organizations fear that if they advocate more than modest changes, no one will listen to them. But the establishment-recommended diets are not nearly as healthy as the diets espoused by Drs. Esselstyn and Ornish. The fact is that a blood cholesterol level of 200 mg/dL is not optimal, a 30% fat diet is not "low-fat," and eating foods containing any cholesterol above 0 mg is unhealthy. Our health institutions are intentionally misleading the public about heart disease, all in the name of "moderation."

Whether scientists, doctors, and policy makers think the public will change or not, the layperson must be aware that a whole foods, plant-based (WFPB) diet is far and away the healthiest diet. In the seminal paper regarding the landmark Lifestyle Heart Trial, the authors, Dr. Ornish and his scientific colleagues, write, *"The point of our study was to determine what is true, not what is practicable* [my emphasis]."[57]

We now know what is true: a WFPB diet can prevent and treat heart disease, saving hundreds of thousands of Americans every year.

Dr. William Castelli, the long-time director of the Framingham Heart Study, a cornerstone of heart disease research, espouses a WFPB diet.

Dr. Esselstyn, who has demonstrated the most significant reversal of heart disease in all of medical history, espouses a WFPB diet.

Dr. Ornish, who has pioneered reversal of heart disease without drugs or surgery and proved widespread economic benefit for patients and insurance providers, espouses a WFPB diet.

Since writing the first edition of this book, I have encountered dozens more doctors who have recommended to their heart patients a WFPB diet and who have, as Drs. Esselstyn and Ornish did, observed spectacular results. Although their numbers are still tiny compared to the full cardiology field, there are far more of them than I knew—and those numbers are growing.

Now is a time of great hope and challenge, a time when people can control their health. One of the best and most caring doctors I have ever met puts it best:

> *The collective conscience and will of our profession*
> *is being tested as never before. Now is the time*
> *for us to have the courage for legendary work.*
> — Dr. Caldwell B. Esselstyn, Jr.[8]

OBESITY

P erhaps you've heard the news.
      Perhaps you've caught a glimpse of the staggering statistics on
   obesity among Americans.

Perhaps you've simply noticed that, compared to a few years ago, more people at the grocery store are overweight.

Perhaps you've been in classrooms, on playgrounds, or at day care centers and noticed how many kids are already burdened with a weight problem and can't run twenty feet without getting winded.

Our struggle with weight is hard to miss these days. Open a newspaper or a magazine, or turn on the radio or TV—you know that America has a weight problem. In fact, more than two out of three adult Americans are at least overweight. One-third of the adult population is obese. Not only are these numbers high, but the rate at which they have been rising is ominous (Chart 1.2, page 5).[1]

But what do the terms *overweight* and *obese* mean? The standard expression of body size is the body mass index (BMI). It represents body weight (in kilograms, kg) relative to body height (in meters squared, m^2). By most official standards, being overweight is having a BMI above twenty-five, and being obese is having a BMI over thirty. The same scale is used for both men and women. You can determine your own BMI using Chart 6.1, which lists the necessary information in pounds and inches for your convenience.

Chart 6.1: Body Mass Index Table

	Normal						Overweight					Obese		
BMI (kg/m)	19	20	21	22	23	24	25	26	27	28	29	30	35	40
Height (in.)	Weight (lb.)													
58	91	96	100	105	110	115	119	124	129	134	138	143	167	191
59	94	99	104	109	114	119	124	128	133	138	143	148	173	198
60	97	102	107	112	118	123	128	133	138	143	148	153	179	204
61	100	106	11	116	122	127	132	137	143	148	153	158	185	211
62	104	109	115	120	126	131	136	142	147	153	158	164	191	218
63	107	113	118	124	130	135	141	146	152	158	163	169	197	225
64	110	116	122	128	134	140	145	151	157	163	169	174	204	232
65	114	120	126	132	138	144	150	156	162	168	174	180	210	240
66	118	124	130	136	142	148	155	161	167	173	179	186	216	247
67	121	127	134	140	146	153	159	166	172	178	185	191	223	255
68	125	131	138	144	151	158	164	171	177	184	190	197	230	262
69	128	135	142	149	155	162	169	176	182	189	196	203	236	270
70	132	139	146	153	160	167	174	181	188	195	202	209	243	278
71	136	143	150	157	165	172	179	186	193	200	208	215	250	286
72	140	147	154	162	169	177	184	191	199	206	213	221	258	294
73	144	151	159	166	174	182	189	197	204	212	219	227	265	302
74	148	155	163	171	179	186	194	202	210	218	225	233	272	311
75	152	160	168	176	184	192	200	208	216	224	232	240	279	319
76	156	164	172	180	189	197	205	213	221	230	238	246	287	328

THE CHILDREN

Perhaps the most depressing element of our supersize mess is the growing number of overweight and obese children. About 18% of six- to eleven-year-olds and 21% of twelve- to nineteen-year-olds in America are overweight.[2] Another 15% are at risk of becoming overweight.[3]

Overweight children face a wide range of psychological and social challenges. As you know, children have a knack for being open and blunt; sometimes the playground can be a merciless place. Overweight children find it more difficult to make friends and are often thought of as lazy and sloppy. They are more likely to have behavioral and learning difficulties, and the low self-esteem likely to be formed during adolescence can last forever.[4]

Young people who are overweight also are highly likely to face a host of medical problems. They often have elevated cholesterol levels, which can be a predictor for any number of deadly diseases. They are more likely to have problems with glucose intolerance, and, consequently, diabetes. Type 2 diabetes, formerly seen only in adults, is skyrocketing among adolescents. (See chapters seven and nine for a more thorough discussion of childhood diabetes.) Elevated blood pressure is *nine times* more likely to occur among obese kids. Sleep apnea, which can cause neurocognitive problems, is found in one in ten obese children. A wide variety of bone problems is more common in obese kids. Most importantly, an obese young person is much more likely to be an obese adult,[4] greatly increasing the likelihood of life-long health problems.

CONSEQUENCES FOR THE ADULT

If you are obese, you may not be able to do many things that could make your life more enjoyable. You may find that you cannot play vigorously with your grandchildren (or your children), walk long distances, participate in sports, find a comfortable seat in a movie theatre or airplane, or have an active sex life. In fact, even sitting still in a chair may be impossible without experiencing back or joint pain. For many, standing is hard on the knees. Carrying around too much weight can dramatically affect physical mobility, work, mental health, self-perception, and social life. So you see, this isn't about death; it really is about missing many of the more enjoyable things in life.[5]

Clearly no one *desires* to be overweight. So why is it that two out of three adult Americans are overweight? Why is one-third of the population obese?

The problem is not a lack of money. In 1999, medical care costs relating to obesity alone were estimated to be $70 billion.[6] In 2002, a mere three years later, the American Obesity Association listed these costs at $100 billion.[7] By 2006, obesity-related medical treatment costs reached between $147 and $210 billion.[8] This is not all. Add another $60 billion or more out-of-pocket expenses that we spend trying to keep off the weight in the first place.[9] Going on special weight-loss diet plans and popping pills to cut our appetites or rearrange our metabolism have become a national pastime.

This is an economic black hole that sucks our money away without offering anything in return. Imagine paying $40 to a plumber to fix your leaky kitchen sink, and then two weeks later, the sink pipes explode and flood the kitchen, and it costs $500 to repair. I bet you wouldn't ask that plumber to fix your sink again! So then why do we endlessly try those weight-loss plans, books, drinks, energy bars, and assorted gimmicks when they don't deliver as promised?

I applaud people for trying to achieve a healthy weight. I don't question the worthiness or dignity of overweight people any more than I question cancer victims. My criticism is of a societal system that allows and even encourages this problem. I believe, for example, that we are drowning in an ocean of very bad information, too much of it intended to put money into someone else's pockets. What we really need, then, is a new solution featuring good information for individual people to use, at a price that they can afford.

THE SOLUTION

The solution to losing weight is a whole foods, plant-based (WFPB) diet, coupled with a reasonable amount of exercise. It is a long-term lifestyle change, rather than a quick-fix fad, and it can provide sustained weight loss while minimizing risk of chronic disease.

Have you ever known anyone who regularly consumes fresh fruits, vegetables, and whole grain foods—and rarely, if ever, consumes meats or junk foods like chips, French fries, and candy bars? What is his or her weight like? If you know many people like this, you have probably noticed that they tend to have a healthy weight. Now think of traditional cultures around the world. Think of traditional Asian cultures (Chinese, Japanese, Indian), where a couple of billion people have been eating a mostly plant-based diet for thousands of years. It's hard to imagine these people—at least until recently—as anything other than slender.

Now imagine a guy buying two hot dogs and ordering his second beer at a baseball game, or a woman ordering a cheeseburger and fries at your local fast-food joint. The people in these images look different, don't they? Unfortunately, the guy munching his hot dogs and sipping his beer is the "all-American" image. I have had visitors from other countries tell me that one of the first things they notice when they arrive in our good land is the exceptional number of fat people.

Solving this problem does not require magic tricks or complex equations involving blood types or carbohydrate counting or soul searching. Simply trust your observations on who is slim, vigorous, and healthy, and who is not. Or trust the findings of some impressive research studies, large and small, showing time and time again that vegetarians and vegans are slimmer than their meat-eating counterparts. People in these studies who are vegetarian or vegan are anywhere from five to thirty pounds slimmer than their fellow citizens.[10–16]

In one intervention study, overweight subjects were told to eat as much as they wanted of foods that were mostly low fat, whole foods, and plant based. In three weeks these people lost an average of seventeen pounds.[17] At the Pritikin Center, 4,500 patients who had gone through their three-week program got similar results. By feeding a mostly plant-based diet and promoting exercise, the Center found that its clients lost 5.5% of their body weight over three weeks.[18]

Published results for still more intervention studies using a low-fat, whole foods, mostly plant-based diet:

- About two to five pounds lost after twelve days[19]
- About ten pounds lost in three weeks[20,21]
- Sixteen pounds lost over twelve weeks[22]
- Twenty-four pounds lost after one year[23]

All of these results show that consuming a WFPB diet will help you to lose weight and, furthermore, it can happen quickly. The only question is how much weight you can lose. In most of these studies, the people who shed the most pounds were those who started with the most excess weight.[24] After the initial weight loss, the weight can be kept off for the long term by staying on the diet. Most importantly, losing weight this way is consistent with long-term health.

Some people, of course, can be on a plant-based diet and still not lose weight. There are a few very good reasons for this. First and foremost, losing body weight on a plant-based diet is much less likely to occur if the diet includes too many refined carbohydrates. *Sweets, pastries, and pastas won't do it.* These foods are high in readily digested sugars and starches and, for the pastries, oftentimes very high in fat as well. As mentioned in chapter four, these highly processed, unnatural foods are not part of a plant-based diet that works to reduce body weight and promote health. This is one of the main reasons that I usually refer to the optimal diet as a *whole foods*, plant-based diet.

Notice that a strict vegetarian diet is not necessarily the same thing as a WFPB diet. Some people become vegetarian only to replace meat with dairy foods, added oils, and refined carbohydrates, including pasta made with refined grains, sweets, and pastries. I refer to these people as "junk-food vegetarians" because they are not consuming a nutritious diet.

The second reason weight loss may be elusive is if a person never engages in any physical activity. A reasonable amount of physical activity, sustained on a regular basis, can pay important dividends.

Thirdly, certain people have a family predisposition for overweight bodies that may make their challenge more difficult. If you are one of these people, I can only say that you probably need to be especially rigorous in your diet and exercise. In rural China, we noticed that obese people simply did not exist, even though Chinese immigrants in Western countries do succumb to obesity. Now, as the dietary and lifestyle practices of people in China are becoming more like ours, so, too, have their bodies become more like ours. Amazing as it may seem, China is now number two behind the U.S. in number of obese people, and this has happened in a very short period of time.[25] For those with genetic predispositions, it doesn't take much bad food before their change in diet starts to cause problems.

Keeping body weight off successfully should be part of a long-term lifestyle. Gimmicks that produce impressively large, quick weight losses often don't work in the long term. Short-term gains should not come along with long-term pain, like kidney problems, heart disease, cancer, bone and joint ailments, and other problems that may be brought on with popular diet fads. If the weight was gained slowly, over a period of months and years, why would you expect to take it off healthily in a matter of weeks? Treating weight loss as a race doesn't work; it only makes the dieter more eager to quit the diet and go back to the eating habits that put them in need of losing weight in the first place. One very large study of 21,105 vegetarians and vegans[16] found that body mass index was "lower among those who had adhered to their diet for five or more years" compared to people who had been on the diet for less than five years.

WHY THIS WILL WORK FOR YOU

So there is a solution to the weight-gain problem. But how can you apply it to your own life?

First of all, throw away ideas about counting calories. Generally speaking, you can eat as much as you want and still lose weight—*as long you eat the right type of food*. (See chapter twelve for details.) Secondly, stop expecting sacrifice, deprivation, or blandness; there's no need. Feeling hungry is a sign that something is wrong, and prolonged hunger causes your body to slow the overall rate of metabolism in defense. Moreover, there are mechanisms in our bodies that naturally allow the right kind of plant-based foods to nourish us, without our having to think about every morsel of food we put in our mouths. It is a worry-free way to eat. Give your body the right food and it will do the right thing.

In some studies, those who follow a whole foods, low-fat, plant-based diet consume fewer calories. It's not because they're starving themselves. In fact, they will likely spend more time eating and eat a larger volume of food than their meat-eating counterparts.[26] That's because fruits, vegetables, and grains—as whole foods—are much less energy-dense than animal foods and added fats. There are fewer calories in each spoonful or cupful of these foods. Remember that fat has nine calories per gram while carbohydrates and protein have only four calories per gram. In addition, whole fruits, vegetables, and grains have a lot of fiber, which makes you feel full[26,27] and yet contribute relatively small amounts of calories to your meal. So by eating a healthy meal, you may reduce the calories that you consume, digest, and absorb, even if you eat significantly more food.

This idea on its own, however, is not yet a sufficient explanation for the benefits of a WFPB diet. The same criticisms I made against the Atkins Diet and the other popular low-carb diets (chapter four) can also be applied to short-term studies in which subjects consume fewer calories while eating a plant-based diet. Over the long term, these subjects will find it very difficult to continue consuming an abnormally low level of calories; weight loss due to calorie restriction rarely leads to long-term weight loss. This is why other studies play such a crucial part in explaining the health benefits of a WFPB diet—these studies show that the weight loss is due to more than simple calorie restriction.

These studies document the fact that *vegetarians consume the same amount or even significantly more calories than their meat-eating counterparts, and yet are still slimmer.*[14,28,29] The China Study demonstrated that rural Chinese consuming a plant-based diet actually consume significantly more calories per pound of body weight than Americans. Most people would automatically assume that these rural Chinese would therefore be heavier than their meat-eating counterparts. But here's the kicker: *the rural Chinese are still slimmer while consuming a greater volume of food and more calories.* Much of this effect is undoubtedly due to greater physical activity . . . but this comparison is between average Americans and the least active Chinese, those who do office work. Furthermore, studies done in Israel[28] and the United Kingdom,[14] neither of which represent primarily agrarian cultures, also show that vegetarians may consume the same or significantly more calories and still weigh less.

What's the secret? One factor that I've mentioned previously is the process of thermogenesis, which refers to our production of body heat during metabolism. Vegetarians have been observed to have a slightly higher rate of metabolism during rest,[30] meaning they burn up slightly more of their ingested calories as body heat rather than depositing them as body fat.[31] A relatively small increase in metabolic rate translates to a large number of calories burned over the course of twenty-four hours. Most of the scientific basis for the importance of this phenomenon was presented in chapter four and in a research publication of my own.[32]

EXERCISE

The slimming effect of physical activity is obvious. Scientific evidence concurs. A recent review of all the credible studies compared the relationship between body weight and exercise[33] and showed that people who were more physically active had less body weight. Another set of studies showed that exercising on a regular basis helped to keep off weight originally lost through exercise programs. No surprise here, either. Starting and stopping an exercise program is not a good idea. It is better to build it into your lifestyle so that you will become and continue to be more fit overall, not just burn off calories.

How much exercise is needed to keep the pounds off? A rough estimate derived from a good review[33] suggested that exercising a mere fifteen to forty-five minutes per day, every day, will maintain a body weight that is eleven to eighteen pounds lighter than it would otherwise be. Interestingly, we should not forget our "spontaneous" physical activity, the kind that is associated with chores of daily life. This can account for 100–800 calories per day (kcal/day).[34,35] People who are regularly "up and about" doing physical things are going to be well ahead of those who get trapped in a sedentary lifestyle.

The advantages of combining diet and exercise to control body weight were brought home to me by a very simple study involving our experimental animals. Recall that our experimental animals were fed diets containing either the traditional 20% casein (cow's milk protein) or the much lower 5% casein. The rats consuming the 5% casein diets had strikingly less cancer, lower blood cholesterol, and longer lives. They also consumed slightly more calories but burned them off as body heat.

Some of us had noticed over the course of these experiments that the 5% casein animals seemed to be more active than the 20% casein animals. To test this idea, we housed rats fed either 5% or 20% casein diets in cages equipped with exercise wheels outfitted with meters to record the number of turns of the wheel. *Within the very first day, the 5% casein-fed animals voluntarily "exercised" in the wheel about twice as much as the 20% casein-fed animals.*[36] Exercise remained considerably higher for the 5% casein animals throughout the two weeks of the study.

Now we can combine some really interesting observations on body weight. A plant-based diet operates on calorie balance to keep body weight under control in two ways. First, it discharges calories as body heat instead of storing them as body fat, and it doesn't take many calories to make a big difference over the course of a year. Second, a plant-based diet encourages more physical activity. And, as body weight goes down, it becomes easier to be physically active. Diet and exercise work together to decrease body weight and improve overall health.

GOING IN THE RIGHT DIRECTION

Obesity is the most ominous harbinger of poor health that Western nations currently face. Tens of millions of people will fall prey to disability, putting our health care systems under greater strain than has previously been seen.

There are many people and institutions working to reduce this problem, but their point of attack is often illogical and misinformed. First, there are the many quick-fix promises and gimmicks. Obesity is not a condition that can be fixed in a few weeks or even a few months, and you should beware of diets, potions, and pills that create rapid weight loss with no promise of good health in the future. *The diet that helps to reduce weight in the short run needs to be the same diet that creates and maintains health in the long run.*

Second, the tendency to focus on obesity as an independent, isolated disease[37,38] is misplaced. Considering obesity in this manner directs our attention to a search for specific cures while ignoring control of the other diseases to which obesity is strongly linked. That is, we sacrifice context.

Also, I would urge that we ignore the suggestion that knowing its genetic basis might control obesity. A few years ago,[39–41] there was great publicity given to the discovery of "the obesity gene." Then there was the discovery of a second gene related to obesity, and a third gene, and a fourth, and on and on. The purpose behind the obesity gene search is to allow researchers to develop a drug capable of knocking out or inactivating the underlying cause of obesity. This is extremely shortsighted, as well as unproductive. Believing that specific identifiable genes are the basis of obesity (i.e., it's all in the family) also allows us to fatalistically blame a cause that we cannot control.

I find it tragic that although the topic of obesity has been researched so long, an explanation is still so far away. PubMed, the search engine for the U.S. National Library of Medicine, reveals approximately *3,700* obesity research reviews, representing 246,000 individual research publications. Every conceivable perspective on this disease seems to have been investigated, from its biological cause, to its genetic basis, prevalence in the world, costs to society, reversal, and relationship to personal behaviors. And in spite of this unfathomable amount of research, there has been very little progress in our efforts to bring this "disease" under control; it seems to have done little to stymie obesity's progression over time and into every society that chooses the Western diet.

Much of this research has sprung from the notion that obesity is an independent disease, formalized with its own specific medical code—a classification choice that was the subject of considerable discussion more than two decades ago. Arguments in favor were that a specific identity would facilitate its diagnosis and treatment, as well as insurance reimbursement. Arguments against were that obesity is primarily a symptom of a constellation of highly correlated, interrelated degenerative diseases and ailments typically observed among people consuming a Western diet. Treating obesity in isolation means ignoring associated diseases that have been shown to arise from the same dietary cause.

But while the science may be complex, the practical answer is simple. We *can* control the cause. It is right at the end of our fork.

DIABETES

Type 2 diabetes, the most common form, often accompanies obesity. As we, as a nation, continue to gain weight, our rate of diabetes spirals out of control. In the eight years from 1990 to 1998, the incidence of diabetes increased 33%.[1] As of 1998, over 8% of American adults were diabetic. As of 2012, 9.3% of adults were diabetic, and over 200,000 kids under twenty had diabetes (though this latter figure includes both Types 1 and 2).[2] That translates to more than 29.1 million Americans. The scariest figure? Just under one-third of those people with diabetes didn't yet know that they had it.[3]

You know the situation is serious when our children, at the age of puberty, start falling prey to the form of diabetes usually reserved for adults over forty. One newspaper recently illustrated the epidemic with the story of a girl who weighed 350 pounds at the age of fifteen, had the "adult-onset" form of diabetes, and was injecting insulin into her body three times a day.[4]

What is diabetes, why should we care about it, and how do we stop it from happening to us?

TWO FACES OF THE SAME DEVIL

Almost all cases of diabetes are either Type 1 or Type 2. Type 1 develops in children and adolescents, and thus is sometimes referred to as juvenile-onset diabetes. This form accounts for 5% to 10% of all diabetes cases. Type 2, which accounts for 90% to 95% of all cases, used to occur primarily in adults age forty and up, and thus was called adult-onset diabetes.[3] But because up to 45% of new diabetes cases in children are Type 2 diabetes,[5] the age-specific names are being dropped, and the two forms of diabetes are simply referred to as Type 1 and Type 2.[5]

In both types, the disease begins with dysfunctional glucose metabolism. Normal metabolism goes like this:

- We eat food.
- The food is digested and the carbohydrate part is broken down into simple sugars, much of which is glucose.
- Glucose (blood sugar) enters the blood, and insulin is produced by the pancreas to manage its transport and distribution around the body.
- Insulin, acting like an usher, opens doors for glucose into different cells for a variety of purposes. Some of the glucose is converted to short-term energy for immediate cell use, and some is stored as long-term energy (fat) for later use.

As a person develops diabetes, this metabolic process collapses. Type 1 diabetics cannot produce adequate insulin because the insulin-producing cells of their pancreas have been destroyed or are dysfunctional. This is the result of the body attacking itself, making Type 1 diabetes an autoimmune disease. (Type 1 diabetes and other autoimmune diseases are discussed in chapter nine.) Type 2 diabetics can produce insulin, but the insulin doesn't do its job effectively: once the insulin starts "giving orders" to dispatch the blood sugar into cells, the body doesn't pay attention, and the blood sugar is not metabolized properly. This is called insulin resistance.

Imagine your body as an airport, complete with vast parking areas. Each unit of your blood sugar is an individual traveler. After you eat, your blood sugar rises. In our analogy, then, that means lots of travelers would start to arrive at the airport. The people would drive in, park in a lot, and walk to the stop where the shuttle bus is supposed to pick them up. As your blood sugar continues to rise, all the airport parking lots would fill to capacity, and all the people would congregate at the shuttle bus stops. The shuttle buses, of course, represent insulin. In the diabetic airport, unfortunately, there are all sorts of problems with the buses. In the Type 1 diabetic airport, the shuttle buses simply don't exist. The only shuttle bus manufacturer in the known universe, Pancreas Company, was shut down. In the Type 2 diabetic airport, there are some shuttle buses, but they don't work very well.

In both cases, travelers never get to where they want to go. The airport system breaks down, and chaos ensues. In real life, this corresponds with a rise in blood sugar to dangerous levels. In fact, diabetes is diagnosed by the observation of elevated blood sugar levels, or its "spillage" into urine.

What are the long-term health risks of glucose metabolism being disrupted? Here's a summary, taken from a Centers for Disease Control report.[3] The italicized data are recent statistics, added in this second edition; the other data are from the first edition.[2]

DIABETES COMPLICATIONS

Heart Disease
- 2–4 times the risk of death from heart disease.
- *1.8 times the risk of heart disease*

Stroke
- 2–4 times the risk of stroke.
- *1.5 times the risk of stroke*

High Blood Pressure
- Over 70% of people with diabetes have high blood pressure.

Blindness
- Diabetes is the leading cause of blindness in adults.
- *28.5% of diabetics have retinopathy that may lead to loss of vision.*

Kidney Disease
- Diabetes is the leading cause of end-stage kidney disease
- In 1999, over 100,000 diabetics underwent dialysis or kidney transplantation.
- *In 2011, there were 228,924 cases of diabetes-related kidney failure in those on chronic dialysis or who had undergone kidney transplant.*

Nervous System Disease
- 60–70% of diabetics suffer mild to severe nervous system damage.

Amputation
- Over 60% of all lower limb amputations occur with diabetics.

Dental Disease
- Increased frequency and severity of gum disease that can lead to tooth loss.

Pregnancy Complications
Increased Susceptibility to Other Illnesses
Death

Modern drugs and surgery offer no cure for diabetics. At best, current drugs allow diabetics to maintain a reasonably functional lifestyle, but these drugs will never treat the cause of the disease. As a consequence, diabetics face a lifetime of drugs and medications, making diabetes an enormously costly disease. The economic toll of diabetes in the U.S.: over $245 billion a year in 2013,[6] up from $130 billion in 2000.[3]

But there is hope. In fact, there is much more than hope, if we simply keep an open mind. The food we eat has enormous influence over this disease. The right diet not only prevents but also treats diabetes. What, then, is the "right" diet? You can probably guess what I'm going to say, but let the research speak for itself.

NOW YOU SEE IT, NOW YOU DON'T

Like most chronic diseases, diabetes shows up more often in some parts of the world than in others. This has been known for a hundred years. It has also been well documented that those populations with low rates of diabetes eat different diets than those populations with high rates of diabetes. But is that just a coincidence, or is there something else at work?

Chart 7.1: Diets and Diabetes Rates, Circa 1925[5, 7]

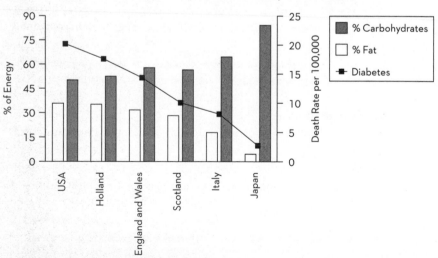

About ninety years ago, H. P. Himsworth compiled all the existing research in a report comparing diets and diabetes rates in six countries. What he found was that some cultures were consuming high-fat diets, while others had diets high in carbohydrates. These fat vs. carbohydrate consumption patterns were the result of animal- vs. plant-food consumption. Chart 7.1 documents the diet and disease conditions for these countries in the early part of the twentieth century.[7]

As carbohydrate intake goes up and fat intake goes down, the number of deaths from diabetes plummets from 20.4 to 2.9 per 100,000 people. The verdict? A high-carbohydrate, low-fat diet—a plant-based diet—is unmistakably associated with lower rates of diabetes.

Thirty years later, the question was reexamined. After examining four countries from Southeast Asia and South America, researchers again found that high-carbohydrate diets were linked to low rates of diabetes. Researchers noted that the country with the highest rate of diabetes, Uruguay, had a diet that was "typically 'Western' in character, being high in calories, animal protein, [total] fat and animal fat." Countries with low rates of diabetes used a diet that was "relatively lower in protein (particularly animal protein), fat and animal fat. A high proportion of calories is derived from carbohydrates, particularly from rice."[8]

These same researchers enlarged their study to eleven countries through Central and South America and Asia. The strongest association they found with diabetes was excess weight.[9] Populations eating the most Western type of diet also had the highest cholesterol levels, which in turn was strongly associated with the rate of diabetes.[9] Is this starting to sound familiar?

WITHIN ONE POPULATION

These old, cross-cultural studies can be crude, resulting in conclusions that are not entirely reliable. Perhaps the difference in diabetes rates in the above studies was not due to diet, but to genetics. Perhaps other unmeasured cultural factors, like physical activity, were more relevant. A better test would be a study of diabetes rates in a single population.

The Seventh-day Adventists population is a good example. They are an interesting group of people to study because of their dietary habits: their religion encourages them to stay away from meat, fish, eggs, coffee, alcohol, and tobacco. As a result, half of them are vegetarian. But 90% of these vegetarians still consume dairy and/or egg products, thus deriving a significant amount of their calories from animal sources. It should also be noted that the meat-eating Adventists are not the meatiest of eaters. They consume about three servings of beef a week, and less than one serving a week of fish and poultry.[10] I know plenty of people who consume this amount of meat (including fish and poultry) every two days.

In dietary studies involving the Adventists, scientists compare "moderate" vegetarians to "moderate" meat eaters. This is not a big difference. *Even so, the Adventist vegetarians are much healthier than their meat-eating counterparts.*[10] *Those Adventists that "deprived" themselves of meat also "deprived" themselves of the ravages of diabetes. Compared to the meat eaters, the vegetarians had about one-half the rate of diabetes.*[10,11] They also had almost half the rate of obesity.[10]

In another study, scientists measured diets and diabetes in a population of Japanese American men in Washington State.[12] These men were the sons of Japanese immigrants to the U.S. Remarkably, they had more than four times the prevalence of diabetes than the average rate found in similar-aged men who stayed in Japan. So what happened?

Those Japanese Americans who developed diabetes also ate the most animal protein, animal fat, and dietary cholesterol, each of which is only found in animal-based foods.[12] Total fat intake also was higher among the diabetics. These same dietary characteristics also resulted in excess weight. These second-generation Japanese Americans ate a meatier diet with less plant-based food than men born in Japan. The researchers wrote, "Apparently, the eating habits of Japanese men living in the United States resemble more the American eating style than the Japanese." The consequence: four times as much incidence of diabetes.[12]

Some other studies:

- Researchers found that increased fat intake was associated with an increased rate of Type 2 diabetes among 1,300 people in the San Luis Valley in Colorado. They said, "The findings support the hypothesis that high-fat, low-carbohydrate diets are associated with the onset of non-insulin-dependent [Type 2] diabetes mellitus in humans."[13]
- In a recent twenty-five-year period, the rate at which children in Japan contracted Type 2 diabetes had more than tripled. Researchers noted that consumption of animal protein and animal fat had drastically increased in the past fifty years. They said that this dietary shift, along with low exercise levels, might be to blame for this explosion of diabetes.[14]
- In England and Wales the rate of diabetes markedly dropped from 1940 to 1950, largely during World War II when food consumption patterns changed markedly. During the war and its aftermath, fiber and grain intake went up and fat intake went down. People ate "lower" on the food chain because of national necessity. Around 1950, though, people gave up the grain-based

diets and returned to eating more fat, more sugar, and less fiber. Sure enough, diabetes rates started going up.[15]

- Researchers studied 36,000 women in Iowa for six years. All were free of diabetes at the start of the study, but more than 1,100 cases of diabetes developed after six years. The women who were least likely to get diabetes were those that ate the most whole grains and fiber[16]—those whose diets contained the most carbohydrates (the complex kind found in whole foods).

All of these findings support the idea that both across and within populations, high-fiber, whole, plant-based foods protect against diabetes, and high-fat, high-protein, animal-based foods promote diabetes.

CURING THE INCURABLE

All of the research cited above was *observational,* and an observed association, even if frequently seen, may only be an incidental association that masks the real cause–effect relationship of environment (including diet) and disease. There is, however, also research of the "controlled" or intervention variety. This involves changing the diets of people who already have either full-blown Type 1 or Type 2 diabetes or mild diabetic symptoms (impaired glucose tolerance).

James Anderson, MD, is one of the most prominent scientists to have studied diet and diabetes in recent decades, garnering dramatic results using dietary means alone. One of his studies examined the effects of a high-fiber, high-carbohydrate, low-fat diet on twenty-five Type 1 diabetics and twenty-five Type 2 diabetics in a hospital setting.[17] None of his fifty patients were overweight and all of them were taking insulin shots to control their blood sugar levels.

His experimental diet consisted mainly of whole plant foods and the equivalent of only a cold cut or two of meat a day. He put his patients on the conservative, American-style diet recommended by the American Diabetes Association for one week and then switched them over to the experimental "veggie" diet for three weeks. He measured their blood sugar levels, cholesterol levels, weight, and medication requirements. The results were impressive.

Type 1 diabetics cannot produce insulin. It is difficult to imagine any dietary change that might aid their predicament. *But after just three weeks, the Type 1 diabetes patients were able to lower their insulin medication by an average of 40%!* Their blood sugar profiles improved dramatically. *Just as importantly, their cholesterol levels dropped by 30%![17]* Remember, one of the dangers of being diabetic is the secondary outcomes, heart disease and stroke. Lowering risk factors for those secondary outcomes by improving the cholesterol profile is almost as important as treating high blood sugar.

Type 2 diabetics, unlike Type 1, are more "treatable" because they haven't incurred such extensive damage to their pancreas. So the results from Anderson's Type 2 patients on the high-fiber, low-fat diet were even more impressive. Of the twenty-five Type 2 patients, twenty-four were able to discontinue their insulin medication! Let me say that again. *All but one person were able to discontinue their insulin medication in a matter of weeks![17]*

One man had a twenty-one-year history of diabetes and was taking thirty-five units of insulin a day. After three weeks of intensive dietary treatment, his insulin dosage dropped to eight units a day. After eight weeks at home, his need for insulin shots vanished.[17] Chart 7.2 shows a sample of patients and how eating a plant-based diet lowered their insulin medications. This is a huge effect.

In another study of fourteen lean diabetic patients, Anderson found that diet alone could lower total cholesterol levels by 32% *in just over two weeks*.[18] Some of the results are shown in Chart 7.3.

These benefits, representing a decrease in blood cholesterol from 206 mg/dL to 141 mg/dL, are astounding—especially considering the speed with which they appear. Dr. Anderson also found no evidence that this cholesterol decrease was temporary as long as people continued on the diet; it remained low for four years.[19]

Chart 7.2: Insulin Dosage Response to Diet

Chart 7.3: Blood Cholesterol on High-Carbohydrate, High-Fiber Diet

Another group of scientists at the Pritikin Center achieved equally spectacular results by prescribing a low-fat, plant-based diet and exercise to a group of diabetic patients. *Of forty patients on medication at the start of the program, thirty-four were able to discontinue all medication after only twenty-six days.*[20] This research group also demonstrated that the benefits of a plant-based diet will last for years if the same diet is continued.[21]

These are examples of some very dramatic research, but they only scratch the surface of all the supporting research that has been done. One scientific paper reviewed nine publications citing the use of high-carbohydrate, high-fiber diets and two more standard-carbohydrate, high-fiber diets to treat diabetic patients.[22] All eleven studies resulted in improved blood sugar and cholesterol levels. (Dietary fiber supplements, by the way, although beneficial, did not have the same consistent effects as a change to a whole foods, plant-based [WFPB] diet.[23])

Since publication of the first edition of this book, many more trials testing the effects of the WFPB diet on diabetics have been conducted.

Perhaps the most impressive finding since this book's first edition is the peer-reviewed report of Dr. Neal Barnard and his colleagues.[24] In a seventy-four-week study—relatively long compared to the usual two- to three-month studies—subjects on a vegan diet fared better than subjects on the diet recommended by the American Diabetes Association (ADA), with some of the differences in response being statistically significant. What made this finding even more impressive was the fact that participants following the vegan diet did not adhere fully to a strict whole food, plant-based diet, and so their diet was not as nutritionally potent as it could have been (see Figure 7.4).

Chart 7.4: Nutrient Composition of Vegan, WFPB, and ADA Diets

	WFPB	Vegan (Barnard's Study)[24]	ADA Equivalent (Barnard's Study)[24]	ADA (Recommended)
Fat, % cal	~10	22.3	33.7	<25–30
Carbohydrate, % cal	~80	66.3	46.5	45–60
Protein, % cal	~10	14.8	21.1	15–20
Cholesterol, mg/day	0	50	242	<200
Total fiber, g/day	50+	29.6	19	25–30

The dietary changes achieved in this real-world trial, factoring in challenges of patient compliance, approach but do not reach the nutrient composition of the WFPB diet. Dietary fat is higher (22.3% vs. ~10%), dietary protein is higher (14.8% vs. ~10%), and dietary carbohydrates are lower (66.3% vs. ~80%). Total fiber consumption (30 g/day) is substantially lower than the 50+ possible in the WFPB diet, as indicated by intakes in China as high as 77 g/day. Also, the participants in the vegan group were consuming a small amount of animal-based foods, as indicated by the recorded cholesterol consumption (plant-based foods have no cholesterol).

Given these differences and based on other clinicians' experiences and previous research, I suspect the benefits would have been larger had there been greater dietary change. For example, a 1976 study demonstrated that a high (75%) "complex" (i.e., whole food) carbohydrate diet allowed nine of thirteen diabetic men to completely discontinue, and two more to halve, the insulin medications they previously needed when eating a 43% complex carbohydrate ADA diet.[25]

(It's also worth noting that the ADA diet in this study was near the margin of the ADA recommendations—low in plant-based carbohydrates and dietary fiber and high in protein and fat, with high consumption of animal-based cholesterol. If this is how Type 2 diabetics interpret ADA guidelines, it is clear that no resolution of disease is possible beyond the peripheral management of symptoms through pills and procedures.)

The diet of the "vegan" Type 2 diabetics was better than that of the ADA Type 2 diabetics, yet still a far cry from the diet shown in earlier research, offered in controlled settings, to have such a very rapid, remarkably profound effect in treating and resolving this disease. The vegan diet is going in the right direction, just not nearly fast enough. And in the meantime, we've spent more than a quarter trillion dollars (as of 2012)[6] pretending to treat a disease—the fourth leading cause of death—that already has a cure.

THE PERSISTENCE OF HABIT

As you can see from these findings, we can beat diabetes. Two studies in the early 2000s considered a combination of diet and exercise effects on this disease.[26,27] One study placed 3,234 nondiabetic people at risk for diabetes (elevated blood sugar) into three different groups.[26] One group, the control, received standard dietary information and a drug placebo (no effect), one received the standard dietary information and the drug metformin, and a third group received "intensive" lifestyle intervention, which included a moderately low-fat diet and an exercise plan to lose at least 7% of their weight. After almost three years, the lifestyle group had 58% fewer cases of diabetes than the control group. The drug group reduced the number of cases only by 31%. Compared to the control, both treatments worked, but clearly a lifestyle change is much safer and more powerful than simply taking a drug. Moreover, the lifestyle change would be effective in solving other health problems, whereas the drug would not.

The second study also found that the rate of diabetes could be reduced by 58% just by modest lifestyle changes, including exercise, weight loss, and a moderately low-fat diet.[27] Imagine what would happen if people fully adopted the healthiest diet: a whole foods, plant-based diet. I strongly suspect that virtually all Type 2 diabetes cases could be prevented.

Unfortunately, misinformation and ingrained habits are wreaking havoc on our health. Our habit of eating hot dogs, hamburgers, and French fries is killing us. Even Dr. James Anderson, who achieved profound results with many patients by prescribing a near-vegetarian diet, is not immune to habitual health advice. He writes, "Ideally, diets providing 70% of calories as carbohydrate and up to 70 gm fiber daily offer the greatest health benefits for individuals with diabetes. However, these diets allow only one to two ounces of meat daily and are impractical for home use for many individuals."[22] Why does Professor Anderson, a very fine researcher, say that such a diet is "impractical" and thereby prejudice his listeners before they even consider the evidence?

Yes, changing your lifestyle may seem impractical. It may seem impractical to give up meat and high-fat foods, but I wonder how practical it is to be 350 pounds and have Type 2 diabetes at the age of fifteen, like the girl mentioned at the start of this chapter. I wonder how practical it is to have a lifelong condition that can't be cured by drugs or surgery; a condition that often leads to heart disease, stroke, blindness, or amputation; a condition that might require you to inject insulin into your body every day for the rest of your life.

Radically changing our diets may be "impractical," but it might also be worth it.

COMMON CANCERS: BREAST, PROSTATE, LARGE BOWEL (COLON AND RECTAL)

M uch of my career concentrated on the study of cancer. My laboratory work focused on several cancers, including those of the liver,
breast, and pancreas, and some of the most impressive data from
China were related to cancer. For this lifetime work, the American Institute
for Cancer Research kindly presented me with their Research Achieve-
ment award in 1998.

An exceptional number of books have summarized the evidence on the
effects of nutrition on a variety of cancers, each with their own particular-
ities. But what I've found is that the nutritional effects on the cancers I've
chosen to discuss here are virtually the same for all cancers, regardless
of whether they are initiated by different factors or are located in different
parts of the body. Using this principle, I can limit my discussion to three cancers, which will allow me space in the rest of the book to address diseases
other than cancer, and to demonstrate the breadth of evidence linking food
to many health concerns.

I have chosen to comment on three cancers that affect hundreds of
thousands of Americans and that generally represent other cancers as well:
two reproductive cancers that get plenty of attention, breast and prostate;
and one digestive cancer, large bowel—the second leading cause of cancer
death, behind lung cancer.

BREAST CANCER

It was spring about twenty years ago. I was in my office at Cornell when I was told that a woman with a question regarding breast cancer was on the phone.

"I have a strong history of breast cancer in my family," the woman, Betty, said. "My mother and grandmother both died from the disease, and my forty-five-year-old sister was recently diagnosed with it. Given this family problem, I can't help but be afraid for my nine-year-old daughter. She's going to start menstruating soon and I worry about her risks of getting breast cancer." Her fear was evident in her voice. "I've seen a lot of research showing that family history is important, and I'm afraid that it's inevitable that my daughter will get breast cancer. One of the options I've been thinking about is a mastectomy for my daughter, to remove both breasts. Do you have any advice?"

This woman was in an exceptionally difficult position. Does she let her daughter grow up into a deathtrap, or grow up without breasts? Although extreme, this question represents a variety of similar questions faced every day by thousands of women around the world.

These questions were especially encouraged by the early reports on the discovery of the breast cancer gene, BRCA-1. Headline articles in the *New York Times* and other newspapers and magazines trumpeted this discovery as an enormous advance. The hoopla surrounding BRCA-1, which now also includes BRCA-2, reinforced the idea that breast cancer was due to genetic misfortune. This caused great fear among people with a family history of breast cancer. It also generated excitement among scientists and pharmaceutical companies. The possibility was high that new technologies would be able to assess overall breast cancer risk in women by doing genetic testing; they hoped they might be able to manipulate this new gene in a way that would prevent or treat breast cancer. Journalists busily started translating selective bits of this information for the public, relying heavily on the fatalistic genetic attitude. No doubt this contributed to the concern of mothers like Betty.

"Well, let me first tell you that I am not a physician," I said. "I can't help you with diagnosis or treatment advice. That's for your physician to do. I can speak about the current research in a more general way, however, if that is of any help to you."

"Yes," she said, "that's what I wanted."

I told her a little bit about the China Study and about the important role of nutrition. I told her that just because a person has the gene for a disease does not mean that they are destined to get the cancer; prominent studies reported that only a tiny minority of cancers can be solely blamed on genes.

I was surprised at how little she knew about nutrition. She thought genetics was the only factor that determined risk. She didn't realize that food was an important factor in breast cancer as well.

We talked for twenty or thirty minutes, a brief time for such an important matter. By the end of the conversation I had the feeling that she was not satisfied with what I told her. Perhaps it was my conservative, scientific way of talking, or my reluctance to give her a recommendation. Maybe, I thought, she had already made up her mind to do the procedure.

She thanked me for my time and I wished her well. I remember thinking about how often I receive questions from people about specific health situations, and that this was one of the most unusual.

But Betty wasn't alone. One other woman also talked to me regarding the possibility of her young daughter undergoing surgery to remove both breasts. Other women who already had one breast removed wondered whether to have the second breast removed as a preventive measure.

It's clear that breast cancer is an important concern in our society. One out of eight American women will be diagnosed with this disease during their lifetimes—one of the highest rates in the world. Grassroots breast cancer organizations are widespread, strong, relatively well funded, and exceptionally active compared to other health activist organizations. This disease, perhaps more than any other, incites panic and fear in many women.

When I think back to that conversation I had with Betty, I now feel that I could have made a stronger statement about the role nutrition plays in breast cancer. I still would not have been able to give her clinical advice, but the information I now know might have been of more use to her. So what would I tell her now?

RISK FACTORS

There are at least four important breast cancer risk factors that are affected by nutrition, as shown in Chart 8.1. Many of these relationships were confirmed in the China Study after being well established in other research.

With the exception of blood cholesterol, these risk factors are variations on the same theme: exposure to excess amounts of female hormones, including estrogen and progesterone, increases breast cancer risk. Women who consume a diet rich in animal-based foods, with a reduced amount of whole, plant-based foods, reach puberty earlier and menopause later, thus extending their reproductive lives. They also have higher levels of female hormones throughout their life span, as shown in Chart 8.2.

Chart 8.1: Breast Cancer Risk Factors and Nutritional Influence

Risk of breast cancer increases when a woman has...	A diet high in animal foods and refined carbohydrates...
...early age of menarche (first menstration)	...lowers the age of menarche
...late age of menopause	...raises the age of menopause
...high levels of female hormones in the blood	...increases female hormone levels
...high blood cholesterol	...increases blood cholesterol levels

Chart 8.2: Dietary Influence on Female Hormone Exposure Over a Woman's Lifetime (Schematic)

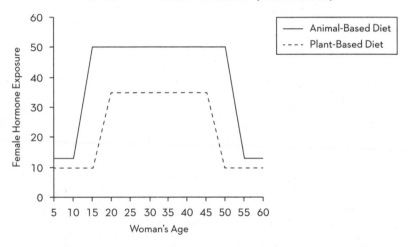

According to our China Study data, lifetime exposure to estrogen[1] is at least 2.5–3.0 times higher among Western women when compared with rural Chinese women. This is a huge difference for such a critically important hormone.[2] To use the words of one of the leading breast cancer research groups in the world,[3] "there is overwhelming evidence that estrogen levels are a critical determinant of breast cancer risk."[4,5] Estrogen directly participates in the cancer process.[6,7] It also tends to indicate the presence of other female hormones[8–12] that play a role in breast cancer risk.[6,7] Increased levels of estrogen and related hormones result from consuming typical Western diets, high in fat and animal protein and low in dietary fiber.[3,13–18]

The difference in estrogen levels between rural Chinese women and Western women[19] is all the more remarkable because a previous report[20] found that a mere 17% decrease in estrogen levels could account for a huge difference in breast cancer rates when comparing different countries. Imagine, then, what 26–63% lower blood estrogen levels and eight to nine fewer reproductive years of blood estrogen exposure could mean, as we found in the China Study.

This idea that breast cancer is centered on estrogen exposure[3,21,22] is profound because diet plays a major role in establishing estrogen exposure. This suggests that the risk of breast cancer is preventable if we eat foods that will keep estrogen levels under control. The sad truth is that most women simply are not aware of this evidence. If this information were properly reported by responsible and credible public health agencies, I suspect that many more young women might be taking very real, very effective steps to avoid this awful disease.

THE COMMON ISSUES

Genes

Understandably, women who are most afraid of this disease have a family history of breast cancer. Family history implies that genes do play a role in the development of breast cancer. But I hear too many people say, in effect, that "it's all in the family" and deny that they can do anything to help themselves. This fatalistic attitude removes a sense of personal responsibility for one's own health and profoundly limits available options.

It is true that if you have a family history of breast cancer, you are at an increased risk of getting the disease.[23,24] However, one research group found that less than 3% of all breast cancer cases can be attributed to family history.[24] Even though other groups have estimated that a higher percentage of cases are due to family history or genes,[25] the vast majority of breast cancer in American women is not due to these factors. But genetic fatalism continues to define the nation's mind-set.

Among the genes that influence breast cancer risk, BRCA-1 and BRCA-2 have received the most attention since their discovery in 1994.[26–29] These genes, when mutated, confer a higher risk both for breast and ovarian cancers.[30,31] These mutated genes may be passed on from generation to generation; that is, they are inherited.

In the excitement over these discoveries, however, other information has been ignored. First, only 0.2% of individuals in the general population (1 in 500) carry the mutated forms of these genes.[25] Because of the rarity of these genetic aberrations, only a few percent of the breast cancer cases in the general population can be attributed to mutated BRCA-1 or BRCA-2 genes.[32,33] Second, these genes are not the only genes that participate in the development of this disease[32]; many more will surely be discovered. Third, the mere presence of BRCA-1, BRCA-2, or any other breast cancer gene does not guarantee disease occurrence. Environmental and dietary factors play a central role in determining whether these genes are expressed.

A later paper[31] reviewed twenty-two studies that assessed the risk of breast (and ovarian) cancer among women who carried mutated BRCA-1 and BRCA-2 genes. Overall, disease risk was 65% for breast cancer and 39% for ovarian cancer by age seventy for BRCA-1 women, and 45% and 11%, respectively, for BRCA-2 women. Women with these genes certainly face high risks for breast cancer. But even among these high-risk women, there is still good reason to believe that more attention to diet is likely to pay handsome rewards. *About half of the women who carry these rare, potent genes do not get breast cancer.*

In short, although the discovery of BRCA-1 and BRCA-2 added an important dimension to the breast cancer story, the excessive emphasis given to these particular genes and genetic causation in general is not warranted.

I do not mean to diminish the importance of knowing all there is to know about these genes for the small minority of women who carry them. But we need to remind ourselves that these genes need to be "expressed" in order for them to participate in disease formation, and nutrition may control this. We've already seen in chapter three how a diet high in animal-based protein alters genetic expression.

Screening and Non-Nutritional Prevention

With all of this new information regarding genetic risk and family history, women are often encouraged to get screened for breast cancer. Screening is a reasonable step, especially for women who may have tested positive for the BRCA genes. But it's important to remember that doing a mammography or getting a genetic test to see if you harbor BRCA genes does not constitute prevention of breast cancer.

Screening is merely an observation to see whether the disease has progressed to an observable state. Some studies[34–36] have found that groups of women who undergo frequent mammography have slightly lower mortality rates than groups of women who do not undergo frequent mammography. This implies that our cancer treatments are more likely to be successful if the cancer is found at an earlier stage. This is likely to be true, but there is some concern over the way statistics are used in this debate.

One of the statistics used to support early detection and the ensuing treatments is that once women are diagnosed with breast cancer, their likelihood of surviving for at least five years is higher than ever before.[37] What this really means is that with the aggressive campaign for regular screening, many women are discovering their breast cancer at an earlier stage of disease. When disease is discovered at an earlier stage, it is less likely to lead to death within five years, regardless of treatment. *As a consequence, we may have an improved five-year survival rate simply because women find out that they have breast cancer earlier in the disease progression, not because our treatments have improved over time.*[38]

Beyond the current screening methods, there are other non-nutritional options for prevention that have been promoted. They are especially of interest to women who have a high risk of breast cancer due to family history and/or the presence of the BRCA genes. These options include taking a drug such as tamoxifen and/or mastectomy.

Tamoxifen is one of the most popular drugs taken to prevent breast cancer,[39,40] but the long-term benefits of this option are not clear. One major U.S. study showed that tamoxifen administered over a period of four years to women at increased risk of breast cancer reduced the number of cases by an impressive 49%.[41] This benefit, however, may be limited to women whose estrogen levels are very high. It was this result that led the U.S. Food and Drug Administration to approve use of tamoxifen by women who met certain criteria.[42] Other studies suggest that the enthusiasm for this drug is not warranted. Two less substantial European trials[43,44] have failed to show any statistically significant tamoxifen benefit, raising some doubt about how dramatic the benefit really is. Moreover, there is the additional concern that tamoxifen raises the risks for stroke, uterine cancer, cataracts, deep vein thrombosis, and pulmonary embolism, although the overall benefits of breast cancer prevention are still believed to outweigh the risks.[42] Other chemicals have also been investigated as alternatives to tamoxifen, but these drugs are encumbered by limited effectiveness and/or some of the same troublesome side effects.[45,46]

Drugs such as tamoxifen and its newer analogues are considered *anti-estrogen* drugs. In effect, they work by reducing the activity of estrogen, which is known to be associated with elevated breast cancer risk.[4,5] My question is quite simple: Why don't we ask why estrogen is so high in the first place, and, once we recognize its nutritional origin, why don't we correct that cause? We now have enough information to show that a diet low in animal-based protein, low in fat, and high in whole plant foods will reduce estrogen levels. Instead of suggesting dietary change as a solution, we spend hundreds of millions of dollars developing and publicizing a drug that may or may not work and that almost certainly will have unintended side effects.

The ability of dietary factors to control female hormone levels has long been known in the research community, but a more recent study was particularly impressive.[47] Several female hormones, which increase with the onset of puberty, were lowered by 20–30% (even by 50% for progesterone!) simply by having girls eight to ten years of age consume a diet modestly low in fat and animal-based food for seven years.[47] These results are extraordinary because they were obtained with a modest dietary change and were produced during a critical time of a young girl's life, when the first seeds of breast cancer were being sowed. These girls consumed a diet of no more than 28% fat and less than 150 mg cholesterol/day: a moderate plant-based diet. I believe that had they consumed a diet devoid of animal-based foods and had they started this diet earlier in life, they would have seen even greater benefits, including a delay in puberty and an even lower risk of breast cancer later in life.

Women at high risk for breast cancer are given three options: watch and wait, take tamoxifen medication for the remainder of their lives, or undergo mastectomy. There should be a fourth option: consuming a diet free of animal-based foods, refined carbohydrates, and added fats; avoiding alcohol (which increases breast cancer risk); and enjoying abundant exercise (which significantly decreases risk), in addition to regular monitoring for those at high risk. I stand by the usefulness of this fourth option even for women who have already had a first mastectomy. Using diet as an effective treatment of already-diagnosed disease has been well documented in human studies with advanced heart disease,[48,49] clinically documented Type 2 diabetes (see chapter seven), early prostate cancer,[50] advanced melanoma[51] (a deadly skin cancer) and, in experimental animal studies,[52] liver cancer.

Environmental Chemicals

Another breast cancer conversation has been taking place for some years now, and has been the subject of increasing interest in the years since the first edition of this book was published. It concerns environmental chemicals. These widely distributed chemicals have been shown to disrupt hormones, although it is not clear which hormones in humans are being disrupted. They may also cause reproductive abnormalities, birth defects, and Type 2 diabetes.

There are many different types of offending chemicals, most of which are commonly associated with industrial pollution. One group, including dioxins and PCBs, persist in the environment because they are not metabolized when consumed. Thus they are not excreted from the body. Because of this lack of metabolism, these chemicals accumulate in the body fat and breast milk of lactating mothers. Some of these chemicals are known to promote the growth of cancer cells, although humans may not be at significant risk unless one consumes excessive quantities of meat, milk, and fish. Indeed, 90–95% of our exposure to these chemicals comes from consuming animal products—yet another reason why consuming animal-based foods can be risky.

A second group of these environmental chemicals is also commonly perceived to be a significant cause of breast[53] and other cancers. They are called PAHs (polycyclic aromatic hydrocarbons) and are found in auto exhaust, factory smokestacks, petroleum tar products, and tobacco smoke, among other processes common to an industrial society. Unlike PCBs and dioxins, when we consume PAHs (in food and water), we can metabolize and excrete them. But there is a snag: when the PAHs are metabolized within the body, they produce intermediate products that react with DNA to form tightly bound complexes, or adducts (see chapter three). This is the first step in causing cancer. In fact, these chemicals later were shown to adversely affect the BRCA-1 and BRCA-2 genes of breast cancer cells grown in the laboratory.[54]

In chapter three, I described studies in my laboratory showing that when a very potent carcinogen is put into the body, the rate at which it causes problems is mostly controlled by nutrition. Thus the rate at which PAHs are metabolized into products that bind to DNA is very much controlled by what we eat. Very simply, consuming a Western-type diet will increase the rate at which chemical carcinogens like PAHs bind to DNA to form products that cause cancer.

So when a 2002 study found slightly increased levels of PAH-DNA adducts in women with breast cancer in Long Island, New York,[55] it may well have been that these women were consuming a more meaty diet, which increased the binding of the PAHs to DNA. It is entirely possible that the quantity of PAHs being consumed had nothing to do with increasing breast cancer risk. In fact, in this study, the number of PAH-DNA adducts in these women seem to be *unrelated* to PAH exposure.[55] How is this possible? Perhaps all of the women in this Long Island study consumed a relatively uniform, low level of PAHs, and the only ones who subsequently got breast cancer were the ones who ate a diet high in fat and animal protein, thus causing more of the ingested PAHs to bind to their DNA.

In this same Long Island study, breast cancer was not associated with PCBs and dioxins, the chemicals that can't be metabolized.[56] This and other findings suggest that environmental chemicals seem to play a far less significant role for breast cancer than the kind of foods we choose to eat.

Many research reports on this topic have been published since the first edition of this book in 2005, but these reports almost uniformly assume that environmental chemicals are the main causal factors for breast cancer, leaving little or no role for nutrition—not even any discussion. At best, they make superficial references to associations of obesity or calorie intake with breast cancer, but even then leave unsaid what causes obesity or what is known about its relationship to calorie intake and expenditure.

One of the most representative examples of this literature, and one that has been substantially referenced, is a Canadian case-control study, in which 1,005 breast cancer cases and 1,146 community controls were surveyed for possible associations of breast cancer with occupations that involved environmental chemical exposure.[57] Only five of twenty-nine occupation categories (agriculture, bars/gambling, automotive plastics manufacturing, food canning, and metal working[58]) showed statistically significant associations with breast cancer risk, and four of those were barely significant. This strikes me as very weak evidence for an association of environmental chemicals with breast cancer. Nonetheless, these researchers still suggested that their findings "support hypotheses linking breast cancer risk and exposures likely to include carcinogens and chemicals that disrupt endocrine [hormone] activities."

While exposure to environmental chemicals based on occupation does appear to play some role in cancer development, blaming the relationship between diet and breast cancer on environmental chemicals in our food has long been used to avoid the far more important role of our food's nutrient composition. To judge which best explains the relationship of diet with breast cancer, consider the following two major studies. The first is a post-2005 review of 439 recent studies on breast cancer and environmental chemicals.[59] Its authors correctly emphasize the enormous complexity of breast cancer causation and illustrate this complexity by presenting many classes of chemicals thought to increase breast cancer risk. But then they fail to take into account a role for nutrition in breast cancer causation; as they say in the report's introduction, "We do not discuss the often complicated and inconclusive literature examining possible relationships between diet, stress or obesity and risk for breast cancer."

A second major report concluded, after carefully reviewing the conclusions of an exhaustive collection of diet and breast cancer studies, that there is "no association [of diet with breast cancer incidence] that is consistent, strong, and statistically significant, with exception of alcohol intake, overweight, and weight gain."[60] But they also suggested, correctly, that this lack of effect may be due to the limited dietary variation typically seen in within-country studies when compared with the much greater dietary variation seen in between-country studies.

Together, these reports would appear to favor environmental chemicals as a more likely explanation for the impressive diet association with breast cancer. But this preference is based on inferences, not empirical findings. In evaluating the nutritional explanation for diet's association with breast cancer, the summary reports draw on the insufficient dietary variation observed for in-country dietary studies rather than the greater variation observed in between-country studies, a choice that reflects either a lack of author knowledge or a lack of sufficient experimental power to detect the nutrition effect likely to exist.

Upon ingestion, environmental chemicals—like their pharmaceutical relatives—are detoxified (sometimes activated) by a major liver enzyme system called the mixed function oxidase. Nutrition can substantially and quickly modify this enzyme activity, a fact that I reviewed over forty years ago.[61] We showed that modest changes in dietary protein, for example, can greatly change the toxicity of a pesticide like heptaclor,[62] a barbiturate like phenobarbital,[63] and the carcinogenicity of even the most potent chemical carcinogens, like aflatoxin (see chapter three). Each may be called an environmental chemical. The observed effects of environmental chemicals in these and other studies may primarily be an expression of nutrition's effect on disease outcomes, with or without environmental chemical intervention.

The same is the case for observations related to the "endocrine disruptor" chemicals, which disrupt the activity of hormones like estrogen that affect a wide variety of biological systems. Breast cancer risk is encouraged with greater estrogen exposure. But convincing evidence shows that nutrition (especially dietary protein,[64] fiber,[65] and fat[66]) can alter the estrogen levels in blood, thus producing estrogen disruptor–like activities.

How much of these environmental chemical associations reported in the literature are due to chemical exposure, per se, and how much to nutritional modifications of these effects? Is it possible that the five communities in the Canadian occupation study that showed an association of environmental chemicals with more breast cancer did so due to the consumption of less nutritious foods? When we scientists refrain from getting data on diet, we cannot know the answer. And I am left with the same conclusion I presented in the first edition of this book: that breast cancer is primarily caused by the same nutrition that elevates risk for other cancers—a diet lacking in whole, plant-based foods.

I want to be abundantly clear: I vigorously oppose exposing ourselves to unnatural environmental chemicals, especially those with demonstrated toxicity. But a narrow focus on adverse effects of environmental chemicals should not be used to sidestep the really important way of reducing disease occurrence—a WFPB diet.

Hormone Replacement Therapy

I must briefly mention one final breast cancer issue: whether to use hormone replacement therapy (HRT), which increases breast cancer risk. HRT is taken by many women to alleviate unpleasant effects of menopause, protect bone health, and prevent coronary heart disease.[67] However, it is now becoming widely acknowledged that HRT is not as beneficial as once thought, and it may have certain severe side effects. So what are the facts?

I wrote this commentary for the first edition of this book at an opportune time, because the results of some large trials of HRT use had just been released in the previous year.[67] Of special interest are two large, randomized intervention trials: the Women's Health Initiative (WHI)[68] and the Heart and Estrogen/Progestin Replacement Study (HERS).[69] Among women who take HRT, after 5.2 years the WHI trial is showing a 26% *increase* in breast cancer cases, while the HERS study is seeing an even greater 30% increase.[70] These studies are consistent. It appears that increased exposure to female hormones, via HRT, does indeed lead to more breast cancer.

It has been thought that HRT is associated with lower rates of coronary heart disease.[67] However, this is not necessarily true. In the large WHI trial, for every 10,000 healthy postmenopausal women who took HRT, there were seven more women with heart disease, eight more with strokes, and eight more with pulmonary embolisms[68]—the opposite of what had been expected. HRT may *increase* cardiovascular disease risk after all. On the other hand, HRT did have a beneficial effect on colorectal cancer and bone fracture rate. Among every 10,000 women, there were six fewer colorectal cancers and five fewer bone fractures.[68]

Since publication of the first edition, reports indicated that breast cancer incidence "fell sharply (by 6.7%) in 2003, as compared with 2002," then leveled off in 2004.[71] The size of this decline closely corresponded to the decline in HRT use over the same period, further supporting the earlier findings cited above that estrogen promotes breast cancer. as well as showing the rapidity of response when HRT exposure is terminated.

So how do you make a decision with such information? Just by adding and subtracting the numbers we can see that HRT may well be the cause of more harm than good. We can tell each individual woman to make her own decision depending on which disease and which unpleasant outcome or symptom she fears the most, as many physicians are likely to do. But this can be a tough decision for women who are having a difficult time with menopause. These women must choose between living unaided through the emotional and physical symptoms of menopause in order to preserve a low risk of breast cancer, or taking HRT to manage their menopause discomforts while increasing their risk of breast cancer and, possibly, cardiovascular disease. To say that this scenario troubles me would be an understatement. We have spent well over a billion dollars on the research and development of these HRT medical preparations, and all we get is some apparent pluses and probably even more minuses. Calling this troubling doesn't begin to describe it.

Instead of relying on HRT, I suggest that there is a better way, using food. The argument goes like this:

- During the reproductive years, hormone levels are elevated, although the levels among women who eat plant-based diets are not as elevated.
- When women reach the end of their reproductive years, it is entirely natural for reproductive hormones of all women to drop to a low "base" level.
- As reproductive years come to an end, the lower hormone levels among plant eaters don't crash as hard as they do among animal eaters. Using hypothetical numbers for circulating estrogen levels to illustrate the concept, the levels of plant eaters may crash from forty to fifteen, rather than sixty to fifteen for animal eaters.
- These abrupt hormone changes in the body are what cause menopausal symptoms.
- Therefore, a plant-based diet leads to a less severe hormone crash and a gentler menopause.

This argument is eminently reasonable based on what we know, although more studies are necessary. But even if future studies fail to confirm these details, a plant-based diet still offers the lowest risk for both breast cancer and heart disease for other reasons. It might just be the best of all worlds, something that no drug can offer.

In each of the various issues involving breast cancer risk (tamoxifen use, HRT use, environmental chemical exposure, preventive mastectomy), I am convinced that these practices are distractions that prevent us from considering a safer and far more useful nutritional strategy. It is critical that we change the way we think about this disease, and that we provide this information to the women who need it.

LARGE BOWEL CANCER
(INCLUDING COLON AND RECTUM)

At the end of June 2002, George W. Bush handed the presidency over to Dick Cheney for a period of roughly two hours while he underwent a colonoscopy. Because of the implications President Bush's colonoscopy had for world politics, the story made national news, and colon and rectal screening were briefly thrust into the spotlight. Across the country, whether the comedians were making jokes or the news anchors were describing the drama, everybody was suddenly, briefly, talking about this thing called a colonoscopy and what it was for. It was a rare moment in which the country turned its focus to some of the most prolific killer diseases, colon and rectal cancers.

Because colon and rectal cancers are both cancers of the large bowel, and because of their other similarities, they often are grouped together under the term *colorectal cancer*. It is the fourth most common cancer worldwide, in terms of overall mortality,[72] and is the second most common in the United States, with 6% of Americans getting it during their lifetime.[37] Some even claim that, by age seventy, one-half of the population of "Westernized" countries will develop a tumor in the large bowel and 10% of these cases will progress to a malignancy.[73]

GEOGRAPHIC DISPARITY

North America, Europe, Australia, and wealthier Asian countries (Japan, Singapore) have very high rates of colorectal cancer, while Africa, Asia, and

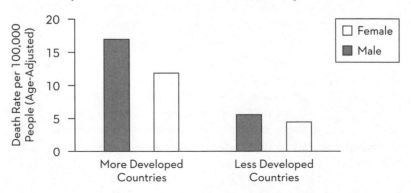

Chart 8.3: Colorectal Cancer Death Rate in "More Developed" Countries and "Less Developed" Countries

most of Central and South America have very low rates. For example, the Czech Republic has a death rate of 34.19 per 100,000 males, while Bangladesh has a death rate of 0.63 per 100,000 males![74,75] Chart 8.3 shows a comparison of average death rates between more developed countries and less developed countries; all these rates are age-adjusted.

The fact that rates of colorectal cancer vary hugely between countries has been known for decades. The question has always been why. Are the differences due to genetics, or to environment?

It seems that lifestyle factors, including diet, play the most important roles in colorectal cancer. Migrant studies have shown that as people move from a low-cancer-risk area to a high-cancer-risk area, they assume an increased risk within two generations.[76] This suggests that diet and lifestyle are important causes of this cancer. Other studies have also found that rates of colorectal cancer change rapidly as a population's diet or lifestyle changes.[76] These rapid changes in cancer rates within one population cannot possibly be explained by changes in inherited genes. In the context of human society, it takes thousands of years to get widespread, permanent changes in the inherited genes that are passed from one generation to the next. Clearly, something about environment or lifestyle is either preventing or enhancing the risk of getting colorectal cancer.

In a landmark paper published almost forty years ago, researchers compared environmental factors and cancer rates in thirty-two countries around the world.[77] One of the strongest links between any cancer and any

Chart 8.4: Female Colon Cancer Incidence and Daily Meat Consumption

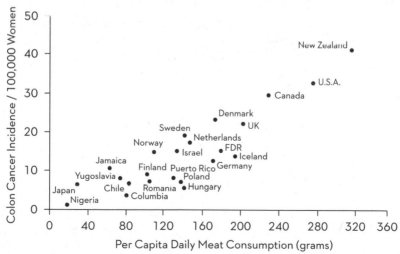

dietary factor was between colon cancer and meat intake. Chart 8.4 shows this link for women in twenty-three different countries.

In this report, countries where more meat, more animal protein, more sugar, and fewer cereal grains were consumed had far higher rates of colon cancer.[77] Another researcher whom I mentioned in chapter four, Denis Burkitt, hypothesized that intake of dietary fiber was essential for digestive health in general. He compared stool samples and fiber intakes in Africa and Europe and proposed that colorectal cancers were largely the result of low fiber intake.[78] Fiber, remember, is only found in plant foods. It is the part of the plant that our body cannot digest. Using data from another famous study that compared diets in seven different countries, researchers found that eating an additional ten grams of dietary fiber a day lowered the long-term risk of colon cancer by 33%.[79] There are ten grams of fiber in one cup of red raspberries, one Asian pear, or one cup of peas. A cup of just about any variety of bean would provide significantly more than ten grams of fiber.

From all this research, it seems clear that something can be said for the importance of diet in colorectal cancer. But what exactly stops colon and rectal cancer? Is it fiber? Is it fruits and vegetables? Is it carbohydrates? Is it milk? Each of these foods or nutrients has been suggested to play a role. The debate has raged, and solid answers are seldom agreed upon.

THE SPECIFIC CURE

Most of the debate over the past thirty-five years on dietary fiber and its link to large bowel cancer began with Burkitt's work in Africa. Because of Burkitt's prominence, many people have believed that fiber is the source of colorectal health. Perhaps you have already heard that fiber is good for preventing colon cancer. At least you probably have heard that fiber "keeps things running well." Isn't that what prunes are known for?

Yet nobody has ever been able to prove that fiber is the magic bullet for preventing colorectal cancer. There are important technical reasons why a definitive conclusion regarding fiber is difficult to make.[80] Each of these reasons is related either directly or indirectly to the fact that dietary fiber is not a single, simple substance producing a single, simple benefit. Fiber represents hundreds of substances, and "its" benefits operate through an exceptionally complex series of biochemical and physiological events. Each time researchers assess the consumption of dietary fiber, they must decide which of the hundreds of fiber sub-fractions to measure and which methods to use. It is nearly impossible to establish a standard procedure because it is virtually impossible to know what each fiber sub-fraction does in the body.

The uncertainty of having a standard procedure prompted us to measure fiber in more than a dozen ways in our China Study. As summarized in chapter four, as consumption of almost all of these fiber types went up, colon and rectal cancer rates went down.[81] But we could make no clear interpretations[82] as to which type of fiber was especially important.

Despite the uncertainties, I continue to believe that Burkitt's[78] initial hypothesis that *fiber-containing diets* prevent colorectal cancers is correct and that some of this effect is due to the aggregate effect of all the fiber types. In fact, the hypothesis that dietary fiber prevents large bowel cancers has become even more convincing. In 1990, a group of researchers reviewed sixty different studies that had been done on fiber and colon cancer.[83] They found that most of the studies supported the idea that fiber protects against colon cancer. They noted that the combined results showed that the people who consumed the most fiber had a 43% lower risk of colon cancer than the people who consumed the least fiber.[83] Those who consume the most vegetables had a 52% lower risk than those who consume the least vegetables.[83] But even in this large review of the evidence, researchers noted, "the data do not permit discrimination between effects due to fiber and non-fiber effects due to vegetables."[83] So is fiber, all by itself, the magic bullet we've been looking for? We still, in 1990, didn't know.

Two years later, a different group of researchers reviewed thirteen studies that had compared people with and without colorectal cancer (case-control design).[84] They found that those who had consumed the most fiber had a 47% lower risk of colorectal cancer than those who consumed the least.[84] In fact, they found that if Americans ate an additional thirteen grams of fiber a day *from food sources* (not as supplements), about a third of all colorectal cancer cases in the U.S. could be avoided.[84] If you'll remember, thirteen grams, in real-world terms, is the amount found in about a cup of any variety of beans.

In recent decades, a mammoth study called the EPIC study collected data on fiber intake and colorectal cancer in 519,000 people across Europe.[85] They found that the 20% of people who consumed the most fiber in their diet, about thirty-four grams per day, had a 42% lower risk of colorectal cancer than the 20% who consumed the least fiber in their diet, about thirteen grams per day.[85] It's important to note once again that, as with all of these studies, dietary fiber was obtained in food, not as supplements. So all we can say is "fiber-containing diets" seem to significantly reduce the risk of colorectal cancer. We still can't say anything definitive about isolated fiber itself. This means that attempts to add isolated fiber to foods may not produce benefits. But consuming plant foods naturally high in fiber is clearly beneficial. These foods include vegetables (the non-root parts), fruits, and whole grains.

In reality, we can't even be sure how much of the prevention of colorectal cancer is due to fiber-containing foods, because as people eat more of these foods, they usually consume fewer animal-based foods. In other words, are fruits, vegetables, and whole grains protective, or is meat dangerous? Or is it both? A 1985 study in South Africa helped to answer these questions. White South Africans have seventeen times more large bowel cancer than black South Africans, and this was first thought to be due to the much higher consumption of dietary fiber among black South Africans provided by unrefined maize.[86] However, black South Africans later were found to be increasingly consuming commercially *refined* maize-meal—maize minus its fiber. They now eat even less fiber than the white South Africans. Yet, colon cancer rates among blacks remain at a low level,[87] which calls into question how much of the cancer-protective effect is due to dietary fiber alone. A later study[88] showed that the higher colon cancer rates among white South Africans could well be due to their elevated consumption of animal protein (77 vs. 25 g/day), total fat (115 vs. 71 g/day), and cholesterol (408 vs. 211 mg/day), as seen in Chart 8.5. The researchers suggested that the much higher colon cancer rates among white South Africans may be more related to the quantity of animal protein and fat in their diets than their lacking the protective factor of dietary fiber.[88]

Chart 8.5: Intake of Animal Protein, Total Fat, and Cholesterol Among Black and White South Africans

What is clear is that diets naturally high in fiber and low in animal-based foods can prevent colorectal cancer. Even in the absence of more specific details, we can still make important public health recommendations. The data clearly show that a whole foods, plant-based (WFPB) diet can dramatically lower colorectal cancer rates. We don't need to know which fiber is responsible, what mechanism is involved, or even how much of the effect is independently due to fiber.

OTHER FACTORS

Studies done through the end of the 1990s have noted that the same risk factors that promote colorectal cancer—a diet low in fruits and vegetables and high in animal foods and refined carbohydrates—can also promote insulin resistance syndrome.[89–91] From there, scientists have hypothesized that insulin resistance may be responsible for colon cancer.[89–94] Insulin resistance was described in chapter six as a diabetic condition. And what's good for keeping insulin resistance under control is also good for colon cancer: a diet of whole, plant-based foods.

This diet happens to be very high in carbohydrates, which have recently been under assault in the marketplace. Because carbohydrate confusion persists, let me remind you that there are two different types of carbohydrates: refined and complex. Refined carbohydrates are the starches and sugars obtained from plants by mechanically stripping off their outer layers, which contain most of the plant's vitamins, minerals, protein, and fiber. This "food" (regular sugar, white flour, etc.) has very little nutritional value. Foods such as pastas made from refined flour, sugary cereals, white bread, candies, and sugar-laden soft drinks should be avoided as much as possible. But do eat whole, complex carbohydrate–containing foods such as unprocessed fresh fruits and vegetables, and whole grain products like brown rice and oatmeal. These unprocessed carbohydrates, especially from fruits and vegetables, are exceptionally health promoting.

You may have heard that calcium is beneficial in fighting colon cancer. This, of course, gets extended to the argument that cow's milk fights colon cancer. It has been hypothesized that high-calcium diets prevent colon cancer in two ways: first, by inhibiting the growth of critical cells in the colon,[95,96] and second, by binding up intestinal bile acids. These acids arise in the liver, move to the intestine, and are thought to get into the large bowel and promote colon cancer development. By binding these bile acids, calcium is said to prevent colon cancer.

One research group demonstrated that high-calcium diets—generally meaning diets high in dairy foods—inhibit the growth of certain cells in the colon,[96] *but this effect was not entirely consistent for the various indicators of cell growth. Furthermore, it is not clear whether these presumably favorable biochemical effects really lead to less cancer growth.*[95,97] Another research group demonstrated that calcium does reduce the presumably dangerous bile acids, but they also observed that a high-wheat diet did an even better job of reducing them.[98] But—and this is the really odd part—when a combination high-calcium and high-wheat diet was consumed, the binding effect on bile acids was weaker than for each individual supplement taken alone.[98] It just goes to show that when individually observed nutrient effects are combined, as in a dietary situation, the expected may become the unexpected.

I doubt that a high-calcium diet, obtained through calcium supplements or through calcium-rich cow's milk, has a beneficial effect on colon cancer. In rural China, where calcium consumption was modest and almost no dairy food was consumed at the time of our survey,[99] colon cancer rates were not higher; instead they were much lower than in the U.S. The parts of the world that consume the most calcium, Europe and North America, have the highest rates of colorectal cancer.

Another lifestyle choice that is clearly important for this disease is exercise. Increased exercise is convincingly associated with less colorectal cancer. In one summary from the World Cancer Research Fund and the American Institute for Cancer Research, seventeen out of twenty studies found that exercise protected against colon cancer.[76]

SCREENING FOR TROUBLE

The benefits of exercise bring me back to former president George W. Bush. He was known to enjoy staying physically fit with a regular running routine, and that is undoubtedly one of the reasons why he received a clean bill of health when he had a colonoscopy. But what is a colonoscopy anyway, and is it really worth the effort to get checked? When people go to the doctor to get a colonoscopy, the doctor inspects the large bowel using a rectal probe and looks for abnormal tissue growth. The most commonly found abnormality is a polyp. Although it is not yet clear exactly how tumors are related to polyps, most scientists would agree[100,101] that they share similar dietary associations and genetic characteristics. Those people who have noncancerous problems in the large bowel, such as polyps, often are the same people who later develop cancerous tumors.

So getting screened for polyps or other problems is a reasonable way to establish risk for large bowel cancer in the future. But what if you have a polyp? What is the best thing to do? Will surgical removal of the polyp lessen colon cancer risk? A nationwide study has shown that, when polyps were removed, there was a 76–90% decrease in the expected cases of colon cancer.[101,102] This certainly supports the idea of routine screening.[101,103] It is commonly recommended that people get a colonoscopy once every ten years starting at the age of fifty. If you have a higher risk of colorectal cancer, it is recommended that you start at the age of forty and screen more frequently.

How do you know if you are at a higher risk for colorectal cancer? We can very roughly assess our personal genetic risk in several ways. We can consider the probability of our getting colon cancer based on the number of immediate family members who already have the disease, we can screen for the presence of polyps, and we now can clinically test for the presence of suspect genes.[104]

This is an excellent example of how genetic research can lead to a better understanding of complex diseases. However, in the enthusiasm for studying the genetic basis for this cancer, two things often get overlooked. First, the proportion of colon cancer cases attributed to known inherited genes is only about 1–3%.[101] Another 10–30%[101] tend to occur in some families more than others (called familial clustering), an effect possibly reflecting a significant genetic contribution. These numbers, however, exaggerate the number of cancers that are solely "due to genes."

Except for the very few people whose colon cancer risk is largely determined by known inherited genes (1–3%), most of the family-connected colon cancer cases (i.e., the additional 10–30%) are still largely determined by environmental and dietary factors. After all, place of residence and diet are often shared experiences within families.

Even if you have a high genetic risk, a healthy plant-based diet is capable of negating most, if not all, of that risk by controlling the expression of these genes. Because a high-fiber diet can only prevent colon cancer—extra fiber won't ever *promote* colon cancer—dietary recommendations should be the same regardless of one's genetic risk.

PROSTATE CANCER

I suspect that most people do not know exactly what a prostate is, even though prostate cancer is commonly discussed. The prostate is a male reproductive organ about the size of a walnut, located between the bladder and the colon. It is responsible for producing some of the fluid that helps sperm on its quest to fertilize the egg.

For such a little thing, it sure can cause a lot of problems. Several of my friends now have prostate cancer or closely related conditions, and they aren't alone. As a 1998 report pointed out, "Prostate cancer is one of the most commonly diagnosed cancers among men in the United States, representing about 25% of all tumors."[105] As many as half of all men seventy years and older have latent prostate cancer,[106] a silent form of the cancer that is not yet causing discomfort. Prostate cancer is not only extremely prevalent, but also slow-growing. Only 7% of diagnosed prostate cancer victims die within five years.[107] This makes it difficult to know how and if the cancer should be treated. The main question for the patient and doctor is: Will this cancer become life threatening before death comes from other causes?

One of the markers used to determine the likelihood of prostate cancer becoming life threatening is the blood level of prostate-specific antigen (PSA). Men are diagnosed as having prostate problems when their PSA levels are above four. But this test alone is hardly a firm diagnosis of cancer, especially if the PSA level is barely above four. The ambiguity of this test leads to some very difficult decision-making. Occasionally my friends ask for my opinion. Should they have a little surgery or a lot? Is a PSA value of 6.0 a serious problem or just a wake-up call? If it's a wake-up call, then what must they do to reduce such a number? While I cannot speak to the clinical condition of an individual, I can speak to the research, and of the research I have seen, there is no doubt that diet plays a key role in this disease.

Although there is debate regarding the specifics of diet and this cancer, let's start with some very safe assumptions that have long been accepted in the research community:

- Prostate cancer rates vary widely between different countries, even more than breast cancer.
- High prostate cancer rates primarily exist in societies with Western diets and lifestyles.
- In developing countries, men who adopt Western eating practices or move to Western countries suffer more prostate cancer.

These disease patterns are similar to those of other diseases of affluence. Mostly this tells us that although prostate cancer certainly has a genetic component, environmental factors play the dominant role. So what environmental factors are important? You can guess that I'm going to say plant-based foods are good and animal-based foods are bad, but do we know anything more specific? Surprisingly, one of the most consistent, specific links between diet and prostate cancer has been dairy consumption.

A 2001 Harvard review of the research could hardly be more convincing:

> *Twelve of . . . fourteen case-control studies and seven of . . . nine cohort studies [have] observed a positive association for some measure of dairy products and prostate cancer; this is one of the most consistent dietary predictors for prostate cancer in the published literature [my emphasis]. In these studies, men with the highest dairy intakes had approximately double the risk of total prostate cancer, and up to a fourfold increase in risk of metastatic or fatal prostate cancer relative to low consumers.*[108]

Let's consider that again: dairy intake is "one of the most consistent dietary predictors for prostate cancer in the published literature," and those who consume the most dairy have double to quadruple the risk.

Another review of published literature done in 1998 reached a similar conclusion:

> *In ecologic data, correlations exist between per capita meat and dairy consumption and prostate cancer mortality rate [one study cited]. In case control and prospective studies, the major contributors of animal protein, meats, dairy products and eggs have frequently been associated with a higher risk of prostate cancer . . . [twenty-three studies cited]. Of note, numerous studies have found an association primarily in older men [six studies cited] though not all [one study cited]. . . . The consistent associations with dairy products could result from, at least in part, their calcium and phosphorous content.*[109]

In other words, an enormous body of evidence shows that animal-based foods are associated with prostate cancer. In the case of dairy, the high intake of calcium and phosphorus also could be partly responsible for this effect.

This research leaves little room for dissent; each of the above studies represents analyses of over a dozen individual studies, providing an impressive bulk of convincing literature.

THE MECHANISMS

As we have seen with other forms of cancer, large-scale observational studies show a link between prostate cancer and an animal-based diet, particularly one based heavily on dairy. Understanding the mechanisms behind the observed link between prostate cancer and dairy clinches the argument.

The first mechanism concerns a hormone that increases cancer cell growth, a hormone that our bodies make, as needed. This growth hormone, insulin-like growth factor 1 (IGF-1), is turning out to be a predictor of cancer just as cholesterol is a predictor for heart disease. Under normal conditions, this hormone efficiently manages the rates at which cells "grow"—that is, how they reproduce themselves and how they discard old cells, all in the name of good health.

Under unhealthy conditions, however, IGF-1 becomes more active, increasing the birth and growth of new cells while simultaneously inhibiting the removal of old cells, both of which favor the development of cancer [seven studies cited[110]]. So what does this have to do with the food we eat? It turns out that consuming animal-based foods increases the blood levels of this growth hormone, IGF-1.[111–113]

With regard to prostate cancer, people with higher than normal blood levels of IGF-I have been shown to have 5.1 times the risk of advanced-stage prostate cancer.[110] There's more: when men also have low blood levels of a protein that binds and inactivates IGF-I,[114] they will have *9.5 times the risk of advanced-stage prostate cancer*.[110] Let's put a few stars by these numbers. They are big and impressive—and fundamental to this finding is the fact that we make more IGF-I when we consume animal-based foods like meat and dairy.[111–113]

The second mechanism relates to vitamin D metabolism. Under most conditions, this "vitamin" is not a nutrient that we need to consume. Our body can make all that we need simply by being in sunlight fifteen to thirty minutes every couple of days. In addition to the production of vitamin D being affected by sunlight, it is also affected by the food that we eat. The formation of the most active form of vitamin D is a process that is closely monitored and controlled by our bodies. This process is a great example of our bodies' natural balancing act, affecting not only prostate cancer, but breast cancer, colon cancer, osteoporosis, and autoimmune diseases like Type 1 diabetes. Because of its importance for multiple diseases, and because of the complexity involved in explaining how it all works, I have provided in Appendix C an abbreviated scheme, just enough to illustrate my point. This web of reactions illustrates many similar and highly integrated reaction networks showing how food controls health.

The main component of this process is an active form of vitamin D produced in the body from the vitamin D that we get from food or sunshine. This active or "supercharged" D produces many benefits throughout the body, including the prevention of cancer, autoimmune diseases, and diseases like osteoporosis. This all-important supercharged D is not something that you get from food or from a drug. A drug composed of isolated supercharged D would be far too powerful and far too dangerous for medical use. Your body uses a carefully composed series of controls and sensors to produce just the right amount of supercharged D for each task at exactly the right time.

As it turns out, our diet can determine how much of this supercharged D is produced and how it works once it is produced. Animal protein that we consume has the tendency to block the production of supercharged D, leaving the body with low levels of this vitamin D in the blood. If these low levels persist, prostate cancer can result. Also, persistently high intakes of calcium create an environment where supercharged D declines, thus adding to the problem.

So what food substance has both animal protein and large amounts of calcium? *Milk and other dairy foods.* This fits in perfectly with the evidence that links dairy consumption with prostate cancer. This information provides what we call biological plausibility and shows how the observational data fit together. To review the potential mechanisms:

- Animal protein causes the body to produce more IGF-1, which in turn throws cell growth and removal out of whack, stimulating cancer development.
- Animal protein suppresses the production of supercharged D.
- Excessive calcium, as found in milk, also suppresses the production of supercharged D.
- Supercharged D is responsible for creating a wide variety of health benefits in the body. Persistently low levels of supercharged D create an inviting environment for different cancers, autoimmune diseases, osteoporosis, and other diseases.

The important story here is how the effects of food—both good and bad—operate through a symphony of coordinated reactions to prevent diseases like prostate cancer. In discovering the existence of these networks, we sometimes wonder which specific function comes first and which comes next. We tend to think of these reactions within the network as independent. But this surely misses the point. What impresses me is the multitude of reactions working together in so many ways to produce the same effect: in this case, to prevent disease.

There is no single "mechanism" that fully explains what causes diseases such as cancer. Indeed, it would be foolish to even think along these lines. But what I do know is this: the totality and breadth of the evidence, operating through highly coordinated networks, supports the conclusions that consuming dairy and meat are serious risk factors for prostate cancer.

DR. ORNISH'S WORK ON PROSTATE CANCER

Since the publication of the first edition of *The China Study*, some of the most compelling new research on the potential impact of a plant-based diet has been on prostate cancer. Dr. Dean Ornish, who demonstrated reversal of advanced heart disease through a plant-based diet in a randomized controlled trial, used the same intervention on men with early-stage prostate cancer. Instead of surgery, radiation, or medication, these men had chosen "watchful waiting," meaning they were simply monitoring markers of cancer for signs of progressing disease. As mentioned, prostate cancer tends to grow slowly, and the treatments we use often have permanent side effects, so some men with early prostate cancer elect to monitor the disease rather than intervene immediately.

Dr. Ornish put one group of these men on a program consisting of a WFPB diet, stress reduction, group support, and exercise, and prescribed standard care for another group. Average PSA levels declined over the course of 12 months in the diet-and-lifestyle group, compared to the standard-care group.[115] Further, their blood actually repressed cancer growth in cell cultures, far, far more than the control group's blood.[115] After three months of the diet-and-lifestyle intervention, these men were noted to have a significant change in the expression of over 500 genes; also, genes known to promote cancer were suppressed.[116] Over the course of two years, 27% of men in the standard-care group required conventional treatment (surgery, radiation, or chemotherapy) while only 5% in the diet-and-lifestyle group required conventional treatment.[117] In short, Dr. Ornish has now shown for early-stage prostate cancer what he demonstrated for advanced heart disease: diet and lifestyle change alone can halt and even reverse this terrible disease.

At this point, it should come as no surprise that recent research has found that men who have been diagnosed with prostate cancer who consume a more Western diet (more processed and red meats, high-fat dairy, and refined grains) have 2.5 times the risk of dying from their cancer within 10 years.[118] Men with prostate cancer consuming three or more servings of dairy products, compared to those consuming less than one serving a day, have a 141% increased risk of dying from their cancer within ten years.[119]

Between Dr. Ornish's powerful intervention research findings, and previous observational research, it has become very difficult to deny a strong effect of diet and lifestyle on prostate cancer prevention and treatment. In Tom's opinion as a medical practitioner, we have such conclusive evidence, including observational, mechanistic, and intervention data, that every doctor should tell every man with prostate cancer to stop consuming dairy immediately and embrace a WFPB diet.

BRINGING IT TOGETHER

Over half a million Americans this year will go to the doctor's office and be told that they have cancer of the breast, prostate, or large bowel. People who get one of these cancers represent 40% of all new cancer patients. These three cancers devastate the lives of not only the victims themselves, but also their family and friends.

When my mother-in-law died of colon cancer at the age of fifty-one, none of us knew very much about nutrition or what it meant for health. It wasn't that we didn't care about the health of our loved ones—of course we did. We just didn't have the information. Yet, over forty years later, not much has changed. Of the people you know who have cancer, or are at risk of having cancer, how many of them have considered the possibility of adopting a WFPB diet to improve their chances? I'm guessing very few of them have done so. Probably they, too, don't have the information.

Our institutions and information providers are failing us. Even cancer organizations, at both the national and local level, are reluctant to discuss or even believe this evidence. Food as a key to health represents a powerful challenge to conventional medicine, which is fundamentally built on drugs, radiation, and surgery (see Part IV). The widespread communities of nutrition professionals, researchers, and doctors are, as a whole, either unaware of this evidence or reluctant to share it. Because of these failings, Americans are being cheated out of information that could save their lives.

There is enough evidence now that doctors should be discussing the option of pursuing dietary change as a potential path to cancer prevention and treatment. There is enough evidence now that the U.S. government should be discussing the idea that the toxicity of our diet is the single biggest cause of cancer. There is enough evidence now that local breast cancer alliances, and prostate and colon cancer institutions, should be discussing the possibility of providing information to Americans everywhere on how a WFPB diet may be an incredibly effective anticancer medicine.

If these discussions were to happen, it is possible that, next year, fewer than 500,000 people would go to the doctor's office and be told they have cancer of the breast, prostate, or large bowel. The year after that, even fewer friends, coworkers, and family members would be given the most dreaded of all diagnoses. And the following year, even fewer.

The possibility that this future could be our reality is real, and as long as this future holds such promise for the health of people everywhere, it is a future worth working for.

AUTOIMMUNE DISEASES

No group of diseases is more insidious than autoimmune diseases. They are difficult to treat, and progressive loss of physical and mental function is a common outcome. Unlike heart disease, cancer, obesity, and Type 2 diabetes, with autoimmune diseases the body systematically attacks itself. The afflicted patient is almost guaranteed to lose.

A quarter million people in the U.S. are diagnosed with one of the more than eighty separate autoimmune diseases each year.[1,2] Women are 2.7 times more likely to be afflicted than are men. As many as 7–10% of people worldwide have an autoimmune disease, amounting to tens of millions in America alone.[3]

The more common of these diseases are listed in Chart 9.1.[2] The first nine comprise 97% of all autoimmune disease cases.[2] The most studied are multiple sclerosis (MS), rheumatoid arthritis, lupus, Type 1 diabetes, and rheumatic heart disease.[2] These are also the primary autoimmune diseases that have been studied in reference to diet.

Others not listed in Chart 9.1 include inflammatory bowel disease,[5] Crohn's disease,[5] rheumatic heart disease,[4] and (possibly) Parkinson's disease.[6]

Each disease name may sound very different, but as one review points out,[2] "It is important to consider . . . these disorders as a group." They show similar clinical backgrounds,[4,7,8] they sometimes occur in the same person, and they are often found in the same populations.[2] MS and Type 1 diabetes, for example, have "near[ly] identical ethnic and geographic distribution."[9] Autoimmune diseases in general become more common the greater the distance from the equator. This phenomenon has been known since 1922.[10] MS, for example, is over 100 times more prevalent in the far north than at the equator.[11]

Chart 9.1: Common Autoimmune Diseases
(From Most Common to Least Common)

1.	Graves' disease (Hyperthyroidism)	10.	Sjogren's disease
2.	Rheumatoid arthritis	11.	Myasthenia gravis
3.	Thyroiditis (Hypothyroidism)	12.	Polymyositis/dermatomyositis
4.	Vitiligo	13.	Addison's disease
5.	Pernicious anemia	14.	Scleroderma
6.	Glomerulonephritis	15.	Primary biliary cirrhosis
7.	Multiple sclerosis	16.	Uveitis
8.	Type 1 diabetes	17.	Chronic active hepatitis
9.	Systemic lupus erythematosus		

Because of some of these common features, it is not too far-fetched to think of the autoimmune diseases as one grand disease living in different places in the body and taking on different names. We refer in this way to cancer, which is specifically named depending on what part of the body it resides in.

All autoimmune diseases are the result of one group of physiological mechanisms gone awry, much like cancer. In this case, the mechanism is the immune system mistakenly attacking cells in its own body. Whether it is the pancreas as in Type 1 diabetes, the myelin sheath as in MS, or joint tissues as in arthritis, all autoimmune diseases involve an immune system that has revolted. It is an internal mutiny of the worst kind, one in which our body becomes its own worst enemy.

IMMUNITY FROM INVADERS

The immune system is astonishingly complex. I often hear people speaking about this system as if it were an identifiable organ like a lung. Nothing could be further from the truth. It is a system, not an organ.

In essence, our immune system is like a military network designed to defend against foreign invaders. The "soldiers" of this network are the white blood cells, which comprise many different sub-groups, each having its own mission. These sub-groups are analogous to a navy, army, air force, and marines, with each group of specialists doing highly specialized work.

The "recruitment center" for the system is in the marrow of our bones. The marrow is responsible for generating specialized cells called stem cells. Some of these cells are released into circulation for use elsewhere in the body; these are called B-cells (for bone). Other cells formed in the bone marrow remain immature, or unspecialized, until they travel to the thymus (an organ in the chest cavity just above the heart) where they become specialized; these are called T-cells (for thymus). These "soldier" cells, along with other specialized cells, team up to create intricate defense plans. They meet at major intersections around the body, including the spleen (just inside the left lower rib cage) and the lymph nodes. These meeting points are like command and control centers, where the soldier cells rearrange themselves into teams to attack foreign invaders.

These cells are remarkably adaptable when they form their teams. They are able to respond to different circumstances and different foreign substances, even those they have never before seen. The immune response to these strangers is an incredibly creative process. It is one of the true wonders of nature.

The foreign invaders are protein molecules called antigens. These foreign cells can be a bacterium or a virus looking to corrupt the body's integrity. So when our immune system notices these antigens, it destroys them. Each of these foreign antigens has a separate identity, which is determined by the sequence of amino acids that comprises its proteins. It is analogous to each and every person having a different face. Because numerous amino acids are available for creating proteins, there are infinite varieties of distinctive "faces."

To counter these antigens, our immune system must customize its defense to each attack. It does this by creating a "mirror image" protein for each attacker. The mirror image is able to fit perfectly onto the antigen and destroy it. Essentially, the immune system creates a mold for each face it encounters. Every time it sees that face after the initial encounter, it uses the custom-made mold to "capture" the invader and destroy it. The mold may be a B-cell antibody or a T-cell-based receptor protein.

Remembering each defense against each invader is what immunization is all about. An initial exposure to chicken pox, for example, is a difficult battle, but the second time your immune system encounters that virus, it will know exactly how to deal with it, and the war will be shorter, less painful, and much more successful. You may not even get sick.

IMMUNITY FROM OURSELVES

Even though this system is a wonder of nature when it is defending the body against foreign proteins, it is also capable of attacking the same tissues that it is designed to protect. This self-destructive process is common to all autoimmune diseases. It is as if the body were to commit suicide.

One of the fundamental mechanisms for this self-destructive behavior is called molecular mimicry. It so happens that some of the foreign invaders that our soldier cells seek out to destroy look the same as our own cells. The immune system molds that fit these invaders also fit our own cells. The immune system then destroys, under some circumstances, everything that fits the mold, including our own cells. This is an extremely complex, self-destructive process involving many different strategies on the part of the immune system, all of which share the same fatal flaw of not being able to distinguish foreign invader proteins from the proteins of our own body.

What does all of this have to do with what we eat? It so happens that the antigens that trick our bodies into attacking our own cells may be in food. During the process of digestion, for example, some proteins slip into our bloodstream from the intestine without being fully broken down into their amino acid parts. The remnants of undigested proteins are treated as foreign invaders by our immune system, which sets about making molds to destroy them and launches the self-destructive autoimmune process.

One of the foods that supplies many of the foreign proteins that mimic our own body proteins is cow's milk. Most of the time, our immune system is quite smart. Just like an army arranges for safeguards against friendly fire, the immune system has safeguards to stop itself from attacking the body it's supposed to protect. Even though an invading antigen looks just like one of the cells in our own body, the system can still distinguish our own cells from the invading antigen. In fact, the immune system may use our own cells to practice making molds against the invader antigen *without actually destroying the friendly cell.*

This is analogous to training camps in preparations for war. When our immune system is working properly, we can use the cells in our body that look like the antigens as a training exercise, without destroying them, to prepare our soldier cells to repulse the invading antigens. It is one more example[1] of the exceptional elegance of nature's ability to regulate itself.

The immune system uses a very delicate process to decide which proteins should be attacked and which should be left alone.[12] The way this incredibly complex process breaks down with autoimmune diseases is not yet understood. We just know that the immune system loses its ability to differentiate between the body's cells and the invading antigen, and instead of using the body's cells for "training," it destroys them along with the invaders.

TYPE 1 DIABETES

In the case of Type 1 diabetes, the immune system attacks the pancreas cells responsible for producing insulin. This devastating, incurable disease mostly strikes children, creating a painful and difficult experience for young families. What most people don't know, though, is that there is strong evidence that this disease is linked to diet and, more specifically, to dairy products. The ability of cow's milk protein to initiate Type 1 diabetes[13-15] is well documented. The possible initiation of this disease goes like this:

- A baby is not nursed long enough and is fed cow's milk protein, perhaps in an infant formula.
- The milk reaches the small intestine, where it is digested down to its amino acid parts.
- For some infants, cow's milk is not fully digested, and small amino acid chains or fragments of the original protein remain in the intestine.
- These incompletely digested protein fragments may be absorbed into the blood.
- The immune system recognizes these fragments as foreign invaders and goes about destroying them.
- Unfortunately, some of the fragments look exactly the same as the cells of the pancreas that are responsible for making insulin.
- The immune system loses its ability to distinguish between the cow's milk protein fragments and the pancreatic cells, and destroys them both, thereby eliminating the child's ability to produce insulin.
- The infant becomes a Type 1 diabetic, and remains so for the rest of his or her life.

This process boils down to a truly remarkable statement: *cow's milk may cause one of the most devastating diseases that can befall a child.* For obvious reasons, this is one of the most contentious issues in nutrition today.

One of the more remarkable reports on this cow's milk effect was published over two decades ago, in 1992, in the *New England Journal of Medicine.*[13] Finnish researchers obtained blood from Type 1 diabetic children, aged four to twelve years. Then they measured the levels of antibodies that had formed in the blood against an incompletely digested protein of cow's milk called bovine serum albumin (BSA). They did the same process with non-diabetic children and compared the two groups (remember, an antibody is the mirror image, or mold, of a foreign antigen). Children who had antibodies to cow's milk protein must have previously consumed cow's milk. It also means that undigested protein fragments of the cow's milk proteins had to have entered the infant's circulation in order to cause antibodies to form in the first place.

The researchers discovered something truly remarkable. Of the 142 diabetic children measured, *every single one had antibody levels higher than 3.55 IgG*. Of the seventy-nine normal children, *every single one had antibody levels less than 3.55*.

In other words, there was no overlap in levels between diabetic and normal children. All of the diabetic children had levels of cow's milk antibodies that were higher than those of all of the non-diabetic children. This implies two things: children with more antibodies consumed more cow's milk, and increased antibodies may cause Type 1 diabetes.

These results sent shock waves through the research community. It was the complete separation of antibody responses that made this study so remarkable. This study,[13] and others done even earlier,[16–18] initiated an avalanche of additional studies over the next several years that continue to this day.[14,19,20]

Several studies have since investigated this effect of cow's milk on BSA antibody levels. All but one showed that cow's milk increases BSA antibodies in Type 1 diabetic children,[19] although the responses were quite variable in their magnitude.

In the decade leading up to the publication of the first edition, scientists had investigated far more than just the BSA antibodies, and a more complete picture is coming into view. Very briefly, it goes something like this[14,20]: infants or very young children of a certain genetic background,[21,22] who are weaned from the breast too early[23] onto cow's milk and who, perhaps, become infected with a virus that may corrupt the gut immune system,[20] are likely to have a high risk for Type 1 diabetes. A study in Chile[24] considered the first two factors, cow's milk and genes. Genetically susceptible children weaned too early onto cow's milk–based formula had a risk of Type 1 diabetes that was 13.1 times greater than children who did not have these genes and who were breast-fed for at least three months (thus minimizing their exposure to cow's milk). Another study in the U.S. showed that genetically susceptible children fed cow's milk as infants had a risk of disease that was 11.3 times greater than children who did not have these genes and who were breast-fed for at least three months.[25] This eleven to thirteen times greater risk is incredibly large (1,000–1,200%!); anything over three to four times is usually considered very important. To put this in perspective, smokers have approximately ten times greater risk of getting lung cancer (still less than the eleven to thirteen times risk here), and people with high blood pressure and cholesterol have a 2.5–3.0 times greater risk of heart disease (Chart 9.2).[19]

So how much of the eleven to thirteen times increased risk of Type 1 diabetes is due to early exposure to cow's milk, and how much is due to genes? These days, there is a popular opinion that Type 1 diabetes is

Chart 9.2: Relative Risks of Various Factors on Various Disease Outcomes

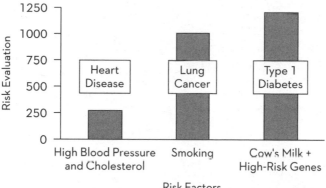

due to genetics, an opinion often shared by doctors as well. But genetics alone cannot account for more than a very small fraction of cases of this disease. Genes do not act in isolation; they need a trigger for their effects to be produced. It has also been observed that after one member of identical twin pairs gets Type 1 diabetes, there is only a 13 33% chance of the second twin getting the disease, even though both twins have the same genes.[14,21,22,26,27] If it were all due to genes, closer to 100% of the identical twins would get the disease. In addition, it is possible that the 13–33% risk for the second twin is due to the sharing of a common environment and diet, factors affecting both twins.

Consider, for example, the observation shown in Chart 9.3, which highlights the link between one aspect of environment, cow's milk consumption, and this disease. Cow's milk consumption by children zero to fourteen years of age in twelve countries[28] shows an almost perfect correlation with Type 1 diabetes.[29] The greater the consumption of cow's milk, the greater the prevalence of Type 1 diabetes. In Finland, Type 1 diabetes is thirty-six times more common than in Japan.[30] Large amounts of cow's milk products are consumed in Finland but very little is consumed in Japan.[28]

As we have seen with other diseases of affluence, when people migrate from areas of the world where disease incidence is low to areas of the world where disease incidence is high, they quickly adopt the high incidence rates as they change their diet and lifestyle.[31–33] This shows that even though individuals may have the necessary gene(s), the disease will occur only in response to certain dietary and/or environmental circumstances.

Disease trends over time show the same thing. The worldwide prevalence of Type 1 diabetes is increasing at an alarming rate of 3% per year.[34]

Chart 9.3: Association of Cow's Milk Consumption and Incidence of Type 1 Diabetes in Different Countries

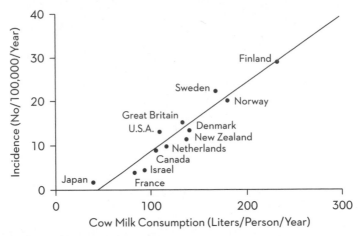

This increase is occurring for different populations even though there may be substantial differences in disease rates. This relatively rapid increase cannot be due to genetic susceptibility. The frequency of any one gene in a large population is relatively stable over time, unless there are changing environmental pressures that allow one group to reproduce more successfully than another group. For example, if all families with Type 1 diabetic relatives had a dozen babies and all families without Type 1 diabetic relatives died off, then the gene or genes that may be responsible for Type 1 diabetes would become much more common in the population. This, of course, is not what is happening, and the fact that Type 1 diabetes is increasing 3% every year is very strong evidence that genes are not solely responsible for this disease.

It seems to me that we now have impressive evidence showing that cow's milk may be an important contributor to Type 1 diabetes. When the results of all these studies are combined (both genetically susceptible and not susceptible), we find that children weaned too early and fed cow's milk have, on average, a 50–60% higher risk of Type 1 diabetes (1.5–1.6 times increased risk).[35]

The earlier information on diet and Type 1 diabetes was impressive enough to cause two significant developments. The American Academy of Pediatrics in 1994 "strongly encouraged" that infants in families where diabetes is more common not be fed cow's milk supplements for their first two years of life. Second, many researchers[20] have developed prospective studies—the kind that follow individuals into the future—to see if a careful monitoring of diet and lifestyle could explain the onset of Type 1 diabetes.

Two of the better known of these studies have been under way in Finland, one starting in the late 1980s[14] and the other in the mid-1990s.[36] One has shown that cow's milk consumption increases the risk of Type 1 diabetes five- to sixfold,[37] while the second[36] tells us that cow's milk increases the development of at least another three to four antibodies in addition to those presented previously. In a separate study, antibodies to beta-casein, another cow's milk protein, were significantly elevated in bottle-fed infants compared to breast-fed infants; children with Type 1 diabetes also had higher levels of these antibodies.[38] In short, of the studies that have reported results, *the findings strongly support the danger of cow's milk, especially for genetically susceptible children.*

Still, a definitive assessment of the association of Type 1 diabetes with cow's milk is difficult because the consumption of cow's milk is so common, leaving only a small range of exposures for experimental investigations. And the research undertaken since the first edition of this book has shown the association of Type 1 diabetes and dietary factors like cow's milk to be even more complex[39]—not surprising!

Recent research has confirmed that the disease mostly begins in genetically susceptible infants and young children,[40] but genes cannot be the sole cause because fewer than 10% of genetically positive infants actually incur Type 1 diabetes. Something more is needed for its development. Cow's milk, especially consumed in place of or shortly after nursing, still appears to be the strongest dietary factor. There has been some evidence that vitamin D supplementation[41] may reduce disease onset, but this evidence has not been entirely consistent.[42]

THE CONTROVERSY OF CONTROVERSY

Imagine looking at the front page of the newspaper and finding the following headline: "Cow's Milk the Likely Cause of Lethal Type 1 Diabetes." Because the reaction would be so strong, and the economic impact monumental, this headline won't be written anytime soon, regardless of the scientific evidence. Stifling this headline is accomplished under the powerful label of "controversy." With so much at stake, and so much information understood by so few people, it is easy to generate and sustain controversy. Controversies are a natural part of science. Too often, however, controversy is not the result of rational scientific debate, but instead reflects a need to delay and distort research results. For example, if I say cigarettes are bad for you and provide a mountain of evidence to support my contention, the tobacco companies might come along and pick out one unsolved detail and then claim that the whole idea of cigarettes being unhealthy is mired in controversy, thereby nullifying all my conclusions. This is easy to do, because there will always be unsolved details; this is the nature of science. Some groups use controversy to stifle certain ideas, impede constructive research, confuse the public, and turn public policy into babble rather than substance. Sustaining and even emphasizing controversy as a means of discrediting findings that cause economic or social discomfort is one of the greatest sins in science.

It can be difficult for the layperson to assess the legitimacy of a highly technical controversy such as that regarding cow's milk and Type 1 diabetes. This is true even if the layperson is interested in reading scientific articles.

Consider, for example, a 1999 scientific review[43] of the cow's milk–Type 1 diabetes association. In ten human studies (all case-control) summarized in a paper published as part of a "controversial topics series,"[43] the authors concluded that five of the ten studies showed a statistically significant positive association between cow's milk and Type 1 diabetes and five did not. Obviously, this at first seems to demonstrate considerable uncertainty, going a long way to discredit the hypothesis.

However, the five studies that were counted as "negative" did not show that cow's milk *decreased* Type 1 diabetes. These five studies showed *no statistically significant effect either way*. In contrast, there are a total of five statistically significant studies and all five showed the same result: early cow's milk consumption is associated with increased risk of Type 1 diabetes. There is only one chance in sixty-four that this was a random or chance result.

There are many, many reasons, some seen and some unseen, why an experiment would find no statistically significant relationship between two factors, even when a relationship really exists. Perhaps the study didn't include enough people, thus decreasing the sensitivity of the study to detect an effect that really exists. Perhaps most of the subjects had very similar feeding practices, limiting detection of the relationship you might otherwise see. Maybe trying to measure infant feeding practices from years ago was inaccurate enough that it obscured the relationship that does exist. Perhaps the researchers were studying the wrong period of time in an infant's life.

The point is, if five of the ten studies did find a statistically significant relationship, and *all five* showed that cow's milk consumption is linked to increasing Type 1 diabetes, and none show that cow's milk consumption is linked to decreasing Type 1 diabetes, I could hardly justify saying, as the authors of this review did, that the hypothesis "has become quite murky with inconsistencies in the literature."[43]

In this same review,[43] the authors summarized additional studies that indirectly compared breast-feeding practices associated with cow's milk consumption and Type 1 diabetes. This compilation involved fifty-two possible comparisons, twenty of which were statistically significant. Of these twenty significant findings, *nineteen favored an association of cow's milk with disease, and only one did not.* Again the odds heavily favored the hypothesized association, something that the authors failed to note.

I cite this example not only to support the evidence showing a cow's milk effect on Type 1 diabetes, but also to illustrate one tactic that is often used to make something controversial when it is not. This practice is more common than it should be and is a source of unnecessary confusion. When researchers do this—even if they do it unintentionally they often have a serious prejudice against the hypothesis in the first place. Indeed, shortly after I wrote this, I heard a brief National Public Radio interview on the Type 1 diabetes problem with the senior author of this review paper.[43] Suffice it to say, the author did not acknowledge the evidence for the cow's milk hypothesis.

Because this issue has mammoth financial implications for American agriculture, and because so many people have such intense personal biases against it, it is unlikely that this diabetes research will reach the American media anytime soon. However, the depth and breadth of evidence now implicating cow's milk as a possible contributor of Type 1 diabetes is impressive, even though the very complex mechanistic details are not yet fully understood. We not only have evidence of the danger of cow's milk, we also have considerable evidence showing that the association between diabetes and cow's milk is biologically plausible. Human breast milk is the perfect food for an infant, and one of the most damaging things a mother can do is to substitute the milk of a cow for her own.

The incidence of Type 1 diabetes is rising rapidly in many parts of the world at an annual rate of 3–5%.[44] It is time to become more vigorous in sharing with the public the evidence we have on cow's milk and its products. Waiting for the evidence to be perfect (it never will be) is an unacceptable strategy, especially when cow's milk protein has long been shown to have other effects of serious concern, including increased blood cholesterol,[45] formation of early atherogenesis (cardiovascular disease[46]), and promotion of experimental cancer,[47] among other effects.

MULTIPLE SCLEROSIS AND OTHER AUTOIMMUNE DISEASES

Multiple sclerosis (MS) is a particularly difficult autoimmune disease, both for those who have it and for those who care for its victims. It is a life-long battle involving a variety of unpredictable and serious disabilities. MS patients often pass through episodes of acute attacks while gradually losing their ability to walk or to see. After ten to fifteen years, they often are confined to a wheelchair, and then to a bed for the rest of their lives.

About 400,000 people in the U.S. alone have the disease, according to the National Multiple Sclerosis Society.[48] It is a disease that is initially diagnosed between twenty and forty years of age and strikes women about three times more often than men.

Even though there is widespread medical and scientific interest in this disease, most authorities claim to know very little about causes or cures. Major multiple sclerosis websites all claim that the disease is an enigma. They generally list genetics, viruses, and environmental factors as possibly playing roles in the development of this disease but pay almost no heed to a possible role for diet. This is peculiar considering the wealth of intriguing information on the effects of food that is available from reputable research reports.[49–51] Once again cow's milk appears to play an important role.

The "multiple" symptoms of this disease represent a nervous system gone awry. In MS patients, the electrical signals carrying messages to and from the central nervous system (brain and spinal cord) and out through the peripheral nervous system to the rest of the body are not well coordinated and controlled. This is because the insulating cover or sheath of the nerve fibers, the myelin, is being destroyed by an autoimmune reaction. Think of what would happen to your household wiring if the electrical insulation became thin or was stripped away, leaving bare wires. The electrical signals would be short-circuited. That is what happens with MS; the wayward electrical signals may destroy cells and "burn" patches of neighboring tissue, leaving little scars or bits of sclerotic tissue. These "burns" can become serious and ultimately destroy the body.

The initial research showing an effect of diet on MS goes back more than half a century to the research of Dr. Roy Swank, who began his work in Norway and at the Montreal Neurological Institute during the 1940s. Later, Dr. Swank headed the Division of Neurology at the University of Oregon Medical School.[52]

Dr. Swank became interested in the dietary connection when he learned that MS appeared to be more common in the northern climates.[52] There is a huge difference in MS prevalence as one moves away from the equator: MS is over 100 times more prevalent in the far north than at the equator,[11] and seven times more prevalent in south Australia (closer to the South Pole) than in north Australia.[53] This distribution is very similar to the distribution of other autoimmune diseases, including Type 1 diabetes and rheumatoid arthritis.[54,55]

Although some scientists speculated that magnetic fields might be responsible for the disease, Dr. Swank thought it was diet, especially animal-based foods high in saturated fats.[52] He found that inland dairy-consuming areas of Norway had higher rates of MS than coastal fish-consuming areas.

Swank conducted his best-known trial on 144 MS patients recruited from the Montreal Neurological Institute. He kept records on these patients for the next thirty-four years.[56] He advised his patients to consume a diet low in saturated fat, most of whom did, but many of whom did not. He then classified them as good dieters or poor dieters, based on whether they consumed less or more than 20 g/day of saturated fat. (For comparison, a bacon cheeseburger with condiments has about sixteen grams of saturated fat. One small frozen chicken pot pie has almost ten grams of saturated fat.)

As the study continued, Dr. Swank found that progression of disease was greatly reduced by the low-saturated-fat diet, which worked even for people with initially advanced conditions. He summarized his work in 1990,[56] concluding that for the sub-group of patients who began the low-saturated-fat diet during the earlier stages of their disease, "about 95% . . . remained only mildly disabled for approximately thirty years." Only 5% of these patients died. *In contrast, 80% of the patients with early-stage MS who consumed the "poor" diet (higher saturated fat) died of MS.* The results from all 144 patients, including those who started the diet at a later stage of disease, are shown in Chart 9.4.

Chart 9.4: MS Death Rate After 144 Patients Dieted for Thirty-Four Years

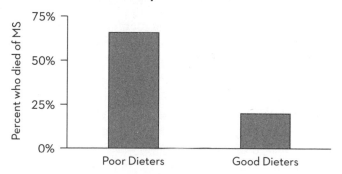

This work is remarkable. To follow people for thirty-four years is an exceptional demonstration of perseverance and dedication. Moreover, if this were a study testing a potential drug, these findings would make any pharmaceutical manufacturer jingle the coins in his or her pocket. Swank's first results were published more than a half century ago,[57] then again[58] and again[59] and again[56] for the next forty years.

Additional studies[51,60,61] have confirmed and extended Swank's observations and gradually have begun to place more emphasis on cow's milk. These new studies show that consuming cow's milk is strongly linked to MS both when comparing different countries[61] and when comparing states within the U.S.[60] Chart 9.5, published by French researchers, compares the consumption of cow's milk with MS for twenty-six populations in twenty-four countries.[61]

Chart 9.5: Association of Cow's Milk Consumption and Multiple Sclerosis

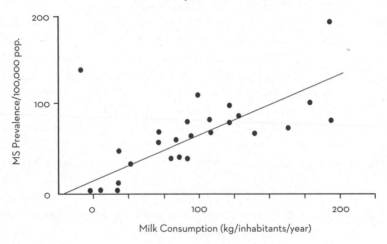

Milk Consumption (kg/inhabitants/year)

This relationship, which is virtually identical to that for Type 1 diabetes, is remarkable, and it is not due to variables such as the availability of medical services or geographic latitude.[60] In some studies[61,62] researchers suggest this strong correlation with fresh cow's milk might be due to the presence of a virus in the milk. These more recent studies also suggest that saturated fat alone probably was not fully responsible for Swank's results. The consumption of meat high in saturated fat, like milk, was also associated with MS in these multi-country studies,[63] while the consumption of fish, containing more omega-3 fat, was associated with low rates of disease.[64]

The association of cow's milk with MS, shown in Chart 9.5, may be impressive, but it does not constitute proof. For example, where do genes and viruses come into play? Either of these, in theory, might account for the unusual geographic distribution of this disease.

In the case of viruses, no definite conclusions are yet possible. A variety of different virus types have been suggested and a variety of effects on the immune system may be involved. However, nothing very convincing has been proven. Some of the evidence is based on finding more viral antibodies in MS patients than in controls, some is based on sporadic outbreaks of MS among isolated communities, and some is based on finding virus-like genes among MS cases.[14,20,65]

With regard to genes, we can begin to puzzle out their association with MS by asking the usual question: What happens to people who migrate from one population to another, keeping their genes the same but changing their diets and their environment? The answer is the same as it was for cancer, heart disease, and Type 2 diabetes. People acquire the risk of the population to which they move, especially if they move before their adolescent years.[66,67] This tells us that this disease is more strongly related to environmental factors than it is to genes.[68]

Specific genes have been identified as possible candidates for causing MS, but, according to a 2001 report,[4] as many as twenty-five genes may be playing such a role. Therefore, it will undoubtedly be a long time before we determine with any precision which genes or combinations of genes predispose someone to MS. Genetic predisposition may make a difference as to who gets MS, but even at best, genes can only account for about one-fourth of the total disease risk.[69]

Although MS and Type 1 diabetes share some of the same unanswered questions on the exact roles of viruses and genes and the immune system, they also share the same alarming evidence regarding diet. For both diseases, a Western diet is strongly associated with disease incidence. Not all studies show that a healthy diet leads to disease improvement. A small one-year trial[70] of a plant-based diet showed no significant benefit in short-term MS symptoms or disability, although there were improvements in the subjects' metabolic health. This illustrates the principle that because a Western diet is so strongly disease-promoting for metabolic conditions and certain cancers, it seems that there is more than enough evidence to prescribe a whole foods, plant-based diet for both the prevention and treatment of these conditions.

THE COMMONALITY OF AUTOIMMUNE DISEASES

What about other autoimmune diseases? There are dozens of autoimmune diseases and I have mentioned only two of the more prominent ones. Can we say anything about them as a whole?

To answer this question, we need to identify how much these diseases have in common. The more they have in common, the greater the probability that they also will share a common cause (or causes). This is like seeing two people you don't know, both of whom have a similar body type, hair color, eye color, facial features, physical and vocal mannerisms, and age, and concluding that they come from the same parents. Just as we hypothesized that diseases of affluence such as cancer and heart disease have common causes because they share similar geography and similar biochemical biomarkers (chapter four), we can also hypothesize that MS, Type 1 diabetes, rheumatoid arthritis, lupus, and other autoimmune diseases may share a similar cause if they exhibit similar characteristics.

First, by definition, each of these diseases involves an immune system that has gone awry in such a way that it attacks "self" proteins that look the same as foreign proteins.

Second, all the autoimmune diseases that have been studied have been found to be more common at the higher geographic latitudes where there is less constant sunshine.[10, 11,71]

Third, some of these diseases have a tendency to afflict the same people. MS and Type 1 diabetes, for example, have been shown to coexist in the same individuals.[72–75] Parkinson's disease, a non-autoimmune disease with autoimmune characteristics, is often found with MS, both within the same geographic regions[76] and within the same individuals.[6] MS also has been associated—either geographically or within the same individuals—with other autoimmune diseases like lupus, myasthenia gravis, Graves' disease, and eosinophilic vasculitis.[73] Juvenile rheumatoid arthritis, another autoimmune disease, has been shown to have an unusually strong association with Hashimoto thyroiditis.[77]

Fourth, of those diseases studied in relation to nutrition, the consumption of animal-based foods—especially cow's milk—is associated with greater disease risk.

Fifth, there is evidence that a virus (or viruses) may trigger the onset of several of these diseases.

A sixth and most important characteristic binding together these diseases is the evidence that their "mechanisms of action" (jargon used to describe the "how to" of disease formation) have much in common. As we consider common mechanisms of action, we might start with sunlight exposure, because this somehow seems linked to the autoimmune diseases. Sunlight exposure, which decreases with increasing latitude, could be important—but clearly there are other factors. The consumption of animal-based foods, especially cow's milk, also increases with distance from the equator. In fact, in one of the more extensive studies, cow's milk was found to be as good of a predictor of MS as latitude (i.e., sunshine).[60] In Dr. Swank's studies in Norway, MS was less common near the coastal areas of the country where fish intake was more common. This gave rise to the idea that the omega-3 fats common to fish might have a protective effect. What is almost never mentioned, however, is that dairy consumption (and saturated fat) was much lower in the fish-eating areas. Is it possible that cow's milk and lack of sunshine are having a similar effect on MS and other autoimmune diseases because they operate through a similar mechanism? This could be very interesting, if true.

As it turns out, the idea is not so crazy. This mechanism involves, once again, vitamin D. There are experimental animal models of lupus, MS, rheumatoid arthritis, and inflammatory bowel disease (e.g., Crohn's disease, ulcerative colitis), each of which is an autoimmune disease.[7,8,78] Vitamin D, operating through a similar mechanism in each case, prevents the experimental development of each of these diseases. This becomes an even more intriguing story when we think about the effect of food on vitamin D.

The first step in the vitamin D process occurs when you go outside on a sunny day. When the sunshine hits your exposed skin, the skin produces vitamin D. The vitamin D then must be activated in the kidney in order to produce a form that helps repress the development of autoimmune diseases. As we've seen before, this critically important activation step can be inhibited by foods that are high in calcium and by acid-producing animal proteins like cow's milk (some grains also produce excess acid). Under experimental conditions, the activated vitamin D operates in two ways: it inhibits the development of certain T-cells and their production of active agents (called cytokines) that initiate the autoimmune response, and/or it encourages the production of other T-cells that oppose this effect.[79,80] (An abbreviated schematic of this vitamin D network is shown in Appendix C.) This mechanism of action appears to be a strong commonality among all autoimmune diseases so far studied.

Knowing the strength of the evidence against animal foods, cow's milk in particular, for both MS and Type 1 diabetes, and knowing how much in common all of the autoimmune diseases have, it is reasonable to begin thinking about food and its relationship to a much broader group of autoimmune diseases. Obviously caution is called for; more research is needed to make conclusive statements about cross–autoimmune disease similarities. But the evidence we have now is already striking.

Today almost no indication of the dietary connection to these diseases has reached public awareness. In 2003, the website of the Multiple Sclerosis International Federation, for example, stated, "There is no credible evidence that MS is due to poor diet or dietary deficiencies." They warned that dietary regimens can be "expensive" and "can alter the normal nutritional balance."[81] If changing your diet is expensive, I don't know what they would say about being bedridden and incapacitated. As far as altering the "normal nutritional balance" is concerned, what is normal? Does this mean the diet that we now eat is "normal"—the diet that is largely responsible for diseases that disable, kill, and make profoundly miserable millions of Americans every year? Are massive rates of heart disease, cancer, autoimmune diseases, obesity, and diabetes "normal"? If this is normal, I propose we start seriously considering the abnormal.

The present Multiple Sclerosis International Federation website does not include this provocative and irresponsible quote. But they still speculate about causes of MS as possibly being due to "environmental" and "genetic" factors, with nary a word about diet. They mention a role for the immune system, MS' inverse relationship with vitamin D, and that MS is not simply a genetic disease, but avoid mentioning that nutrition could account for all three of these observations. Is this progress? I don't think so.

There are 400,000 Americans who are victims of multiple sclerosis, and millions more with other autoimmune diseases. While statistics, research results, and clinical descriptions form the basis for much of my discussion of diet and disease, the importance of the information comes down to the *intimate experience of individual people*. Any one of these serious diseases I've talked about in this chapter can forever alter the life of any person—a family member, a friend, a neighbor, a coworker, or you yourself.

It is time to sacrifice our sacred cows. Reason must prevail. Professional societies, doctors, and government agencies need to stand up and do their duty, so that children being born today do not face tragedies that otherwise could be prevented.

WIDE-RANGING EFFECTS: BONE, KIDNEY, EYE, AND BRAIN DISEASES

10

One of the most convincing arguments for a plant-based diet is the fact that it prevents a broad range of diseases. If I have a conversation with someone about a single study showing the protective effect of fruits and vegetables on heart disease, they may agree that it's all very nice for fruits and vegetables, but they will probably still go home to meatloaf and gravy. It doesn't matter how big the study, how persuasive the results, or how reputable the scientists who conducted the investigation. The fact is that most people have a healthy skepticism about one study standing alone—as well they should.

But if I tell them about dozens and dozens of studies showing that the countries with low rates of heart disease consume low amounts of animal-based foods, and dozens and dozens of studies showing that individuals who eat more whole, plant-based foods get less heart disease, and I go on to document still more studies showing that a diet low in animal-based foods and high in unprocessed plant-based foods can slow or reverse heart disease, then people are more inclined to pay some attention.

If I keep talking and go through this process not only for heart disease, but also obesity, Type 2 diabetes, breast cancer, colon cancer, prostate cancer, multiple sclerosis, and other autoimmune diseases, it's quite possible that people may never eat meatloaf and gravy again.

What has become so convincing about the effect of a diet on health is the breadth of the evidence. While a single study might be found to support almost any idea under the sun, what are the chances that hundreds, even thousands, of different studies show a protective benefit of plant-based foods and/or harmful effects of animal-based foods for so many different diseases? We can't say it's due to coincidence, bad data, biased research, misinterpreted statistics, or "playing with numbers." This has got to be the real deal.

I have so far presented only a small sample of the breadth of evidence that supports plant-based diets. To show you just how broad this evidence is, I will cover five more seemingly unrelated diseases common in America: osteoporosis, kidney stones, blindness, cognitive dysfunction, and Alzheimer's disease. These disorders are not often fatal and are frequently regarded as the inevitable consequences of aging. Therefore, we don't think it's unnatural when Grandpa gets blurry spots in his vision, can't remember the names of his friends, or needs a hip replacement operation. But, as we shall see, even these diseases have a dietary link.

OSTEOPOROSIS

Did you ever have an elementary school teacher tell you that if you didn't have bones, you would just be a shapeless blob on the floor? Or maybe you learned about the human skeleton from that popular song, ". . . the ankle bone is connected to the shin bone, the shin bone is connected to the knee bone," etc. At the same time in your life, you probably were told to drink milk to build strong bones and teeth. Because none of us want to be shapeless blobs, and because our celebrities have been paid to advertise milk's presumed benefits, we drank it. Milk is to bone health as bees are to honey.

Americans consume more cow's milk and its products per person than most populations in the world. So Americans should have wonderfully strong bones, right? Unfortunately not. A recent study showed that American women aged fifty and older have one of the highest rates of hip fractures in the world.[1] The only countries with higher rates are in Europe and in the south Pacific (Australia and New Zealand)[1] where they consume even more milk than the United States. What's going on?

An excess rate of hip fractures is often used as a reliable indicator of osteoporosis, a bone disease that especially affects women after menopause. It is often claimed to be due to an inadequate intake of calcium. Therefore, health policy people often recommend higher calcium consumption. Dairy products are particularly rich in calcium, so the dairy industry eagerly supports efforts to boost calcium consumption. These efforts have something to do with why you were told to drink your milk for strong bones—the politics of which are discussed in Part IV.

Something is amiss, though, because those countries that use the most cow's milk and its products also have the highest fracture rates and the worst bone health. One possible explanation is found in a report showing an impressively strong association between animal protein intake and bone fracture rate for women in different countries.[2] Authored in 1992 by researchers at Yale University School of Medicine, the report summarized data on protein intake and fracture rates taken from thirty-four separate surveys in sixteen countries that were published in twenty-nine peer-reviewed research publications. All the subjects in these surveys were women fifty years and older. It found that a very impressive 70% of the fracture rate was attributable to the consumption of animal protein.

These researchers explained that animal protein, unlike plant protein, increases the acid load in the body.[3] An increased acid load means that our blood and tissues become more acidic. The body does not like this acidic environment and begins to fight it. In order to neutralize the acid, the body uses calcium, which acts as a very effective base. This calcium, however, must come from somewhere. It ends up being pulled from the bones, and the calcium loss weakens them, putting them at greater risk for fracture. We have had evidence for well over a hundred years that animal protein decreases bone health. The explanation of animal protein causing excess metabolic acid, for example, was first suggested in the 1880s[4] and was documented as long ago as 1920.[5] We also have known that animal protein is more effective than plant protein at increasing the metabolic acid load in the body.[6, 7, 8]

When animal protein increases metabolic acid, the amount of calcium in the urine is increased. This effect has been established for over eighty years[5] and has been studied in some detail since the 1970s. Summaries of these studies were published in 1974,[9] 1981,[10] and 1990.[11] Each of these summaries clearly shows that the amount of animal protein consumed by many of us on a daily basis is capable of causing substantial increases in urinary calcium. Chart 10.1 is taken from the 1981 publication.[10] Doubling protein intake (mostly animal-based) from 35–78 g/day causes an alarming 50% increase in urinary calcium. This effect occurs well within the range of protein intake that most of us consume; average American intake is around 70–100 g/day. Incidentally, as mentioned in chapter four, a six-month study funded by the Atkins Center found that those people who adopted the Atkins Diet excreted 50% more calcium in their urine after six months on the diet.[12]

The initial observations on the association between animal protein consumption and bone fracture rates are very impressive, and now we have a plausible explanation as to how the association might work, a mechanism of action.

Chart 10.1: Association of Urinary Calcium Excretion with Dietary Protein Intake

Disease processes are rarely as simple as "one mechanism does it all," but the work being done in this field makes a strong argument. A more recent study comes from the Department of Medicine at the University of California at San Francisco. Using eighty-seven surveys in thirty-three countries, it compares the ratio of vegetable to animal protein consumption to the rate of bone fractures (Chart 10.2).[1] A high ratio of vegetable to animal protein consumption was found to be impressively associated with a virtual disappearance of bone fractures.

These studies are compelling for several reasons. They were published in leading research journals, the authors were careful in their analyses and interpretation of data, they included a large number of individual research reports, and the statistical significance of the association of animal protein with bone fracture rates is truly exceptional. They cannot be dismissed as just another couple of studies; the most recent study represents a summary of eighty-seven separate surveys!

The Study of Osteoporotic Fractures Research Group at the University of California at San Francisco published yet another study[13] of over 1,000 women aged sixty-five and up. Like the multi-country study, researchers characterized women's diets by the proportions of animal and plant protein. After seven years of observations, the women with the highest ratio of animal protein to plant protein had 3.7 times more bone fractures than the women with the lowest ratio. Also during this time the women with the high ratio lost bone almost four times as fast as the women with the lowest ratio.

Experimentally, this study is high quality because it compared protein consumption, bone loss, and broken bones for the same subjects. This

Chart 10.2: Association of Animal Versus Plant Protein Intake and Bone Fracture Rates for Different Countries

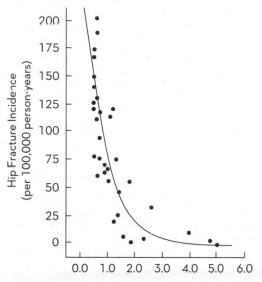

Vegetable-to-Animal Protein Intake Ratio (g/g)

3.7-fold effect is substantial, and is very important because the women with the lowest bone fracture rates still consumed, on average, about half of their total protein from animal sources. I can't help but wonder how much greater the difference might have been had they consumed not 50% but 0–10% of their total protein from animal sources. In our rural China study, where the animal to plant ratio was about 10%, the fracture rate is only about one-fifth that of the U.S. Nigeria shows an animal-to-plant protein ratio only about 10% that of Germany, and the hip fracture incidence is lower by over 99%.[1]

These observations raise a serious question about the widely advertised claim that protein-rich dairy foods protect our bones. And yet we still are warned almost daily about our need for dairy foods to provide calcium for strong bones. An avalanche of commentary warns that most of us are not meeting our calcium requirements, especially pregnant and lactating women. This calcium bonanza, however, is not justified. In one study of ten countries,[14] a higher consumption of calcium was associated with a higher—not lower—risk of bone fracture (Chart 10.3). Much of the calcium intake shown in this chart, especially in high-consumption countries, is due to dairy foods, rather than calcium supplements or non-dairy food sources of calcium.

Mark Hegsted, who produced the results in Chart 10.3, was a long-time Harvard professor. He worked on the calcium issue beginning in the early 1950s, was a principal architect of the nation's first dietary guidelines in

1980, and in 1986 published this graph. Professor Hegsted believed that excessively high calcium intake over a long time impaired the body's ability to control how much calcium it uses and when. Under healthy conditions, the body uses an activated form of vitamin D, calcitriol, to adjust how much calcium it absorbs from food and how much it excretes and distributes to the bone. Calcitriol is considered a hormone; when more calcium is needed, it enhances calcium absorption and restricts calcium excretion. If too much calcium is consumed over a long period of time, the body may lose its ability to regulate calcitriol, permanently or temporarily disrupting the regulation of calcium absorption and excretion. Ruining the regulatory mechanism in this way is a recipe for osteoporosis in menopausal and post-menopausal women. Women at this stage of life must be able to enhance their utilization of calcium in a timely manner, especially if they continue to consume a diet high in animal protein. The fact that the body loses its ability to control finely tuned mechanisms when they are subjected to continuous abuse is a well-established phenomenon in biology.

Chart 10.3: Association of Rates of Hip Fractures with Calcium Intake for Different Countries

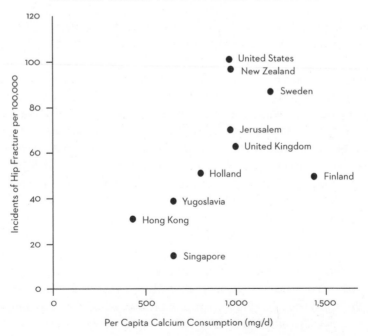

Given these findings, it seems perfectly plausible that animal protein and even calcium—when consumed at excessive levels—are capable of increasing the risk of osteoporosis. Dairy, unfortunately, is the only food that is rich in both of these nutrients. Hegsted, backed by his exceptional experience in calcium research, said in his 1986 paper, "Hip fractures are more frequent in populations where dairy products are commonly consumed and calcium intakes are relatively high."

Years later, the dairy industry still suggests that we should be consuming more of its products to build strong bones and teeth. The confusion, conflict, and controversy rampant in this area of research allow anybody to say just about anything. And of course, huge amounts of money are at stake as well. One of the most cited osteoporosis experts—one funded by the dairy industry—angrily wrote in a prominent editorial[15] that the findings cited above favoring a diet with a higher ratio of plant-to-animal protein could have been "influenced to some extent by currents in the larger society." The "currents" he was referring to were the animal rights activists opposed to the use of dairy foods.

Much of the debate regarding osteoporosis, whether it is conducted with integrity or otherwise, resides in the research concerning the details. As you shall see, the devil lurks in the details, the primary detail being that of bone mineral density (BMD).

Many scientists have investigated how various diet and lifestyle factors affect BMD. BMD is a measure of bone density that is often used to diagnose bone health. If your bone density falls below a certain level, you may be diagnosed with osteoporosis. In practical terms, this means that if you have a low BMD, you are at a higher risk for a fracture.[16–18] But there are some devilishly contradictory and confusing details in this great circus of osteoporosis research. To name a few:

- A high BMD increases the risk of osteoarthritis.[19]
- A high BMD has been linked to a higher risk of breast cancer.[20,21]
- Although high BMD is linked to both increased breast cancer risk and decreased osteoporotic risk, breast cancer and osteoporosis nonetheless cluster together in the same areas of the world and even in the same individuals.[22]
- Rate of bone loss matters just as much as overall BMD.[23]
- There are places where overall bone mass, bone mineral density, or bone mineral content measurements are lower than they are in Western countries, but the fracture rate also is lower, defying accepted logic of how we define "big, strong bones."[24–26]
- Being fat is linked to greater BMD,[24,27] even though areas of the world that have higher rates of obesity also have higher rates of osteoporosis.

Something is wrong with the idea that BMD is the only biomarker that matters in osteoporosis and, by inference, indicates the kind of diet that would lower fracture rates. In contrast, an alternative but much better predictor of osteoporosis is the dietary ratio of animal-to-plant protein.[1,13] The higher the ratio, the higher the risk of disease. And guess what? BMD is not significantly associated with this ratio.[13]

Clearly the conventional recommendations regarding animal foods, dairy, and bone mineral density, which are influenced and advertised by the dairy industry, are besieged by serious doubts in the literature. Here is what I would recommend you do, based on the research, to minimize your risk of osteoporosis:

- Stay physically active. Take the stairs instead of the elevator, go for walks, jogs, bicycle rides. Swim, do yoga or aerobics every couple of days, and don't be afraid to buy barbells to use once in a while. Play a sport or join a social group that incorporates exercise. The possibilities are endless, and they can be fun. You'll feel better, and your bones will be much healthier for the effort.
- Eat a variety of whole plant foods, and avoid animal foods, including dairy. Plenty of calcium is available in a wide range of plant foods, including beans and leafy vegetables and most non-dairy "milks." As long as you stay away from refined carbohydrates, like sugary cereals, candies, plain pastas, and white breads, you should have no problem with calcium deficiency.
- Keep your salt intake to a minimum. Avoid highly processed and packaged foods, which contain excess salt. There is some evidence that excessive salt intake can be a problem.

KIDNEYS

At the website for the UCLA Kidney Stone Treatment Center,[28] you will discover that kidney stones may cause the following symptoms:

- Nausea, vomiting
- Restlessness (trying to find comfortable position to ease the pain)
- Dull pain (ill-defined, lumbar, abdominal, intermittent pain)
- Urgency (urge to empty the bladder)
- Frequency (frequent urination)
- Bloody urine with pain (gross hematuria)
- Fever (when complicated by infection)

- Acute renal colic (severe colicky flank pain radiating to groin, scrotum, labia)

Acute renal colic deserves some explanation. This agonizing symptom is the result of a crystallized stone trying to pass through the thin tube in your body (ureter) that transports urine from the kidney to the bladder. In describing the pain involved, the website states, "This is probably one of the worst pains humans experience. Those who have had it will never forget it . . . The severe pain of renal colic needs to be controlled by potent pain killers. Don't expect an aspirin to do the trick. Get yourself to a doctor or an emergency room."[28]

I don't know about you, but just thinking about these things gives me a shiver. Unfortunately, up to 15% of Americans, more men than women, will be diagnosed with having a kidney stone in their lifetime.[29]

There are several kinds of kidney stones. Although one is a genetically rare type[30] and another is related to many urinary infections, the majority involve stones made of calcium and oxalate. These calcium oxalate stones are relatively common in developed countries and relatively rare in developing countries.[31] Again, this illness falls into the same global patterns as all the other Western diseases.

I first was made aware of the dietary connection with this disease at the Faculty of Medicine of the University of Toronto. I was invited to give a seminar on our China Study findings, and while there I met Professor W. G. Robertson from the Medical Research Council in Leeds, England. This chance encounter was extremely rewarding. Dr. Robertson, as I have come to learn, is one of the world's foremost experts on diet and kidney stones. Dr. Robertson's research group has investigated the relationship between food and kidney stones with great depth and breadth, both in theory and in practice. Their work began more than thirty years ago and continues to the present day. A search of the scientific publications authored or co-authored by Robertson shows at least 100 papers published since the mid-1960s.

One of Robertson's charts, based on a 1968–1973 U.K. study, depicts a stunning relationship between animal protein consumption and the formation of kidney stones (Chart 10.4).[32] The study shows that consuming animal protein at levels above twenty-one grams per person per day (slightly less than one ounce)—on top of a background of protein from plants—is closely correlated with the formation of a high number of kidney stones. This is an impressive relationship.

Few researchers have worked out the details of a research question more thoroughly than Robertson and his colleagues. They have developed a model for estimating the risk of stone formation with remarkable accuracy.[33] Although they have identified six risk factors for kidney stones,[34,35] animal protein consumption was the major culprit. Consumption of animal protein at levels commonly seen in affluent countries leads to the development of four of the six risk factors.[34,35]

Not only is animal protein linked to risk factors for future formation of stones, but it affects recurring stones as well. Robertson published findings showing that, among the patients who had recurrent kidney stones, he was able to resolve their problem simply by shifting their diet away from animal protein foods.[36]

Chart 10.4: Association Between Animal Protein Intake and Formation of Urinary Calculi

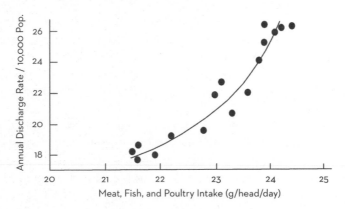

How does this work? When enough animal-protein-containing foods are consumed, the concentrations of calcium and oxalate in the urine increase sharply, usually within hours. Chart 10.5 shows these impressive changes, published by Robertson's group.[35]

The individuals in this study consumed only fifty-five grams per day of land-based animal protein, to which was added another thirty-four grams per day of animal protein in the form of tuna fish. This amount of animal protein consumption is well within the levels most Americans regularly eat. Men consume around 90–100 grams of total protein per day, the majority of which comes from animal foods; women consume about 70–90 grams per day.

When the kidney is under a persistent, long-term assault from increased calcium and oxalate in the urine, kidney stones may result.[35] The following, excerpted from a 1987 review by Robertson,[37] emphasizes the role of diet, especially foods containing animal proteins:

Urolithiasis [kidney stone formation] is a worldwide problem which appears to be aggravated by the high dairy-produce, highly energy-rich and low-fibre diets consumed in most industrialized countries . . . Evidence points, in particular, to a high-meat protein intake as being the dominant factor . . . On the basis of epidemiological and biochemical studies a move toward a more vegetarian, less energy-rich diet would be predicted to reduce the risk of stone in the population.

Chart 10.5: Effect of Animal Protein Intake on Calcium and Oxalate in the Urine

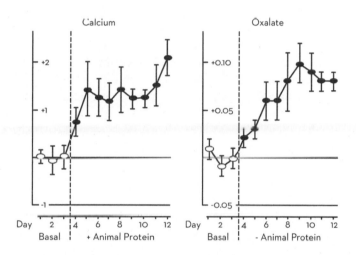

A substantial and convincing effect on stone formation has been demonstrated for animal-based foods. Research also shows that kidney stone formation can be initiated by the activity of free radicals,[38] and may thus be prevented by consumption of antioxidant-containing plant-based foods (see chapter four). For yet another organ and another disease, we see opposing effects (in this case on stone formation) by animal- and plant-based foods.

Incidence of kidney stones has been rising quite rapidly. As of 2012, 10.6% of men and 7.1% of women in the U.S. had developed kidney stones, a 70% increase since 1994.[39] Not surprisingly, increasing fluid intake (i.e., water) helps to reduce kidney stone formation.[40] And high animal protein intake is still being documented as one of the most significant causes of kidney stone formation.[41]

EYE PROBLEMS

People who can see well often take vision for granted. We treat our eyes more as little bits of technology than as living parts of the body, and are all too willing to believe that lasers are the best course of action for maintaining healthy eyes. But during the past couple of decades, research has shown that these bits of "technology" are actually greatly affected by the foods we eat. Our breakfasts, lunches, and dinners have a particular effect on two common eye diseases, cataracts and macular degeneration—diseases that afflict millions of older Americans.

Yes, that's right. I'm about to tell you that if you eat animal foods instead of plant foods, you just might go blind.

Macular degeneration is the leading cause of irreversible blindness among people over age sixty-five. Over 1.6 million Americans suffer from this disease, many of whom become blind.[42] As the name implies, this condition involves destruction of the macula, which is the biochemical intersection in the eye—where the energy of the light coming in is transformed into a nerve signal. The macula occupies center stage, so to speak, and it must be functional for sight to occur.

Around the macula there are fatty acids that can react with incoming light to produce a low level of highly reactive free radicals.[43] These free radicals (see chapter four) can destroy, or degenerate, neighboring tissue, including the macula. But fortunately for us, free radical damage can be repressed thanks to the antioxidants in vegetables and fruits.

Two studies, each involving a team of experienced researchers at prestigious institutions, provide compelling evidence that food can protect against macular degeneration. Both studies were published two decades ago. One evaluated diet[44] and the other assessed nutrients in blood.[45] The findings of these two studies suggested that as much as 70–88% of blindness caused by macular degeneration could be prevented if the right foods are eaten.

The study on dietary intakes[44] compared 356 individuals fifty-five to eighty years of age who were diagnosed with advanced macular degeneration (cases) with 520 individuals with other eye diseases (controls). Five ophthalmology medical centers collaborated on the study.

Researchers found that a higher intake of total carotenoids was associated with a lower frequency of macular degeneration. Carotenoids are a group of antioxidants found in the colored parts of fruits and vegetables. When carotenoid intakes were ranked, those individuals who consumed the most had 43% less disease than those who consumed the least. Not surprisingly, five out of six plant-based foods measured also were associated with lower rates of macular degeneration (broccoli, carrots, spinach or collard greens, winter squash, and sweet potato). Spinach or collard greens conferred the most protection. There was 88% less disease for people who ate these greens five or more times per week when compared with people who consumed these greens less than once per month. The only food group not showing a preventive effect was the cabbage/cauliflower/Brussels sprout group, which sports the least color of the six food groups.[46]

These researchers also looked at the potential protection from disease as a result of the consumption of five of the individual carotenoids consumed in these foods. All but one of these five showed a highly significant protective effect, especially the carotenoids found in the dark green leafy vegetables. In contrast, supplements of a few vitamins, including retinol (preformed "vitamin" A), vitamin C, and vitamin E showed little or no beneficial effects. Yet again, we see that while supplements may give great wealth to supplement manufacturers, they will not give great health to you and me.

When all was said and done, this study found that *macular degeneration risk could be reduced by as much as 88%, simply by eating the right foods.*[44]

At this point you may be wondering, "Where can I get some of those carotenoids?" Green leafy vegetables, carrots, and citrus fruits are all good sources. Herein lies a problem, however. Among the hundreds (maybe thousands) of antioxidant carotenoids in these foods, only a dozen or so have been studied in relation to their biological effects. The abilities of these chemicals to scavenge and reduce free radical damage are well established, but the activities of the individual carotenoids vary enormously depending on dietary and lifestyle conditions. Such variations make it virtually impossible to predict their individual activities, either good or bad. The logic of using them as supplements is much too particular and superficial. It ignores the dynamic of nature. It's much safer to consume these carotenoids in their natural context, in highly colored fruits and vegetables.

The second study[45] compared a total of 421 macular degeneration patients (cases) with 615 controls. Five of the leading clinical centers specializing in eye diseases and their researchers participated in this study. The researchers measured the levels of antioxidants in the blood, rather than the antioxidants consumed. Four kinds of antioxidants were measured: carotenoids, vitamin C, selenium, and vitamin E. Except for selenium, each of these nutrient groups was associated with fewer cases of macular degeneration, although only the carotenoids showed statistically significant results. Risk of macular degeneration was reduced by two-thirds for those people with the highest levels of carotenoids in their blood, when compared with the low-carotenoid group.

This reduction of about 65–70% in this study is similar to the reduction of upwards of 88% in the first study. These two studies consistently demonstrated the benefits of antioxidant carotenoids consumed as food. Given experimental limitations, we can only approximate the proportion of macular degeneration caused by poor dietary habits, and we cannot know which antioxidants are involved. What we can say, however, is that eating antioxidant-containing foods, especially those containing the carotenoids, may prevent macular degeneration. This in itself is a remarkable statement.

Cataracts are slightly less serious than macular degeneration because there are effective surgical options available to restore vision loss caused by this disease. But when you look at the numbers, cataracts are a much larger burden on our society. By the age of eighty, half of all Americans will have cataracts.[42] Currently there are 20 million Americans age forty and older with the disease.

Cataract formation involves the clouding of the eye lens. Corrective surgery involves removing the cloudy lens and replacing it with an artificial lens. The development of the opaque condition, like the degeneration of the macula and so many other disease conditions in our body, is closely associated with the damage created by an excess of reactive free radicals.[47] Once again, it is reasonable to assume that eating antioxidant-containing foods should be helpful.

Starting in 1988, researchers in Wisconsin began to study eye health and dietary intakes in over 1,300 people. Ten years later, they published a report[48] on their findings. The people who consumed the most lutein, a specific type of antioxidant, had one-half the rate of cataracts as the people who consumed the least lutein. Lutein is an interesting chemical because, in addition to being readily available in spinach, along with other dark leafy green vegetables, it also is an integral part of the lens tissue itself.[49,50] Similarly, those who consumed the most spinach had 40% fewer cataracts. In 2014, Chinese scientists reported that consumption of lutein and another antioxidant found in high quantities in green leafy vegetables, zeaxanthin, significantly improved macular degeneration. This can only be considered preliminary but it suggests an ability of antioxidants to help prevent progression of this difficult disease.

These two eye conditions, macular degeneration and cataracts, both occur when we fail to consume enough of the highly colored green and leafy vegetables. In both cases, excess free radicals, increased by animal-based foods and decreased by plant-based foods, are likely to be responsible for these conditions.

MIND-ALTERING DIETS

By the time the first edition of this book hit the shelves ten years ago, I was seventy years old. At the last writing, I had recently attended my high school's fiftieth reunion, where I learned that many of my classmates had died. I was already receiving the AARP magazine, getting discounts on various products for being advanced in age, and receiving social security checks every month. Some euphemists might have called me a "mature adult." I just say old. What does it mean to be old? At seventy, I ran every morning, sometimes six or more miles a day; today, at eighty-two, I am still exercising daily: running or walking three to five miles a day, golfing in the summer, or cross-country skiing in the winter. I still have an active work life, perhaps more active than ever. I still enjoy all the same leisure activities, whether visiting grandchildren, dining with friends, gardening, traveling, golfing, lecturing, or making outdoor improvements like building fences or tinkering with this or that as I used to do on the farm. Some things have changed, though. Clearly there is a difference between the eighty-two-year-old me and the twenty-year-old me. I am slower, not as strong, work fewer hours every day, and am prone to taking naps more frequently than I used to.

We all know that growing old brings with it diminished capacities compared with our younger days. But there is good science to show that thinking clearly well into our later years is not something we need to give up. Memory loss, disorientation, and confusion are not inevitable parts of aging, but problems linked to that all-important lifestyle factor: diet.

There is now good dietary information for the two chief conditions referring to mental decline. On the modest side, there is a condition called "cognitive impairment" or "cognitive dysfunction." This condition describes the declining ability to remember and think as well as one once was able to. It represents a continuum of disease ranging from cases that only hint at declining abilities to those that are much more obvious and easily diagnosed.

Then there are mental dysfunctions that become serious, even life threatening. These are called dementia, of which are there two main types: vascular dementia and Alzheimer's disease. Vascular dementia is primarily caused by multiple little strokes resulting from broken blood vessels in the brain. It is common for elderly people to have tiny, "silent" strokes in their later years. A stroke is considered silent if it goes undetected and undiagnosed. Each little stroke incapacitates part of the brain. The other type of dementia, Alzheimer's, occurs when a protein substance called beta-amyloid accumulates in critical areas of the brain as a plaque, rather like the cholesterol-laden plaque that builds up in cardiovascular diseases.

Alzheimer's is surprisingly common. It is said that 1% of people at age sixty-five have evidence of Alzheimer's, a figure that doubles every five years thereafter.[51] More than five million people are living with the disease and a half million people die each year because they have the disease; it's listed as the sixth leading cause of death in the U.S. By 2050, it is expected that there will be 14 million people with the disease.[52] I suppose this is why we blandly accept "senility" as part of the aging process.

It has been estimated that 10–12% of individuals with mild cognitive impairment progress to the more serious types of dementia, whereas only 1–2% of individuals without cognitive impairment acquire these diseases.[53,54] This means that people with cognitive impairment have about a tenfold risk of Alzheimer's.

Not only does cognitive impairment often lead to more serious dementia, it is also associated with cardiovascular disease,[55–57] stroke,[58] and adult-onset Type 2 diabetes.[59,60] All of these diseases cluster in the same populations, oftentimes in the same people. This clustering means that they share some of the same risk factors. Hypertension (high blood pressure) is one factor[55,61,62]; another is high blood cholesterol.[57] Both of these, of course, can be controlled by diet.

A third risk factor is the amount of those nasty free radicals, which wreak havoc on brain function in our later years. Because free radical damage is so important to the process of cognitive dysfunction and dementia, researchers believe that consuming dietary antioxidants can shield our brains from this damage, as in other diseases. Animal-based foods lack antioxidant shields and tend to activate free radical production and cell damage, while plant-based foods, with their abundant antioxidants, tend to prevent such damage. It's the same dietary cause and effect that we saw with macular degeneration.

Of course, genes play a role, and specific genes have been identified that may increase the risk of cognitive decline.[56] But environmental factors also play a key role, most probably the dominant one.

Earlier, we reported that Japanese American men living in Hawaii had a higher rate of Alzheimer's disease than Japanese living in Japan.[63] Another study found that native Africans had significantly lower rates of dementia and Alzheimer's than African Americans in Indiana.[64] Both of these findings clearly support the idea that environment plays an important role in cognitive disorders.

Worldwide, prevalence patterns of cognitive disorders appear to be similar to other Western diseases. Rates of Alzheimer's are low in less-developed areas.[65] One study compared Alzheimer's rates to dietary variables across eleven different countries and found that populations with a high fat intake and low cereal and grain intake had higher rates of the disease.[66,67]

We seem to be on to something. Clearly, diet has an important voice in determining how well we think in our later years. But what exactly is good for us?

With regard to the more mild cognitive impairment condition, recent research has shown that high vitamin E levels in the blood are related to less memory loss.[68] Less memory loss also is associated with higher levels of vitamin C and selenium, both of which reduce free radical activity.[69] Vitamins E and C are antioxidants found almost exclusively in plant foods, while selenium is found in both animal- and plant-based foods.

In a study of 260 elderly people aged sixty-five to ninety years, it was reported that "[a] diet with less fat, saturated fat and cholesterol, and more carbohydrate, fiber, vitamins (especially folate, vitamins C and E and beta-carotenes) and minerals (iron and zinc) may be advisable not only to improve the general health of the elderly but also to improve cognitive function."[70] This conclusion advocates plant-based foods and condemns animal-based foods for optimal brain function. Yet another study on several hundred older people found that scores on mental tests were higher among those people who consumed the most vitamin C and beta-carotene.[71] Other studies have also found that a low level of vitamin C in the blood is linked to poorer cognitive performance in old age,[72,73] and some have found that B vitamins,[73] including beta-carotene,[74] are linked to better cognitive function.

The seven studies mentioned above all show that one or more nutrients found almost exclusively in plants are associated with a lower risk of cognitive decline in old age. Experimental animal studies have not only confirmed that plant foods are good for the brain, but they also show the mechanisms by which these foods work.[75,76] Although there are important variations in some of these study findings—for example, one study only finds an association for vitamin C, and another only finds an association for beta-carotene and not vitamin C—we shouldn't miss the forest by focusing on one or two trees. No study has ever found that consuming more dietary antioxidants increases memory loss. When associations are observed, it is always the other way around. Furthermore, the association appears to be significant, although more substantial research must be done before we can know exactly how much cognitive impairment is due to diet.

What about the more serious dementia caused by strokes (vascular dementia) and Alzheimer's? How does diet affect these diseases? The dementia that is caused by the same vascular problems that lead to stroke is clearly affected by diet. In a publication from the famous Framingham Study, researchers conclude that for every three additional servings of fruits and vegetables a day, the risk of stroke will be reduced by 22%.[77] Three servings of fruits and vegetables is less than you might think. The following examples count as one serving in this study: 1/2 cup peaches, 1/4 cup tomato sauce, 1/2 cup broccoli, or one potato.[77] Half a cup is not much food. In fact, the men in this study who consumed the most fruits and vegetables consumed as many as nineteen servings a day. If every three servings lower the risk by 22%, the benefits can add up fast (risk reduction approaches but cannot exceed 100%).

This study provides evidence that the health of the arteries and vessels that transport blood to and from your brain is dependent on how well you eat. By extension, it is logical to assume that eating fruits and vegetables will protect against dementia caused by poor vascular health. Research again seems to prove the point. Scientists conducted mental health exams and assessed food intake for over 5,000 older people and monitored their health for over two years. They found that the people who consumed the most total fat and saturated fat had the highest risk of dementia due to vascular problems.[78]

Alzheimer's disease is also related to diet and is often found in conjunction with heart disease,[57] which suggests that they share the same causes. We know what causes heart disease, and we know what offers the best hope of reversing heart disease: diet. Experimental animal studies have convincingly shown that a high-cholesterol diet will promote the production of the beta-amyloid common to Alzheimer's.[57] In confirming these experimental animal results, a study of more than 5,000 people found that greater dietary fat and cholesterol intake tended to increase the risk of Alzheimer's disease specifically,[79] and all dementia in general.[78]

In another study on Alzheimer's,[80] the risk of getting the disease was 3.3 times greater among people whose blood folic acid levels were in the lowest one-third range and 4.5 times greater when blood homocysteine levels were in the highest one-third. What are folic acid and homocysteine? Folic acid is a compound derived exclusively from plant-based foods such as green and leafy vegetables. Homocysteine is an amino acid that is derived primarily from animal protein.[81] This study found that it was desirable to maintain low blood homocysteine and high blood folic acid. In other words, the combination of a diet high in animal-based foods and low in plant-based foods raises the risk of Alzheimer's.[82]

When the first edition of this book was published, the then existing evidence on the causes of Alzheimer's was only suggestive, though it did indicate a causal pathway—and thus solution—similar to that of other Western diseases.

Due to the recent surge in interest in Alzheimer's, about 90% of the available research on Alzheimer's disease has been conducted in the past fifteen years. Much of that has been geared toward better understanding of some basic cellular mechanisms that lead to an entanglement of twisted nerve fibers mostly affecting the memory center of the brain. I must confess that I am not that impressed. This devastating disease is upon us and few, if any, research leads are suggesting how people can avoid it. The only dietary recommendation being advanced is to adhere to a heart-healthy diet, based on the hypothesis that the Western diet causes a buildup of the beta-amyloid protein plaque in the brain the same way cholesterol builds up and causes plaque in our arteries. More specifically, the Alzhemier's Association recommends the Mediterranean and DASH (Dietary Approaches to Stop Hypertension) diets—the latter of which, in particular, is only a very modest improvement compared to the standard American diet. The WFPB diet is much more effective in reversing heart disease than the Mediterranean and DASH diets; the same could be true for Alzheimer's as well.

Mild cognitive impairment, the stuff jokes are made of, still permits the afflicted person to maintain an independent, functional life, but dementia and Alzheimer's are tragic, imposing almost impossibly heavy burdens on victims and their loved ones. Across this spectrum, from minor difficulties in keeping your thoughts in order to serious degeneration, the food you eat can drastically affect the likelihood of mental decline.

The diseases I've covered in this chapter take a heavy toll on most of us in our later years, even though they may not be fatal. Because they are not usually fatal, many people afflicted with these illnesses still live a long life. Their quality of life, however, deteriorates steadily, until the illness renders them largely dependent on others and unable to function in most capacities.

I've talked to so many people who say, "I may not live as long as you health nuts, but I sure am going to enjoy the time I have by eating steaks whenever I want, smoking if I so choose, and doing anything else I want." I grew up with these people. Not long ago, one my best friends suffered a difficult surgery for cancer and spent his last years paralyzed in a nursing home. During the many visits I made to the nursing home, I never failed to come away with a deep appreciation for the health I still possess in my old age. It was not uncommon for me to go to the nursing home to visit my friend and hear that one of the new patients in the home was someone whom my friend and I knew from our earlier days. Too often, they had Alzheimer's and were housed in a special section of the facility.

The enjoyment of life, especially the second half of life, is greatly compromised if we can't see, if we can't think, if our kidneys don't work, or if our bones are broken or fragile. I, for one, hope that I am able to fully enjoy not only the time in the present, but also the time in the future, with good health and independence.

PART III

THE GOOD NUTRITION GUIDE

I was in a restaurant, looking at the menu, when I noticed a very peculiar "low-carb" meal option: a massive plate of pasta topped with vegetables, otherwise known as pasta primavera. The vast majority of calories in the meal clearly came from carbohydrates. How could it be "low-carb"? Was it a misprint? I didn't think so. At various other times I've noted salads, breads, and even cinnamon buns labeled "low-carb," even though their ingredient lists demonstrate that, in fact, the bulk of calories are provided by carbohydrates. What's going on?

This "carb" mania is largely the result of the late Dr. Atkins and his dietary message. Later, *Dr. Atkins' New Diet Revolution* was toppled and replaced by *The South Beach Diet* as the king of the diet books. *The South Beach Diet* is pitched as being more moderate, easier to follow, and safer than Atkins, but from what Tom and I can tell, the weight-loss "wolf" has just put on a different set of sheep's clothing. Both diets are divided into three stages, both severely limit carbohydrate intake during the first phase, and both are heavily based on meat, dairy, and eggs. The South Beach Diet, for example, prohibits bread, rice, potatoes, pasta, baked goods, sugar, and even fruit during the first two weeks. After that, you can be weaned back onto carbohydrates until you are eating what looks like a fairly typical American diet. Perhaps this is why *The South Beach Diet* has been such a hot seller. Before the first edition of *The China Study* was published, *Newsweek* wrote of *South Beach*, "The real value of the book is its sound nutritional advice. It retains the best part of the Atkins regime—meat—while losing the tenet that all carbs should be avoided."[1]

Who at *Newsweek* reviewed the literature to know whether this is sound nutritional advice or not? And if you have the Atkins Diet plus some carbs, how different is this diet from the standard American diet, the toxic diet that has been shown to make us fat, give us heart disease, destroy our kidneys, make us blind, and lead us to Alzheimer's, cancer, and a host of other medical problems?

These are merely examples of the current state of nutrition awareness in the United States. Every day we are reminded that Americans are drowning in a flood of horrible nutrition information. Remember the adage from several decades ago: Americans love hogwash. Another one: Americans love to hear good things about their bad habits. It would appear from a quick glance that these two sayings are true. Or are they?

We have more faith in the average American than that. It's not true that Americans love hogwash—it's that hogwash inundates Americans, whether they want it or not! Some Americans want the truth—they just haven't been able to find it because it is drowned out by hogwash. Very little of the nutrition information that makes it to the public consciousness is soundly based in science, and we pay a grave price. One day olive oil is terrible, the next it is heart healthy. One day eggs will clog your arteries, the next they are a good source of protein. One day potatoes and rice are great, the next they are the gravest threats to your weight you will ever face.

At the beginning of the book we said our goal was to redefine how we think about nutrition information—to eliminate confusion, make health simple, and base our claims on the evidence generated by peer-reviewed nutrition research published in peer-reviewed, professional publications. So far, you have seen a broad sample—and it's only a sample—of that evidence. You have seen that there is overwhelming scientific support for one simple, optimal diet—a whole foods, plant-based diet (WFPB).

We want to condense the nutritional lessons learned from this broad range of evidence and from my forty-plus years of experiences into a simple guide to good nutrition. We have whittled this knowledge down to several core principles, ones that will illuminate how nutrition and health truly operate. Furthermore, we have translated the science into dietary recommendations that you can begin to incorporate into your own life. Not only will you gain a new understanding of nutrition and health, but you will also see exactly which foods you should eat and which foods you should avoid. What you decide to do with this information is up to you, but you can at least know that you, as a reader and a person, have finally been told something other than hogwash.

EATING RIGHT: EIGHT PRINCIPLES OF FOOD AND HEALTH

11

The benefits of a healthy lifestyle are enormous. We want you to know that, based on the information presented in this book, you can increase the odds that you will:

- live longer
- look and feel younger
- have more energy
- lose weight
- lower your blood cholesterol
- prevent and even reverse heart disease
- lower your risk of prostate, breast, and other cancers
- preserve your eyesight in your later years
- prevent and treat diabetes
- avoid surgery in many instances
- vastly decrease the need for pharmaceutical drugs
- keep your bones strong
- avoid impotence
- avoid stroke
- prevent kidney stones
- keep your baby from getting Type 1 diabetes
- alleviate constipation
- lower your blood pressure
- avoid Alzheimer's
- beat arthritis

These are only some of the benefits, and all of them can be yours. The price? Simply changing your diet. It has never been so easy or so relatively effortless to achieve such profound benefits.

We have given you a sampling of the evidence and told you the journey that we have taken to come to our conclusions. Now we want to summarize the lessons about food, health, and disease that we have learned along the way in the following eight principles. These principles should inform the way we do science, the way we treat the sick, the way we feed ourselves, the way we think about health, and the way we perceive the world.

PRINCIPLE #1

Nutrition represents the combined activities of countless food substances. The whole is greater than the sum of its parts.

To illustrate this principle, we need only take you through the biochemical perspective of a meal. Let's say you prepare sautéed spinach with ginger and whole grain ravioli stuffed with butternut squash and spices, topped with a walnut tomato sauce.

The spinach alone is a cornucopia of various chemical components. Chart 11.1 is only a *partial* list of what you might find in your mouth after a bite of spinach.

As you can see, you've just introduced a bundle of nutrients into your body. In addition to this extremely complex mix, when you take a bite of that ravioli with its tomato sauce and squash filling, you get thousands and thousands of additional chemicals, all connected in different ways in each different food—truly a biochemical bonanza.

As soon as this food hits your saliva, your body begins working its magic, and the process of digestion starts. Each of these food chemicals interacts with the other food chemicals and your body's chemicals in very specific ways. It is an infinitely complex process, and it is literally impossible to understand precisely how each chemical interacts with every other chemical. We will never discover exactly how it all fits together.

The main message we're trying to get across is this: the chemicals we get from the foods we eat are engaged in a series of reactions that work in concert to produce good health. These chemicals are carefully orchestrated by intricate controls within our cells and all through our bodies, and these controls decide what nutrient goes where, how much of each nutrient is needed, and when each reaction takes place. This is nature at work.

Chart 11.1: Nutrients in Spinach

Macronutrients	
Water	Fat (many kinds)
Calories	Carbohydrate
Protein (many kinds)	Fiber
Minerals	
Calcium	Sodium
Iron	Zinc
Magnesium	Copper
Phosphorus	Manganese
Potassium	Selenium
Vitamins	
C (Ascorbic Acid)	B-6 (Pyridoxine)
B-1 (Thiamin)	Folate
B-2 (Riboflavin)	A (as carotenoids)
B-3 (Niacin)	E (tocopherols)
Pantothenic acid	
Fatty Acids	
14:0 (Myristic acid)	18:1 (Oleic acid)
16:0 (Palmitic acid)	20:1 (Eicosenoic acid)
18:0 (Stearic acid)	18:2 (Linoleic acid)
16:1 (Palmitoleic acid)	18:3 (Linoleic acid)
Amino Acids	
Tryptophan	Valine
Threonine	Arginine
Isoleucine	Histidine
Leucine	Alanine
Lysine	Aspartic acid
Methionine	Glutamic acid
Cystine	Glycine
Phenylalanine	Proline
Tyrosine	Serine
Phytosterols (many kinds)	

Our bodies have evolved with this infinitely complex network of reactions in order to derive maximal benefit from whole foods, as they appear in nature. The misguided may trumpet the virtues of one specific nutrient or chemical, but this thinking is too simplistic. Our bodies have learned how to benefit from the chemicals in food as they are packaged together, discarding some and using others as they see fit. We cannot stress this enough, as it is the foundation of understanding what good nutrition means.

PRINCIPLE #2

Dietary supplements are not a panacea for good health.

First, let us define what we mean by a "dietary supplement." The FDA states that a dietary supplement, taken orally, may be a "tablet, capsule, soft-gel, gelcap, liquid, or powders."[1] It may include vitamins, minerals, herbs or other botanicals, amino acids and/or concentrates, metabolites, constituents, or extracts. This definition is very broad. When we use "dietary supplement" here, we mean products composed of nutrients (vitamins, minerals, amino acids), and not necessarily herbal and other similar products, which may consist of complex concentrates of whole foods (e.g., in China, watermelon is an herb!).

Because nutrition operates as an infinitely complex biochemical system involving thousands of chemicals and thousands of effects on your health, it makes little or no sense that isolated nutrients taken as supplements can substitute for whole foods. Supplements will not lead to long-lasting health and may cause unforeseen side effects. Furthermore, for those relying on supplements, beneficial and sustained diet change is postponed. The dangers of a Western diet cannot be overcome by consuming nutrient pills.

I have followed the development of the nutrient supplements business from its modern beginning during the mid-1980s, since which time it has become a $32-billion-a-year industry.[2] Two pieces of congressional legislation set the table for this explosion. The first was the 1976 Proxmire Amendment to the government's official food and drug regulations that allowed the industry to sell nutrient supplements without a doctor's prescription. The second was the 1994 Dietary Supplement Health and Education Act (DSHEA),[3] which established standards for these products, thus adding some marketplace credibility. In the interim, the industry also got a huge scientific boost from the highly publicized 1982 National Academy of Sciences report on diet, nutrition, and cancer that I co-authored, although that boost was unintended. We recommended increased consumption of fruits, vegetables, and whole grains because they contained certain beneficial nutrients, but we also explicitly said that this was not to be interpreted as a recommendation to use isolated nutrients in dietary supplements. The industry aggressively argued otherwise, and pushed on, in spite of a decision by the U.S. Federal Trade Commission that their health claims were deemed inappropriate.[4] This aggressive behavior eventually paid off in what must be one of the biggest health hoaxes of all time: the nutrient supplement industry.

It's abundantly clear to us why this massive industry has emerged. Huge profits are an excellent incentive. Furthermore, consumers want to continue eating their customary foods, and popping a few supplements makes people feel better about the potentially adverse health effects their diet causes. Embracing supplements means the media can tell people what they want to hear, and doctors have something to offer their patients. As a result, a multibillion-dollar supplement industry is now part of our nutritional landscape, and the majority of consumers have been duped into believing that they are buying health. This was the late Dr. Atkins' formula. He advocated a high-protein, high-fat diet—sacrificing long-term health for short-term gain (his followers', but especially his own)—and then advocated taking his supplements to address what he called, in his own words, the "common dieters' problems" including constipation, sugar cravings, hunger, fluid retention, fatigue, nervousness, and insomnia.[5]

This strategy of gaining and maintaining health with nutrient supplements, however, started to unravel in 1994–1996 with the large-scale investigation of the effects of supplemental beta-carotene (a precursor to vitamin A) on lung cancer and other diseases.[6,7] After four to eight years of supplement use, patients' lung cancer had not decreased as expected; it had increased! No benefit was found from vitamins A and E for the prevention of heart disease, either.

Since then, numerous additional trials costing hundreds of millions of dollars have been conducted to determine if vitamins A, C, and E prevent heart disease and cancer. Two major reviews of these trials were published shortly before the first edition of *The China Study*.[8,9] The researchers, in their words, "could not determine the balance of benefits and harms of routine use of supplements of vitamins A, C or E; multivitamins with folic acid; or antioxidant combinations for the prevention of cancer or cardiovascular disease."[8] Indeed, they even recommended against the use of beta-carotene supplements.

In the decade since this book was first published, the main science-based findings have agreed: supplements are overrated, with little or no redeeming value.

It is not that all these nutrients aren't important. They are—but only when consumed as food, not as supplements. Isolating nutrients and trying to get benefits equal to those of whole foods reveals an ignorance of how nutrition operates in the body. A 2003 special article in the *New York Times*[10] documents this failure of nutrient supplements to provide any proven health benefit. We are confident that as time passes, we will continue to "discover" that relying on the use of isolated nutrient supplements to maintain health, while consuming the usual Western diet, is not only a waste of money but is also potentially dangerous.

There are, however, two possible exceptions to this. The first is vitamin B_{12}. Many clinicians have been advocating regular vitamin B_{12} for individuals consuming the WFPB diet, which does not contain this vitamin. A variety of hematologic and neurologic symptoms attributed to B_{12} deficiency have been noted and they are readily treated by supplementation.[11]

It is difficult to make firm quantitative recommendations on B_{12} needs given the current state of research. However, there is no evidence that B_{12} supplementation causes adverse health effects, and clinicians have found that B_{12} administration resolves apparent B_{12} deficiency symptoms. Thus it makes common sense that regular B_{12} supplementation should be encouraged. (See more on B_{12} in the next section.)

The second possible exception is vitamin D, though a similar incomplete story exists here. Vitamin D is not a vitamin. It is not a nutrient that we need to consume. Instead, it is a hormone—our bodies *can* make it, when we get enough sunlight exposure. The amount of sunlight generally considered necessary is only fifteen to thirty minutes per day, though admittedly, this can be problematic in the northern climates (where there is much less daylight during the winter months), especially for children who fail to go outdoors. The original research on vitamin D showed that a deficiency was associated with rickets in children, although since then it has been shown to be critically involved in several other aspects of health.

In spite of the media attention that vitamin D has received in recent years, the scientific literature supporting supplementation is not as impressive as one might think. A highly reputable research task force[12] recently concluded, based on a survey of the research literature, that little or no benefit for bone fracture risk was obtained when marginally D-deficient people were treated with vitamin D (although they urged that more research was needed). Another task force report on vitamin D questioned its benefits, reporting that there is, at the moment, no firm evidence that vitamin D supplementation increases or decreases cancer risk.[13]

Whether someone has enough vitamin D is assessed by measuring the 25-hydroxyvitamin D metabolite (calcidiol) stored in the liver. This is not the most active metabolite involved in vitamin D function; that would be the metabolite 1,25-dihydroxyvitamin D (calcitriol), derived from the metabolism of calcidiol. Calcitriol is, according to some estimates,[14] about three orders of magnitude (1000×) more potent than calcidiol, and the body decides how much of this powerful hormone to produce as needed on a microsecond by microsecond basis. Furthermore, it is questionable to assume that the amount of vitamin D you have in reserve relates to functionality. When your "natural gas tank" is only 20% full, does this slow down the flame at the stovetop? The flame can be equally robust until the amount in the tank is virtually gone. Even when stored D (calcidiol) is relatively low, the body should still be able to produce the amount of calcitriol it needs for healthy function.

There are still cases of rickets and osteomalacia (softening of the bones)—in which vitamin D deficiency is so great that bone growth and maintenance becomes dysfunctional—in North America. This illustrates that, for at least a small number of people, the consequences of vitamin D deficiency are very real. Risk is determined by several factors, including location, lifestyle, skin color, and clothing choices. For those at risk, small daily doses of vitamin D can prevent frank deficiency. Too much vitamin D, however, can be toxic, so please consult your doctor before beginning supplementation on your own.

PRINCIPLE #3

There are virtually no nutrients in animal-based foods that are not better provided by plants.

Overall, it is fair to say that any plant-based food has many more similarities in terms of nutrient composition to other plant-based foods than it does to animal-based foods. The same is true the other way around; all animal-based foods are more like other animal-based foods than they are to plant-based foods. For example, even though fish is significantly different from beef, fish has many more similarities to beef than it has to rice. Even the foods that are "exceptions" to these rules, such as nuts, seeds, and processed low-fat animal products, remain in distinct plant and animal "nutrient" groups.

Eating animals is a markedly different nutritional experience from eating plants. The amounts and kinds of nutrients in these two types of foods, shown in Chart 11.2,[6,15–17] illustrate these striking nutritional differences.

As you can see, plant foods have dramatically more antioxidants, fiber, vitamins, and minerals than animal foods. In fact, animal foods are almost completely devoid of several of these nutrients—but they have much more cholesterol and fat. They also have slightly more protein than plant foods,

Chart 11.2: Nutrient Composition of Plant- and Animal-Based Foods (Per 500 Calories of Energy)

Nutrient	Plant-Based Foods*	Animal-Based Foods
Cholesterol (mg)	—	137
Fat (g)	4	36
Protein (g)	33	34
Beta-carotene (mcg)	29,919	17
Dietary Fiber (mg)	31	—
Vitamin C (mg)	293	4
Folate (mcg)	1,168	19
Vitamin E (mg_ATE)	11	0.5
Iron (mg)	20	2
Magnesium (mg)	548	51
Calcium (mg)	545	252

* Equal parts of tomatoes, spinach, lima beans, peas, and potatoes
** Equal parts of beef, pork, chicken, and whole milk

along with more B_{12} and vitamin D, although the vitamin D is largely added to milk. Of course, there are some exceptions: some nuts and seeds are high in fat and protein (e.g., peanuts, sesame seeds), while some animal-based foods are low in fat, usually because it is stripped by artificial processing (e.g., skim milk). But if one looks a little more closely, the fat and the protein of nuts and seeds are different: they are more healthful than the fat and protein of animal foods. They also are accompanied by some interesting antioxidant substances. On the other hand, processed, low-fat, animal-based foods still have some cholesterol, lots of protein, and very little or no antioxidants and dietary fiber, just like other animal-based foods. Because nutrients are primarily responsible for the healthful effects of foods, and because of these major differences in nutrient composition between animal- and plant-based foods, isn't it therefore reasonable to assume that we should expect to see distinctly different effects on our bodies depending on which variety of foods we consume?

By definition, for a food chemical to be an essential nutrient, it must meet two requirements:

- the chemical is necessary for healthy human functioning
- the chemical must be something our bodies cannot make on their own, and therefore must be obtained from an outside source

One example of a chemical that is not essential is cholesterol, a component of animal-based food that is nonexistent in plant-based food. While cholesterol is essential for health, our bodies can make all that we require; we do not need to consume any in food. Therefore, it is not an essential nutrient.

There are four "nutrients" that animal-based foods have that plant-based foods, for the most part, do not: cholesterol and vitamins A, D, and B_{12}. Three of these are nonessential nutrients. Cholesterol our bodies make naturally. Vitamin A our bodies can readily make from beta-carotene, and vitamin D we produce simply by exposing our skin to about fifteen minutes of sunshine every couple of days. Both of these vitamins are toxic if they are consumed in high amounts. This is one more indication that it is better to rely on the vitamin precursors, beta-carotene and sunshine, so that our bodies can readily control the timing and quantities of vitamins A and D that are needed.

As discussed in Principle #2, Vitamin B_{12} is more problematic. Vitamin B_{12} is made by microorganisms found in soil and the intestines of animals, including our own. The amount made in our intestines is not adequately absorbed, so it is recommended that we consume B_{12} in food. Research has shown that plants grown in healthy soil that has a good concentration of vitamin B_{12} will absorb this nutrient.[18] However, in the United States, plants are not a reliable source of B_{12}. We live in such a sanitized world that we rarely come into direct contact with the soil-borne microorganisms that produce B_{12}. At one point in our history, we may have gotten some B_{12} from vegetables that hadn't been scoured of all soil, in addition to any animal food we consumed. Therefore, it is a good assumption that modern Americans who eat highly cleansed plant products and no animal products will not get enough vitamin B_{12}.

Though our society's obsession with nutrient supplements seriously detracts from other, far more important nutrition information, this is not to say that supplements should always be avoided. It is estimated that we hold a three-year store of vitamin B_{12} in our bodies. If you do not eat any animal products, particularly if you are pregnant or breastfeeding, you should take a small B_{12} supplement regularly and consider getting tested for B_{12} levels. If they are on the low side, consider getting confirmatory tests for methylmalonic acid and homocysteine, which are considered to be better indicators of vitamin adequacy, as well. Likewise, if you never get sun exposure, especially during the winter months, you might wish to take a vitamin D supplement and make more of an effort to get outside.

PRINCIPLE #4

Genes do not determine disease on their own. Genes function only by being activated, or "expressed," and nutrition plays a critical role in determining which genes, good and bad, are expressed. We can safely say that the origin of every single disease is genetic. Our genes are the code for everything in our bodies, good and bad. Without genes, there would be no cancer. Without genes, there would be no obesity, diabetes, or heart disease. And without genes, there would be no life.

This might explain why we are spending hundreds of millions of dollars trying to figure out which gene causes which disease and how we can silence the dangerous genes. This also explains why some perfectly healthy young women have had their breasts removed simply because they were found to carry genes that are linked to breast cancer. This further explains why the bulk of resources in science and health in the past decade has shifted to genetic research. At Cornell University alone $500 million is being raised to create a "Life Sciences Initiative." This initiative promises to "forever change the way life-science research is conducted and taught at the university." What is one of the main thrusts of the program? Integrating each scientific discipline into the all-encompassing umbrella of genetic research. It is the largest scientific effort in Cornell's history.[19]

Much of this focus on genes, however, misses a simple but crucial point: not all genes are fully expressed all the time. If they aren't expressed, they remain biochemically dormant. Dormant genes do not have any effect on our health. This idea is obvious to most scientists and many laypeople, but its significance is seldom understood. What causes some genes to remain dormant, and others to express themselves? The answer: environment, especially diet.

To reuse a previous analogy, it is useful to think of genes as seeds. As any good gardener knows, seeds will not grow into plants unless they have nutrient-rich soil, water, and sunshine. Neither will genes be expressed unless they have the proper environment. In our body, nutrition is the environmental factor that determines the activity of genes. As we saw in chapter three, the genes that cause cancer were profoundly affected by the consumption of protein. In Colin's research group, they learned that they could turn the bad genes on and off simply by adjusting animal protein intake.

Furthermore, the China research findings showed that people of roughly the same ethnic background have hugely varying disease rates. Described by some observers as having similar genes, still they get different diseases depending on their environment. Dozens of studies have documented that as people migrate, they assume the disease risk of the country to which they move. They do not change their genes, and yet they fall prey to diseases and illnesses at rates that are rare in their homeland population. (We refer to what others say about the Chinese having "similar genes" in deference to these "others"; we do not agree with this assessment. We believe that gene variance among the Chinese is as great as among any other ethnic group, although we are not aware whether this has been scientifically demonstrated. The main point, however, is still the same—migrants incur diseases of the country to which they move, without changing their genes, however much those genes may vary within the migratory population itself.)

Furthermore, we have seen disease rates change over time so drastically that it is biologically impossible to put the blame on genes. In twenty-five years, the percentage of our population that is overweight or obese has doubled, from 15% to 30%. In addition, diabetes, heart disease, and many other diseases of affluence were rare until the most recent century, and our genetic code simply could not have changed significantly in the past 25, 100, or even 500 years.

So while we can say that genes are crucial to every biological process, we have some very convincing evidence that gene expression is far more important, and gene expression is controlled by environment, especially nutrition.

A further folly of this genetic research is assuming that understanding our genes is simple. It is not. Researchers reported in 2003 their studies of genetic regulation of weight in a tiny worm species.[20] The scientists went through 16,757 genes, turning each one off, and observed the effect on weight. They discovered 417 genes that affect weight. How these hundreds of genes interact over the long term with one another and their ever-changing environment to alter weight gain or loss is an incredibly complex mystery. Goethe once said, "We know accurately only when we know little; with knowledge doubt increases."[21]

Expression of our genetic code represents a universe of biochemical interactions of almost infinite complexity. This biochemical "universe" interacts with many different systems, including nutrition, which itself represents whole systems of complex biochemistry. With genetic research, we suspect we are embarking on a massive quest to shortcut nature only to end up worse off than when we started.

Does all this mean we think that genes don't matter? Of course not. If you take two Americans living in the same environment and feed them exactly the same meaty food every day for their entire lives, it would not be surprising if one died of a heart attack at age fifty-four and the other died of cancer at the age of eighty. What explains the difference? Genes. Genes give us our predispositions. We all have different disease risks due to our different genes. But while we will never know every risk to which we are predisposed, we do know how to control those risks. Regardless of our genes, we can all optimize our chances of expressing the right genes by providing our bodies with the best possible environment—that is, the best possible nutrition. Even though the two Americans in our example succumbed to different diseases at different ages, it is entirely possible that both could have lived many more years with a higher quality of life if they had practiced optimal nutrition.

PRINCIPLE #5

Nutrition can substantially control the adverse effects of noxious chemicals.

Stories of cancer-causing chemicals regularly appear in the press. Acrylamide, artificial sweeteners, nitrosamines, nitrites, Alar, heterocyclic amines, and aflatoxin have all been linked to cancer in experimental studies.

There is a widely held perception that cancer is caused by toxic chemicals that make their way into our bodies in a sinister way. For example, people often cite health concerns to justify their opposition to pumping antibiotics and hormones into farm animals. The assumption is that the meat would be safe to eat if it didn't have those unnatural chemicals in it. The real danger of the meat, however, is the nutrient imbalances, regardless of the presence or absence of those nasty chemicals. Long before modern chemicals were introduced into our food, people still began to experience more cancer and more heart disease when they started to eat more animal-based foods.

A great example of a misunderstood "public health concern" regarding chemicals is the lengthy, $30 million investigation of minimally higher rates of breast cancer in Long Island, New York, referred to in chapter eight. Here, it seemed that chemical contaminants from certain industrial sites were causing breast cancer in women living nearby. But this ill-conceived story has proven to have no merit.

Another chemical carcinogen concern surrounds acrylamide, which is primarily found in processed or fried foods like potato chips. The implication is that if we could effectively remove this chemical from potato chips, they would be safe to eat, even though they continue to be highly unhealthy, processed slices of potatoes drenched with fat and salt.

So many of us seem to want a scapegoat. We do not want to hear that our favorite foods are a problem simply because of their nutritional content.

In chapter three, we saw that the potential effects of aflatoxin, a chemical touted as being highly carcinogenic, could be entirely controlled by nutrition. Even with large doses of aflatoxin, rats could be healthy, active, and cancer-free if they were fed low-protein diets. We also saw how small findings can make big news every time cancer is mentioned. For example, if experimental animals have an increased incidence of cancer after gargantuan exposures, the chemical agent is trumpeted as a cause of cancer, as was the case for NSAR (see chapter three) and nitrites. However, like genes, the activities of these chemical carcinogens are primarily controlled by the nutrients that we eat.

So what do these examples tell us? In practical terms, you aren't doing yourself much good by eating organic beef instead of conventional beef that's been pumped full of chemicals. The organic beef might be marginally healthier, but we would never say that it was a safe choice. Both types of beef have a similar nutrient profile.

It is useful to think of this principle in another way: a chronic disease like cancer takes years to develop. Those chemicals that initiate cancer are often the ones that make headlines. What does not make headlines, however, is the fact that the disease process continues long after initiation, and can be accelerated or repressed during its promotion stage by nutrition. In other words, nutrition primarily determines whether the disease will ever do its damage.

PRINCIPLE #6

The same nutrition that prevents disease in its early stages (before diagnosis) can also halt or reverse disease in its later stages (after diagnosis).

It is worth repeating that chronic diseases take several years to develop. For example, it is generally thought that breast cancer can be initiated in adolescence and not become detectable until after menopause! *So we very well may have lots of middle-aged women walking around with breast cancer initiated during their teens that will not be detectable until after menopause.*[22] For many people this translates into the fatalistic notion that little can be done later in life. Does this mean that these women should start smoking and eating more chicken-fried steak because they're doomed anyway? What do we do, given that many of us may already have an initiated chronic disease lurking in our bodies, waiting to explode decades from now?

As we saw in chapter three, cancer that is already initiated and growing in experimental animals can be slowed, halted, or even reversed by good nutrition. Luckily for us, *the same good nutrition maximizes health at every stage of a disease*. In humans, we have seen research findings showing that a WFPB diet reverses advanced heart disease, helps obese people lose weight, and helps diabetics get off their medication and return to a more normal, pre-diabetes life. Research has also shown that early-stage prostate cancer may be attenuated or reversed by lifestyle changes.[23]

Some diseases, of course, appear to be irreversible. The autoimmune diseases are perhaps most frightening because once the body turns against itself, they may become unstoppable. And yet, amazingly, even some of these diseases may be slowed or attenuated by diet. Recall the research showing that even Type 1 diabetics can lower their medication requirements by eating the right food. Evidence also shows that rheumatoid arthritis can be slowed by diet,[24] as can multiple sclerosis.[25,26]

We believe that an ounce of prevention does equal a pound of cure, and the earlier in life good foods are eaten, the better one's health will be. But for those who already face the burden of disease, we must not forget that nutrition still can play a vital role.

PRINCIPLE #7

Nutrition that is truly beneficial for one chronic disease will support health across the board.

When I was trying to get the first edition of this book published, I had a meeting with an editor at a major publishing house, and described to her my intent to create disease-specific chapters that related diet to particular ailments or groups of ailments. The editor asked, in effect, "Can you make specific diet plans for each disease, so that every chapter doesn't have the same recommendations?" In other words, could I tell people to eat a specific way for heart disease and a different way for diabetes? The implication, of course, was that the same eating plan for multiple diseases simply wasn't catchy enough, wasn't sufficiently "marketable."

Although this might be good marketing, it is not good science. As I have come to understand more about the biochemical processes of various diseases, I have also come to see how these diseases have much in common. Because of these impressive commonalities, it only makes sense that the same good nutrition will generate health and prevent diseases *across the board*. Even if a WFPB diet is more effective at treating heart disease than brain cancer, you can be sure that this diet will not promote one disease while it stops another. It will never be "bad" for you. This one good diet can only help across the board.

So I'm afraid Tom and I don't have a different, catchy formula for each disease—just a single dietary prescription. But rather than be forlorn about its effect on book sales, we'd prefer to remain excited about telling you how simple food and health really is. It is a chance to clear away much of the incredible public confusion. *Quite simply, you can maximize health for diseases across the board with one simple diet.*

PRINCIPLE #8

Good nutrition creates health in all areas of our existence. All parts are interconnected.

Much has been made of "holistic" health in recent times. This concept can mean a variety of things to different people. Many people lump all of the "alternative" medicines and activities into this concept, so holistic health comes to mean acupressure, acupuncture, herbal medicines, meditation, vitamin supplements, chiropractic care, yoga, aromatherapy, feng shui, massage, and even sound therapy.

Conceptually, Tom and I believe in holistic health, but not as a catch-phrase for every unconventional and oftentimes unproven medicine around. Food and nutrition, for example, are of primary importance to our health. The process of eating is perhaps the most intimate encounter we have with our world: what we eat becomes part of our body. But other experiences also are important, such as physical activity, emotional and mental health, and the well-being of our environment. Incorporating these various spheres into our concept of health is important because they are all interconnected. Indeed, this is a holistic concept.

These expanding interconnections became apparent to me through animal experimentation. Rats fed low-protein diets were not only spared liver cancer, but also had lower blood cholesterol and noticeably more energy, and voluntarily exercised twice as much as the high-protein rats. The evidence regarding increased energy levels has been supported by an enormous amount of anecdotal evidence I have encountered over the years: people have more energy when they eat well. This synergy between nutrition and physical activity is extremely important, and is evidence that these two parts of life are not isolated from each other. Good nutrition and regular exercise combine to offer more health per person than the sum of each part alone.

We also know that physical activity has an effect on emotional and mental well-being. Much has been said about the effect physical activity has on various chemicals in our bodies, which in turn affects our moods and our concentration.[27] And experiencing the rewards of feeling better emotionally and being more mentally alert provides the confidence and motivation to treat ourselves to optimal nutrition, which reinforces the entire cycle. Those who feel good about themselves are more likely to respect their health by practicing good nutrition.

Sometimes people try to play these different parts of their lives against each other. People wonder if they can erase bad eating habits by being a runner. The answer to this is no. The benefits and risks of diet are crucially important, and more sizable, than the benefits and risks of other activities. Besides, why would anyone want to try and balance benefits and risks when they could have all the benefits working together? People also wonder whether a perceived health benefit is because of the exercise or because of a good diet. In the end, that's simply an academic question. The fact is that these two spheres of our lives are intimately interconnected, and what's important is that *it all works together to promote or derail health.*

Furthermore, it turns out that if we eat the way that promotes the best health for ourselves, we promote the best health for the planet. By eating a WFPB diet, we use less water, less land, and fewer resources, produce less pollution, and inflict less suffering on our farm animals. John Robbins has done more than any other person to bring this issue to the front of American consciousness, and we strongly recommend reading his 2010 book, *The Food Revolution.*

Our food choices have an incredible impact not only on our metabolism, but also on the initiation, promotion, and even reversal of disease; on our energy; on our physical activity; on our emotional and mental well-being; and on our world environment. *All of these seemingly separate spheres are intimately interconnected.*

We have mentioned the wisdom of nature at various points in this book, and we have come to see the power of the natural world's workings. It is a wondrous web of health, from molecules, to people, to other animals, to forests, to oceans, to the air we breathe. This is nature at work, from the microscopic to the macroscopic.

WHOLE AND WHOLISM

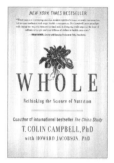

Principle #8 is central to the main theme of my 2013 book, *Whole: Rethinking the Science of Nutrition*, written with Howard Jacobson.[28] I found I was not satisfied with writing just these few words in the first edition of this book as to why and how metabolic events work together the way they obviously do, and wanted to delve further into this question, as well as the related question of why people haven't heard this information about nutrition before.

I did not especially like the common spelling of *holism* for that "working together" concept. Instead I prefer *wholism* (as opposed to *reductionism*). It is not clear how or when historically the very sensible concept of wholeness lost its "w," but in my world of science, holism is anathema, for it conveys a view that gaining knowledge is faith-based or irrational rather than a matter of collecting and describing a set of observations as "facts" that have shape and logical form.

The best biological illustration of this concept of wholism is the indescribably vast universe of coordinated events, activities, and components of the cell, sometimes referred to as the basic unit of biology. We have between 10 and 100 trillion cells in our bodies, each drawing on the same genetic blueprint to do its special thing. The cell's complexity, both in space and time, like a micro-universe, is infinite, and we only see more of that same complexity all the way up the ladder of life and to the far reaches of the universe.

WHO CARES, ANYWAY?

The principles outlined here began, for Colin, with a narrowly focused question on diet and cancer in rats, then expanded into a universe of questions about human and societal health around the world. In large measure, these principles are his attempt to answer the far-reaching questions that he was forced to ask during his career.

The applicability of these principles should not be underestimated. Most importantly, they can help to reduce public confusion regarding food and health. The latest fads, the newest headlines, and the most recent study results are put into a useful context. We need not leap from our seats every time a chemical is called a carcinogen, every time a new diet book hits the shelf, or every time a headline screams about solving disease through genetic research.

Simply put, we can relax. We can take a much-needed deep breath and sit back. Moreover, we can do science more intelligently, and ask better questions, because we have a sound framework relating nutrition to health. In effect, we can interpret new findings with a broader context in mind. With these newly interpreted findings, we can enrich or modify our original framework and invest our money and resources where they matter to increase our society's health. The benefits of understanding these principles are wide ranging and profound for individuals, societies, our fellow animals, and our planet.

HOW TO EAT

When Tom, my youngest son and collaborator on this book, was thirteen years old, our family was in the final stages of a slow shift to becoming vegetarian. One Sunday morning, Tom came home from a sleepover at a close friend's house and told us a memorable story.

The night before, Tom was being grilled, in a friendly way, on his eating habits. The sister of Tom's friend had asked him, rather incredulously, "You don't eat meat?" He had never justified his eating habits; he had just gotten used to eating what was on the dinner table. As a consequence, Tom was not practiced at answering such a question. So he simply answered, "No, I don't," without offering any explanations.

The girl probed a bit more. "So what do you eat?" Tom answered, with a few shrugs, "I guess just . . . plants." She said, "Oh," and that was the end of that.

The reason we enjoy this story is because Tom's response, "plants," was so simple. It was a truthful answer, but couched in an entirely untraditional manner. When someone asks for the glazed ham across the table, she doesn't say, "Pass the flesh of the pig's butt, please," and when someone tells his children to finish their peas and carrots, he doesn't say, "Finish your plants." But since our family changed its eating habits, we've come to enjoy thinking of food as either plants or animals. It fits well into the philosophy of keeping the information on food and health as simple as possible.

Food and health are anything but simple in our country. We often marvel at the complexity of various weight-loss plans. Although the writers always advertise their plan's ease of use, in reality it's never easy. Followers of these diets have to count calories, points, servings, or nutrients or eat specific amounts of certain foods based on specific, mathematical ratios. There are tools to be used, supplements to be taken, and worksheets to be completed. It is no wonder that dieting seldom succeeds.

Eating should be an enjoyable and worry-free experience, and shouldn't rely on deprivation. Keeping it simple is essential if we are to enjoy our food.

One of the most fortunate findings from the mountain of nutritional research we've encountered is that good food and good health is simple. The biology of the relationship of food and health is exceptionally complex, but the message is still simple. The recommendations coming from the published literature are so simple that we can state them in one sentence: eat a whole foods, plant-based diet, while minimizing the consumption of refined foods, added salt, and added fats. (See table on the next page.)

SUPPLEMENTS

Daily supplements of vitamin B_{12}, and perhaps vitamin D for people who spend most of their time indoors and/or live in the northern climates, are encouraged. For vitamin D, you shouldn't exceed RDA recommendations.

That's it. That's the diet science has found to be consistent with the greatest health and the lowest incidence of heart disease, cancer, obesity, and many other Western diseases.

What Does Minimize Mean? Should You Eliminate Meat Completely?

The findings from the China Study indicate that the lower the percentage of animal-based foods that are consumed, the greater the health benefits—even when that percentage declines from 10% to 0% of calories. So it's not unreasonable to assume that the optimum percentage of animal-based products is zero, at least for anyone with a predisposition for a degenerative disease.

But this has not been absolutely proven. It is true that most of the health benefits described in this book have been realized at low but non-zero levels of animal-based foods.

My advice is to try to eliminate all animal-based products from your diet, but not obsess over it. If a tasty vegetable soup has a chicken stock base, or if a hearty loaf of whole wheat bread includes a tiny amount of egg, don't worry about it. These quantities, very likely, are nutritionally unimportant. Even more importantly, the ability to relax about very minor quantities of animal-based foods makes applying this diet much easier—especially when eating out or buying already-prepared foods.

While we recommend that you not worry about small quantities of animal products in your food, we are not suggesting that you deliberately plan to incorporate small portions of meat into your daily diet. My recommendation is that you try to avoid all animal-based products.

Eat All You Want (While Getting Lots of Variety) of Any Whole, Unrefined, Plant-Based Food

General Category	Specific Examples
Fruits	orange, okra, kiwi, red pepper, apple, cucumber, tomato, avocado, zucchini, blueberries, strawberries, green pepper, raspberries, butternut squash, pumpkin, blackberries, mangoes, eggplant, pear, watermelon, cranberries, acorn squash, papaya, grapefruit, peach
Vegetables	
Flowers	broccoli, cauliflower (not many of the huge variety of edible flowers are commonly eaten)
Stems and Leaves	spinach, artichokes, kale, lettuce (all varieties), cabbage, Swiss chard, collard greens, celery, asparagus, mustard greens, Brussels sprouts, turnip greens, beet greens, bok choi, arugula, Belgian endive, basil, cilantro, parsley, rhubarb, seaweed
Roots	potatoes (all varieties), beets, carrots, turnips, onions, garlic, ginger, leeks, pinto beans, white beans
Legumes (seed-bearing nitrogen-fixing plants)	green beans, soybeans, peas, peanuts, adzuki beans, black beans, black-eye peas, cannellini beans, garbanzo beans, kidney beans, lentils, pinto beans, white beans
Mushrooms	white button, baby bella, cremini, Portobello, shiitake, oyster
Nuts	walnuts, almonds, macadamia, pecans, cashew, hazelnut, pistachio
Whole grains (in breads, pastas, etc.)	wheat, rice, corn, millet, sorghum, rye, oats, barley, teff, buckwheat, amaranth, quinoa, kamut, spelt
Minimize	
Refined carbohydrates	pastas (except whole grain varieties), white bread, crackers, sugars, and most cakes and pastries
Added vegetable oils	corn oil, peanut oil, olive oil
Fish	salmon, tuna, cod
Avoid	
Meat	steak, hamburger, lard
Poultry	chicken, turkey
Dairy	cheese, milk, yogurt
Eggs	eggs and products with a high egg content (i.e., mayonnaise)

There are three excellent reasons to go all the way. First, following this diet requires a radical shift in your thinking about food. It's more work to just do it halfway. If you plan for animal-based products, you'll eat them—and you'll almost certainly eat more than you should. Second, you'll feel deprived. Instead of viewing your new food habit as being able to eat all the plant-based food you want, you'll be seeing it in terms of having to limit yourself, which is not conducive to staying on the diet long-term. And third, you will, within a month or so, perhaps a little more, actually break the physiological addiction that we acquire from eating large amounts of fat and refined carbohydrates. If your friend had been a smoker all of his or her life and looked to you for advice, would you tell them to cut down to only two cigarettes a day, or would you tell them to quit smoking altogether? It's in this way that we're telling you that moderation, even with the best intentions, sometimes makes it more difficult to succeed.

CAN YOU DO THIS?

For most Americans, the idea of giving up virtually all meat products—including beef, chicken, fish, cheese, milk, and eggs—seems impossible. You might as well ask Americans to stop breathing. The whole idea seems strange, fanatical, or fantastic.

This is the biggest obstacle to the adoption of a plant-based diet: most people who hear about it don't seriously consider it, despite the truly impressive health benefits.

If you are one of these people—if you are curious about these findings but know in your heart that you will never be able to give up meat—then no amount of talk will ever convince you to change your mind.

You have to try it and see it for yourself.

Give it one month. You've been eating cheeseburgers your whole life; a month without them won't kill you.

A month isn't enough time to give you any long-term benefits, but it is long enough for you to discover four things:

1. There are some great foods you can eat in a plant-based diet that you otherwise may never have discovered. You may not be eating everything you want (desire for meat may last longer than a month), but you will be eating lots of great, delicious foods.
2. It's not all that bad. Some people take to this diet quite quickly and love it. Many take months to fully adjust to it, at which point they

often discover some new tastes. But almost everyone will find that it's a lot easier than they thought.

3. You'll feel better. Even after only a month, most people will feel better and likely lose some weight, too. Try having your blood work done both before and after. Odds are, you'll see significant improvement in even that period of time if you've been eating the standard American diet. (Since we made the one-month recommendation in the first edition of this book, several groups have organized relatively formal opportunities to use the diet for periods of 7–10 days only, with blood work done before and after. My eldest son, Nelson, and his consulting physician have done it six times, for groups as large as 130 people. Depending on what diet and numbers people begin with, it is possible to see total cholesterol drop by 100 points or more, LDL cholesterol by 50–75 points, and body weight by 5–10 pounds in as few as seven days. Also, blood pressure generally decreases more than with antihypertensive drugs.)

4. Most important, you'll discover that it's possible. You may love the diet, or you may not, but at the very least you'll come away from your one-week or one-month trial knowing that it's possible. *You can do it, if you choose to.* All the health benefits discussed in this book are not just for Tibetan monks and fanatical Spartans. You can have them, too. It's your choice.

The first month can be challenging (more on this shortly), but it gets much easier after that. And for many, it becomes a great pleasure.

We know this is hard to believe until you experience it for yourself, but your tastes change when you are on a plant-based diet. You not only lose your taste for meat, you begin to discover new flavors in much of your food, flavors that were dulled when you ate a primarily animal-based, sugar-and-fat-laced diet. A friend once described it as like being dragged to an independent film when you wanted to go to the latest Hollywood action flick. You go in muttering, but you discover, to your surprise, that the film is great—and much more fulfilling than the "shoot 'em up" movie would have been.

THE TRANSITION

If you take us up on our suggestion to try a plant-based diet for one month, you'll likely face five main challenges:

- In the first week, you may have some stomach upset as your digestive system adjusts. This is natural; it is nothing to worry about and doesn't usually last long.
- You'll need to put some time into this. Don't begrudge this time—heart disease and cancer take time, too. Specifically, you'll need to learn some new recipes, be willing to try new dishes, and discover new restaurants. You'll need to pay attention to your tastes and come up with meals that you really enjoy. This is key.
- You'll need to adjust psychologically. No matter how full the plate is, many of us were trained to think that without meat, it's not a real meal—especially at dinner. You'll need to overcome this prejudice.
- You may not be able to go to the same restaurants you used to, and if you can, you certainly won't be able to order the same things. This takes some adjustment.
- Your friends, family, and colleagues may not be supportive. For whatever reasons, many people will find it threatening that you are eating a plant-based diet. Perhaps it's because, deep down, they know their diet isn't very healthy and find it threatening that someone else is able to give up unhealthy eating habits when they cannot.

VEGETARIAN AND VEGAN VERSUS WHOLE FOOD, PLANT-BASED

You'll notice we use the phrase "eating a whole food, plant-based diet" rather than "vegan" or "vegetarian." We intentionally do not use these words. Most people who choose to become a vegetarian or vegan have done so for ideological reasons. Although this reason is entirely satisfactory, the diet that results may be limited in nutrient composition. About 90% of vegetarians still consume dairy, as well as eggs; some occasionally eat fish and chicken. A vegan diet doesn't use foods of animal origin but can still include a lot of processed foods, and is often high in fat, sugar, and salt, which compromise human health.

We believe that the health value of a diet is best indicated by the relative amounts of fat, protein, and carbohydrate it contains, and that the optimal diet gets approximately 10% of calories from fat, 10% from protein, and 80% from total carbohydrate (although we also believe that it is permissible for most healthy people to stray somewhat from these benchmarks, as long as their diet still relies on whole, intact fruits, grains, legumes, and vegetables). We don't support sharp boundaries because, for example, we know that calories from protein can be higher than 10%, perhaps even 15% or so, even in a diet consisting solely of whole foods—if a large amount of legumes are consumed, for example. The experimental results on protein and cancer presented in chapter three suggest that 10% is a threshold for cancer occurrence, but keep in mind that this 10% figure refers to animal protein being fed in isolation. It is, however, a level that meets our physiological needs, and that can be easily provided by a diverse plant-based diet.

Take a look at the nutrient profiles of vegan and vegetarian diets and how they compare with other dietary practices in Chart 12.1.

Chart 12.1: Nutrient Profiles of Various Diets

Items	Meat Eaters	Fish Eaters	Vegetarians	Vegans	WFPB
Total protein	17.2	15.5	14.0	13.1	10.0
Dairy protein	3.6	3.9	4.1	—	—
Total fat	31.3	30.3	30.0	30.5	10.0
Total carb	48.0	50.7	52.8	54.0	80.0
Vegetables	216	254	264	308	*
Total dairy	337	160	365	—	—

There is no upper limit on vegetable consumption in a WFBP diet.

Note: All entries are % of total energy except foods (g/day).

These data are for England.[1] Most surveys of the standard American diet (SAD) show it to be higher in fat (about 35%–40% vs. 31.5%) and meat consumption (more than twice as high).[1] The average fat content of the first four diets here is close to 30% of total calories, not very different from the standard American diet at about 35%–40%. In contrast, the WFPB diet strives for about 10% fat. It is quite clear that the nutrient profiles of the "V" diets are not very different from the SAD diet in the U.S. or the "Meat Eater" diet in England. And all four diets, including the "V" diets, are substantially different from the WFPB diet.

We'd also like to offer you a few pieces of advice for your first month:

- In the long term, plant-based eating is cheaper than an animal-based diet, but as you learn, you may spend a little extra money trying things. Do it. It's worth it.
- Eat well. If you eat out, try lots of restaurants to find some great plant-based dishes (looking for ones marked "vegan" is a great place to start). Ethnic restaurants often offer the most options for plant-based meals, and the unique tastes are exquisite. Learn what's out there.
- Eat enough. One of your health goals may be to lose weight. That's fine, and on a WFPB diet you likely will. But don't hold back—whatever you do, don't go hungry.
- Eat a variety. Mixing it up is important both for getting all the necessary nutrients and for maintaining your interest in the diet.

The bottom line is that you can eat a plant-based diet with great pleasure and satisfaction. But making the transition is a challenge. There are psychological barriers and practical ones. It takes time and effort. You may not get support from your friends and family. But the benefits are nothing short of miraculous. And you'll be amazed at how easy it becomes once you form new habits.

Take the one-month challenge. You'll not only do great things for yourself, you'll be part of the vanguard working toward moving America into a healthier, leaner future.

Glenn is an associate of ours who had been a dedicated meat eater before the first edition of *The China Study* was published. In fact, he had recently tried the Atkins Diet, lost some weight, but dropped off the diet when his cholesterol went through the roof. He was forty-two and overweight. Colin gave him a draft of his manuscript and Glenn agreed to take the one-month challenge. Here are a few of his observations:

GLENN'S TIPS

The first week is quite challenging. It's hard to figure out what to eat. I'm not much of a cook, so I got some recipe books out and tried creating some vegan dishes. As someone who would swing through McDonald's or heat up a frozen dinner, I found it annoying to have to cook meals each evening. At least half of them were a disaster and had to be thrown out. But over time I found a few that were fantastic. My sister gave me a recipe for West African peanut stew that was incredible and like nothing I ever tasted. My mom gave me a vegetarian chili recipe that was great. And I stumbled on a great whole wheat spaghetti dish with lots of vegetables and a faux meat sauce (made from soy) that was amazing. I challenge anyone to know that this was a vegan dish. But all of this does take time.

I'm rediscovering fruit. I've always loved fruit, but for some reason I don't really eat much of it. Maybe it's not eating meat, but I'm finding that I'm enjoying fruit more than ever. I now cut up a grapefruit and eat it as a snack. I really like it! I would have never done that before; I actually think my tastes are getting more sensitive.

I was avoiding eating out—something I used to do constantly—for fear of not having a vegan option. But I'm getting more adventurous now. I've found some new restaurants that have some great vegan side dishes, including a wonderful local Vietnamese place (I know that most Vietnamese food isn't strictly vegan, since they use a fish sauce in many dishes, but for nutritional purposes it's very close). The other day I got dragged into a pizza place with a large group; there was nothing I could do, and I was starved. I ordered a cheese-less pizza with lots of vegetables. They even made it with a whole wheat crust. I was prepared to choke it down but actually it was surprisingly good. I've brought that home a few times since.

I'm finding that cravings for meat products are pretty much gone, particularly if I don't let myself get hungry. And, honestly, I'm eating like a pig. Being overweight, I've always been self-conscious about what I eat. Now I eat like a madman, and feel virtuous to boot. I can honestly say I'm enjoying the food I'm eating now a lot more than before, partly because I'm fussier now in what I eat. I only eat foods I really like.

The first month went by quicker than I thought it would. I've lost eight pounds and my cholesterol has dropped dramatically. I'm spending a lot less time on this now, particularly since I've found so many restaurants I can eat at, plus I cook huge meals and then freeze them. My freezer is stocked with vegan goodies.

The experiment is over but I stopped thinking of it as an experiment weeks ago. I can't imagine why I would go back to my old eating patterns.

THE CHINA STUDY SOLUTION— FROM THOMAS M. CAMPBELL, MD

Having been part of the care provided to thousands of patients over several years in traditional primary-care offices and specialized diet and lifestyle programs, I've seen people's short- and long-term struggles with making healthy choices. I have come to believe that supporting behavior change ought to be the holy grail of modern medicine, though our current paradigm mostly seems to ignore this facet of patient care (more on that in Part IV).

All of us are masters of rationalization. We find all sorts of ways to justify doing things we know we shouldn't be doing. And our social connections and the environment in which we live have a profound effect on our lifestyle choices, more than many would like to believe.

With these thoughts in mind, I encourage you to draw "bright lines" as you try to change your diet. For example, draw a bright line by making a choice for the week or month that you simply won't eat any food other people bring in to your workplace. Devise an explanation, tell people publicly about what you're trying, and commit fully to not crossing the bright line you've drawn. For many people, it's actually harder to embrace "moderate" changes. It's harder to try to limit yourself to just one bite of a cookie in the break room now and then than not to have any cookies at all; it's a losing strategy and demands more willpower. Moderation means something different to each person, and allows the power of rationalization to creep in and keep you from your goals. I also encourage you to pay attention to your social connections and environment. You can put some effort into these parts of your life in a way that supports your dietary changes.

After writing the first edition of this book, I, and my dad in particular, have given many lectures on a WFPB diet. Although the general eating plan is simple, certain questions commonly arise as someone is thinking of trying it. "What about soy? What about fish? I thought some oils were healthy? Does it need to be organic? And what about gluten? And sugar?" After encountering these questions over and over, I wrote *The China Study Solution* (titled *The Campbell Plan* in hardcover). If you want a specific eating plan for two weeks with recipes and evidence-based answers to the common questions about what exactly you should be eating with a nod to behavior-change strategies, I encourage you to pick up and use that book as a starting point.

I have seen many patients become healthier by changing their diet and lifestyle. There are usually stumbles along the way, and it's obviously true that a healthy diet and lifestyle will not prevent and reverse all disease, but I have never seen any other medical intervention with such a broad range of benefits. As I tell patients, for many of our most common chronic diseases, diet and lifestyle choices are more important than anything I can give them or do to them.

PART IV

WHY HAVEN'T YOU HEARD THIS BEFORE?

Often when people hear of scientific information that justifies a radical shift in diet to plant foods, they can't believe their ears. "If all that you say is true," they wonder, "why haven't I heard it before? In fact, why do I usually hear the opposite of what you say: that milk is good for us, that we need meat to get protein, and that cancer and heart disease are all in the genes?" These are legitimate questions, and the answers are a crucial part of this story. To get to these answers, however, we believe it is essential to know how information is created and how it reaches the public consciousness.

As you will come to see, much is governed by the Golden Rule: he who has the gold makes the rules. There are powerful, influential, and enormously wealthy industries that stand to lose a vast amount of money if Americans start shifting to a plant-based diet. Their financial health depends on controlling what the public knows about nutrition and health. Like any good business enterprise, these industries do everything in their power to protect their profits and their shareholders.

You might be inclined to think that industry pays scientists under the table to "cook the data," bribes government officials, or conducts illegal activities. Many people love a sensational story. But the powerful interests that maintain the status quo do not usually conduct illegal business. As far as we know, they do not pay scientists to cook the data. They do not bribe elected officials or make sordid underhanded deals.

The situation is much worse.

The entire system—government, science, medicine, industry, media, and academia—promotes profits over health, technology over food, and confusion over clarity. Most, but not all, of the confusion about nutrition is created in legal, fully disclosed ways and is disseminated by unsuspecting, well-intentioned people, whether they are researchers, politicians, or journalists. The most damaging aspect of the system is not sensational, nor is it likely to create much of a stir upon its discovery. It is a silent enemy that few people see and understand.

My experiences within the scientific community illustrate how the entire system generates confusing information and why you haven't heard the message of this book before. In the following chapters, we have divided the "system" of problems into the entities of science, industry, government, medicine, and academia, but, as you will come to see, there are instances where it is nearly impossible to distinguish science from industry, government from science and academia, or government from industry. With the exception of the new chapter that considers academia, the chapters that follow remain largely as they appeared in the first edition of this book. But this section only scratches the surface in its attempt to answer the question *Why haven't you heard this before?*

When *The China Study* was first published, it was met with a few hostile, even vitriolic reactions. Why? Because a message that encourages a diet only of plants and describes its effects as wholistic is a virtually unparalleled one-two punch that challenges the status quo on multiple fronts. Powerful interests whose livelihoods are threatened by the WFPB message were (and continue to be) eager to resist *The China Study*'s message, and that resistance is often subtle, not easily seen by the general public. And while there has been increasing interest in this idea from the public, too many people (including believers) concern themselves with trivial questions concerning individual nutrients, individual mechanisms, and/or individual disease endpoints that divert attention from the much more important message: the unique nutritional properties of whole foods.

As this section of the book attests, I have long sought explanations for why such an exciting and hopeful message was not yet common knowledge. But after *The China Study*'s initial publication, I found myself searching for a more profound explanation for what motivated the intensely negative reactions the book provoked. My second book, *Whole*,[1] published in 2013, was the result of that search. In it, I examine some of the fundamental assumptions we make about nutrition, biomedical research, medical practice, and the application of biomedical science in the entire socioeconomic-political system in which we live. I also explore the complex interconnections between the parts of that system, and how they work together (some intentionally, some unwittingly) to create confusion and spread misinformation. This exploration also includes the media, a subject on which the first edition of *The China Study* did not comment, although they often have great influence over the public discussion on diet and health—influence that, due to market constraints, can be very damaging indeed.

Whole's writing was driven not only by the negative reactions to *The China Study*, and their increase during the past decade as the WFPB message has gained more and more prominence, but by the discouraging changes I was seeing even in institutions and professional societies whose missions I once believed were the same as mine. I have spent a lifetime assuming, somewhat naïvely, that those of us who spend public money had a shared mission to serve the public—or so we proudly said. I was wrong. The professional societies to which I belong or have belonged have become even more entrenched in their staid, comfortable, worn-out missions. Even members of the academic institution that I served for so long, Cornell University, have made clear their objections to the path I've taken; certain administrators have done everything they can to sidetrack or discredit this message.

I have seen enough misbehavior within the health research and practice communities to last for several lifetimes—enough to etch cynicism into my very soul. Still, we must find ways to tell with hope our story about the impact food could have on our lives, so that we might solve the incredible societal problems described in this book: poor personal health, destructive health care costs, environmental degradation, political corruption. Make no mistake—these problems are massive. If they are not resolved, they will, no doubt, destroy our society and our planet with it. But they can be solved, and we have sufficient evidence not only that nutrition can do so, but also that it can do so far more effectively than any other means available to us. Many of us know the seriousness of the problem, but few, even now, know its most promising solution.

Much has been done already in the last ten years, despite the naysayers who protect the status quo at any cost—including the sacrifice of truth. But we have a big challenge still ahead of us in elevating the public's consciousness about the connection between food and personal health, the environment, and the rest of society, and an even greater one in connecting this multifaceted problem with its solution. The first step is understanding the players.

SCIENCE—
THE DARK SIDE

13

When I was living in a mountain valley outside of Blacksburg, Virginia, my family enjoyed visiting a retired farmer down the road, Mr. Kinsey, who always had a funny story to tell. We used to look forward to evenings listening to his stories on his front porch. One of my favorites was the great potato bug scam.

He told us of his farm days before pesticides, and recounted that when a potato crop became infested with potato bugs, the bugs had to be removed and killed, one by one, by hand. One day, Mr. Kinsey noticed an advertisement in a farm magazine for a great potato bug killer, on sale for five dollars. Although five dollars was no small sum of money in those days, Mr. Kinsey figured the bugs were enough of a hassle to warrant the investment. A short while later, when he received the great potato bug killer, he opened the package and found two blocks of wood and a short list of three instructions:

- Pick up one block of wood.
- Place the potato bug on the flat face of the wood.
- Pick up the second block of wood and press firmly onto the potato bug.

Scams, tricks, and outright deception for personal gain are as old as history itself, and perhaps no discipline in our society has suffered more from this affliction than the discipline of health. Very few experiences are as personal and as powerful as those of people who have lost their health prematurely. Understandably, they are willing to believe and try just about anything that might help. They are a highly vulnerable group of consumers.

In the mid-1970s, along came a prime example of a health scam, at least according to the medical establishment. It concerned an alternative cancer treatment called Laetrile, a natural compound made largely from apricot pits. If you had cancer and had been unsuccessfully treated by your regular doctors here in the United States, you may have considered heading to Tijuana, Mexico. *Washington Post Magazine* documented the story of Sylvia Dutton, a fifty-three-year-old woman from Florida, who had done just that as a last attempt to thwart a cancer that had already spread from her ovaries to her lymph system.[1] Friends and fellow churchgoers had told her and her husband about the Laetrile treatment and its ability to cure advanced cancer. In the magazine article,[1] Sylvia's husband said, "There are at least a dozen people in this area who were told they were going to be dead from cancer who used Laetrile and now they're out playing tennis."

The catch, however, was that Laetrile was a highly contentious treatment. Some people in the medical establishment argued that animal studies had repeatedly shown Laetrile to have no effect on tumors.[1] Because of this, the U.S. Food and Drug Administration had decided to suppress the use of Laetrile, which gave rise to the popular clinics south of the border. One famous hospital in Tijuana treated "as many as 20,000 American patients a year."[1] One of those patients was Sylvia Dutton, for whom Laetrile unfortunately did not work.

But Laetrile was only one of many alternative health products. By the end of the 1970s, Americans were spending $1 billion a year on various supplements and potions that promised magical benefits.[2] These included pangamic acid, which was touted as a previously undiscovered vitamin with virtually unlimited powers; various bee concoctions; and other supplement products including garlic and zinc.[2]

At the same time in the scientific community, more and more health information, specifically nutrition information, was being generated at a furious pace. In 1976, Senator George McGovern had convened a committee that drafted dietary goals recommending decreased consumption of fatty animal foods and increased consumption of fruits and vegetables because of their effects on heart disease. The first draft of this report, linking heart disease and food, caused such an uproar that a major revision was required before it was released for publication. In a personal conversation, McGovern told me that he and five other powerful senators from agricultural states lost their respective elections in 1980 in part because they had dared to question the animal foods industry.

At the end of the 1970s, the McGovern report succeeded in prodding the government to produce its first-ever dietary guidelines, which were rumored to promote a message similar to that of McGovern's committee.

At about the same time, there were widely publicized government debates about whether food additives were safe, and whether saccharin caused cancer.

PLAYING MY PART

In the late 1970s I found myself in the middle of this rapidly changing environment. By 1975 my program in the Philippines had ended, and I was well into my experimental laboratory work here in the United States, after having accepted a full professorship with tenure at Cornell University. Some of my early work on aflatoxin and liver cancer in the Philippines (chapter two) had garnered widespread interest, and my subsequent laboratory work investigating nutritional factors, carcinogens, and cancer (chapter three) was attracting national attention. At that time, I had one of only two or three laboratories in the country doing basic research on nutrition and cancer. It was a novel endeavor.

From 1978 to 1979 I took a year-long sabbatical from Cornell to go to the epicenter of national nutritional activity: Bethesda, Maryland. The organization that I was working with was the Federation of American Societies for Experimental Biology and Medicine, or FASEB. Six individual research societies made up the federation, representing pathology, biochemistry, pharmacology, nutrition, immunology, and physiology. FASEB sponsored annual joint meetings of all six societies, and upwards of 20,000 scientists attended. I was a member of two of these societies, nutrition and pharmacology, and was particularly active in the American Institution of Nutrition (now named the American Society for Nutritional Sciences). My principle work was to chair, under contract to the Food and Drug Administration, a committee of scientists investigating potential hazards of using nutrient supplements.

While there, I also was invited to be on a public affairs committee that served as liaison between FASEB and Congress. The committee's charge was to stay on top of congressional activity and represent our societies' interests in dealings with lawmakers. We reviewed policies, budgets, and position statements, met with congressional staffs, and held meetings around big, impressive "boardroom" tables in distinguished, august meeting rooms. I often got the feeling I was in the citadel of science.

As a prerequisite to representing my nutrition society on this public affairs committee, I first had to decide, for myself, how nutrition is best defined. It's a far more difficult question than you may think. We had scientists who were interested in applied nutrition, which involves people and communities. We had medical doctors interested in isolated food compounds as pharmacological drugs and research scientists who only worked with isolated cells and well-identified chemicals in the laboratory. We even had people who thought nutrition studies should focus on livestock as well as people. The concept of nutrition was far from clear; clarification was critical. The average American's view of nutrition was even more varied and confused. Consumers were constantly being duped by fads, yet remained intensely interested in nutrient supplements and dietary advice coming from any source, whether that source was a diet book or a government official.

One day in late spring of 1979, while doing my more routine work, I got a call from the director of the public affairs office at the FASEB, Walter Ellis, who coordinated the work of our congressional liaison committee.

Ellis informed me that there was yet another new committee being formed within one of the FASEB societies, the American Institute of Nutrition, that might interest me.

"It's being called the Public Nutrition Information Committee," he told me, "and one of its responsibilities will be to decide what is sound nutritional advice to give to the public.

"Obviously," he added, "there's a big overlap between what this new committee wants to do and what we do on the public affairs committee."

I agreed.

"If you're interested, I would like to have you join this new committee as a representative of the public affairs office," he said.

The proposal sounded good to me because it was early in my career and it meant getting a chance to hear the scholarly views of some of the "big name" nutrition researchers. It also was a committee, according to its organizers, that could evolve into a "supreme court" of public nutrition information. It might serve, for example, to identify nutrition quackery.

A BIG SURPRISE

At the time that this new Public Nutrition Information Committee (PNIC) was being formed, a maelstrom was developing across town at the prestigious National Academy of Sciences (NAS). A public dispute was taking place between the NAS president, Phil Handler, and the internal NAS Food and Nutrition Board (FNB). Handler wanted to bring in a group of distinguished scientists from outside the NAS organization to deliberate on the subject of diet, nutrition, and cancer and write a report. This did not please the FNB, which wanted control over this project. Handler's NAS was being offered congressional funding to produce a report on a subject that had not been previously considered in this way.

Within the scientific community it was widely known that the FNB was strongly influenced by the meat, dairy, and egg industries. Two of its leaders, Bob Olson and Alf Harper, had strong connections to these industries. Olson was a well-paid consultant to the egg industry, and Harper acknowledged that 10% of his income came from offering his services to food companies, including large dairy corporations.[3]

Ultimately Handler, as president of the NAS, went around his FNB and arranged for a panel of expert scientists from outside of his organization to write the 1982 report *Diet, Nutrition, and Cancer*.[4] As it turned out, I was one of thirteen scientists chosen to be on the panel to write the report.

As could be expected, Alf Harper, Bob Olson, and their FNB colleagues were not happy about losing control of this landmark report. They knew it could greatly influence national opinion about diet and disease. Mostly they feared that the great American diet was going to be challenged, perhaps even called a possible cause of cancer.

James S. Turner, chairman of a related Consumer Liaison Panel within the NAS, was critical of the FNB and wrote, "We can only conclude that the [Food and Nutrition] Board is dominated by a group of change-resistant scientists who share a rather isolated view about diet and disease."[3]

After being denied control of this promising new report on diet, nutrition, and cancer, the pro-industry FNB needed to do some damage control. An alternate group was quickly established: the new PNIC. Who were its leaders? Bob Olson, Alfred Harper, and Tom Jukes (a long-time industry scientist), each of whom held a university faculty position. I was initially innocent of the group's purpose, but by our first meeting in the spring of 1980, I had discovered that, of the eighteen members on that committee, I was the only individual who did not have ties to the commercial world of food and drug companies and their coalitions.

This committee was a stacked deck; its members were entrenched in the status quo. Their professional associations, their friends, the people they fraternized with, were all pro-industry. They enjoyed the meaty American diet themselves and were unwilling to consider the possibility that their views were wrong. In addition, some of them enjoyed handsome benefits, including first-class travel expenses and nice consulting fees, paid by animal foods companies. Although there was nothing illegal about any of these activities, it certainly laid bare a serious conflict of interest that put most of the committee members at odds with the public interest.

This is analogous to the situation, as it unfolded, surrounding cigarettes and health. When scientific evidence first emerged to show that cigarettes were dangerous, hordes of health professionals vigorously defended smoking. For example, the *Journal of the American Medical Association* continued to advertise tobacco products, and many doctors played their part to staunchly defend tobacco use. In many cases, these scientists were motivated by understandable caution. But there were quite a few others, particularly as the evidence against tobacco mounted, whose motivations were clearly personal bias and greed.

So there I was, on a committee that was to judge the merit of nutrition information, a committee composed of some of the most powerful pro-industry scientists. I was the only one not handpicked by the industry cronies, as I was there at the behest of the director of the FASEB public affairs office. At that point in my career, I had not formed any particularly strong views for or against the standard American diet. More than anything, I was interested in promoting honest, open debate—something that would immediately put me at odds with this new organization.

THE FIRST MEETING

From the first moment of the first PNIC meeting in April 1980, I knew I was the chicken who had wandered into a fox's den, although I went in with high hopes and an open, though naïve, mind. After all, lots of scientists, myself included, have consulted with companies while working to maintain an objective mind in the best interest of public health.

In the second session of our first committee meeting, the chairman, Tom Jukes, passed around a proposed news release, handwritten by himself, regarding the mission of the committee. In addition to announcing our formation, the news release listed examples of the kind of nutrition frauds that our committee intended to expose.

As I scanned the list of so-called frauds, I was stunned to see the 1977 McGovern dietary goals[5] on the list. First drafted in 1976, these relatively modest goals suggested that less meat and fat consumption and more fruit and vegetable consumption might prevent heart disease. In this proposed news release, they were described as nothing more than simple quackery, just like the widely condemned Laetrile and pangamic acid preparations. In essence, the recommendation to shift our eating habits to more fruits and vegetables and whole grains was being called a fraud. This was the committee's attempt to demonstrate their ability to be the supreme arbiter of reliable scientific information!

Having looked forward to my membership on this new committee, I was shocked to see what was emerging. Although I had no particular predilection toward any one type of diet at the time, I knew that the land-mark diet, nutrition, and cancer panel that I was on at the NAS would likely recommend something similar to McGovern's goals, this time citing can-cer research instead of heart disease research. The scientific results with which I was familiar very clearly seemed to justify the moderate recommen-dations made by McGovern's dietary goals committee.

Sitting next to me at our first meeting was Alf Harper, whom I had held in high esteem since our days at MIT where he was the General Foods Pro-fessor of Nutritional Sciences. Early in the meeting, when this handwritten proposed news release was passed out to the committee members, I leaned over to Harper and pointed to the place where it listed McGovern's dietary goals among other common scams and whispered incredulously, "Do you see this?"

Harper could sense my unease, even disbelief, and so quickly spoke up. In a patronizing tone, he said to the group, "There are honorable people in our society who may not necessarily agree with this list. Perhaps we should put it on hold." A reluctant discussion ensued, and they decided to forgo the proposed press release.

With the conclusion of the news release issue, the meeting came to an end. As far as I was concerned, it was a dubious beginning at best.

A couple of weeks later, back in upstate New York, I turned on a morn-ing TV news show and Tom Brokaw appeared on the screen and started talking about nutrition with Bob Olson, of all people. They were discuss-ing a recent report that Olson and friends had produced at the NAS called "Toward Healthful Diets." This report, which was one of the briefest, most superficial reports on health ever produced by the NAS, extolled the virtues of the high-fat, high-meat American diet and basically confirmed that all was well with how America was eating.

From a scientific point of view, the message was a doozy. I remember one exchange where Tom Brokaw asked about fast food, and Olson con-fidently stated that McDonald's hamburgers were fine. With millions of viewers watching this "expert" praise the health value of McDonald's ham-burgers, it's no wonder that consumers around the country were confused. Only a handful of insiders could possibly know that his views did not even come close to reflecting the best understanding of the science at the time.

THE SECOND MEETING

We were back for round two in Atlantic City at our annual meeting in late spring of 1981. From our correspondence over the past year, the PNIC already had an informal agenda in place. First, we were to establish the proposition that nutrition scams were eroding the public's trust in the nutrition research community. Second, we needed to publicize the idea that advocating more vegetable and fruit consumption and less meat and high-fat foods was, itself, a scam. Third, we intended to position our committee as a permanent, standing organization. Up to this point, our group had only served in a temporary capacity, as an exploratory committee. Now it was time to get on with our job of becoming the permanent, principal source of reliable nutrition information in the U.S.

Within the first few days of arriving at the convention, a fellow member of the committee, Howard Applebaum, told me of the developing gossip. "Did you hear?" he whispered. "Olson's decided that they're going to reconstitute the committee and you are going to be removed." At that time, Olson was still serving his one-year term as president of the parent society, the American Institute of Nutrition, and had the power to do such things.

I remember thinking that this news was neither surprising nor disappointing. I knew I was the black sheep of the committee and had already stepped out of line at our inaugural meeting the previous year. My continued involvement in this particular group was going to amount to nothing more than trying to swim up Niagara Falls. The only reason I was involved in the first place was because the director of the public affairs office at FASEB had secured me the spot.

I had thought the first year's committee meeting was dubious, but I ran into an even more bizarre beginning at that second meeting a year later, before Olson had the chance to remove me. When the proposal to become a permanent organization within our society was put forth, I was the only one to challenge the idea. I expressed concern that this committee and its activities reeked of McCarthyism, which had no place in a scientific research society. What I was saying made the chair of the committee intensely angry and physically hostile, and I decided it was best to just leave the room. I was clearly a threat to everything the committee members wanted to achieve.

After the whole ordeal was related to the newly elected incoming president, Professor Doris Calloway of UC Berkeley, the PNIC was abolished and reformed, with me as the chair. Fortunately, I persuaded our six-member committee to disband after less than a year, and the whole sorry affair came to an end.

To stay and "fight the good fight," so to speak, was not an option. It was early in my career and the awesome power wielded by the senior members of my society was stark and intellectually brutal. For many of these characters, searching for a truth that promoted public health over the status quo was not an option. I am absolutely convinced that had I busied myself with tackling these issues so early in my career, I would not be writing this book. Research funding and publications would have been difficult if not impossible to obtain.

Meanwhile, Bob Olson and some of his colleagues turned their attention elsewhere, focusing on a relatively new organization founded in 1978 called the American Council on Science and Health (ACSH). Headquartered in New York City, the ACSH bills itself, still today, as a "consumer education consortium concerned with issues related to food, nutrition, chemicals, pharmaceuticals, lifestyle, the environment and health." The group also claims to be an "independent, nonprofit, tax-exempt organization,"[6] but they receive 76% of their funding from corporations and corporate donors, according to the National Environmental Trust who cite *Congressional Quarterly*'s Public Interest Profiles.[7]

According to the National Environmental Trust,[7] the ACSH has claimed in their reports that cholesterol is not related to coronary heart disease, "the unpopularity of food irradiation . . . is not based in science," "endocrine disruptors" (e.g., PCBs, dioxins, etc.) are not a human health problem, saccharin is not carcinogenic, and implementation of fossil-fuel restrictions to control global warming should not be implemented. Searching for a serious critique of the food industry from the ACSH is like searching for a needle in a haystack. Although I believe that some of their arguments may have merit, I seriously question their claim to be an objective broker of "consumer education."

FALLING ON MY PETARD

During the entire experience with the PNIC, I continued to work on the NAS report on diet, nutrition, and cancer, which was released in June 1982.[4] As might have been expected, when this report was published, all hell broke loose. Being the first such report on diet and cancer, it received extensive publicity, fast becoming the most sought-after report in NAS history. It was establishing high-profile goals for the dietary prevention of cancer, which were very similar to those of the 1976 McGovern Committee report on diet and heart disease. We were principally encouraging the consumption of fruits, vegetables, and whole grain cereal products, while decreasing total fat intake. The fact that this report was concerned with cancer instead of heart disease, however, elevated emotions. The stakes were high and getting higher; cancer incites a far greater fear than heart disease.

Given the stakes, some powerful enemies came out of the woodwork. Within two weeks, the Council on Agriculture, Science, and Technology

(CAST), an influential lobbying group for the livestock-based farming industry, produced a report summarizing the views of fifty-six "experts" who were concerned about the effect of our NAS report on the agriculture and food industries. Olson, Jukes, Harper, and their like-minded colleagues on the now defunct PNIC weighed in as experts. Their report was quickly published, then placed in the hands of all 535 U.S. congressional members. It was clear that CAST was deeply concerned about the possible impact that our report might have on the public.

CAST wasn't the only group that stepped up to criticize the report. In addition, there were the American Meat Institute, National Broiler Council, National Cattlemen's Association, National Livestock and Meat Board, National Meat Association, National Milk Producers Federation, National Pork Producers Council, National Turkey Federation, and United Egg Producers.[3] I wouldn't presume to know how much cancer research the National Turkey Federation conducts, but I'm guessing that their criticism of our report was not born out of their desire for truth in science.

It was ironic that I had learned some of my most valuable lessons growing up on a dairy farm, and yet the work I was doing was portrayed as being at odds with agricultural interests. Of course, these mammoth corporate interests were far removed from the farmers I knew growing up—the hardworking, honest families that maintained small farms, just big enough to get by comfortably. I often have wondered whether these Washington agricultural interests truly represent America's great farming tradition, or whether they only represent agricultural conglomerates with operations worth tens of millions of dollars.

Alf Harper, who had written a strong letter of support for my first faculty position after leaving MIT, wrote me a stern personal letter in which he declared that I had "fallen on [my] own petard." A petard is a type of bomb or firecracker. Apparently, my involvement in the PNIC and the NAS *Diet, Nutrition, and Cancer* report was finally too much for even him to bear.

Times were hot, to be sure. Congressional hearings, in which I testified, were held on the NAS report itself; *People* magazine featured me in a prominent article, and an endless series of news media reports continued over the next year.

AMERICAN INSTITUTE FOR CANCER RESEARCH

It seemed that for the first time in our history, the government was seriously thinking about what we eat as a means of controlling cancer. This was fertile territory for doing something new, and something new did indeed fall into my lap. I was invited to assist a new organization called the American Institute for Cancer Research (AICR) in Falls Church, Virginia. The founders of this organization were fundraisers and had learned that it was possible to raise, through mailing campaigns, large sums of money for cancer research. It seemed that many people were interested in learning something new about cancer beyond the usual model of surgery, radiation, and cytotoxic drugs.

This budding organization was well aware of our 1982 NAS report[4] that focused on diet and cancer, and so invited me to join them as their senior science advisor. I encouraged them to focus on diet because the nutrition connection with cancer was becoming an important area of research, yet was receiving very little, if any, support from the major funding agencies. I especially encouraged them to emphasize whole foods as a source of nutrition, not nutrient supplements, partly because this was the message of the NAS report.

As I began to work with the AICR, two challenges simultaneously arose. First, the AICR needed to get established as a credible organization to promote the message and support research. Second, the NAS recommendations needed to be publicized. Therefore, I thought it made sense for the AICR to help publicize the NAS recommendations. Dr. Sushma Palmer, executive director of the NAS project,[4] and Harvard professor Mark Hegsted, who was the key advisor to the McGovern Committee, agreed to join me in endorsing this AICR project. Simultaneously, the AICR president, Marilyn Gentry, suggested that the AICR could publish the NAS report and send free copies to 50,000 physicians in the U.S. These projects, which seemed to me to be logical, useful, and socially responsible, were also highly successful. The associations we were making and the exposure we were generating were aimed at increasing the public's health. As I was quick to find out, however, creating an organization focused on diet as a central link in cancer causation was seen as a threat to a great many people. It was clear that the AICR's projects were beginning to hit the mark because of the hostile feedback coming from the food, medical, and drug industries. It seemed that every effort was being made to discredit them.

I was surprised that government interference was particularly harsh. National and state attorney general offices questioned the AICR's status and its fundraising procedures. The U.S. Post Office joined in the fray, questioning whether the AICR could use the mail to spread "junk" information. We all had our suspicions as to who were encouraging these government offices to quash the dissemination of this diet and cancer information. Collectively, these public agencies were making life very difficult. Why were they attacking a nonprofit organization promoting cancer research? It all came down to the fact that the AICR, like the NAS, was advancing an agenda that connected diet and cancer.

The American Cancer Society (ACS) became an especially vigorous detractor. In its eyes, the AICR had two strikes against it: it might compete for the same funding donors, and it was trying to shift the cancer discussion toward diet. The ACS had not yet acknowledged that diet and nutrition were connected to cancer. (It wasn't until many years later in the early 1990s that it developed dietary recommendations to control cancer when the idea was receiving considerable currency with the public.) It was very much a medically based organization invested in the conventional use of drugs, radiation, and surgery. A short while before, the ACS had contacted our NAS committee about the possibility of our joining them to produce dietary recommendations to prevent cancer. As a committee, we declined, although a couple of the people on our committee did offer their individual services. The ACS seemed to sense a big story on the horizon and didn't like the idea that another organization, the AICR, might get the credit.

MISINFORMATION

It may seem that I am coming down a tad harsh on an organization that most people regard as purely benevolent, but the ACS acted differently behind the scenes than it did in public.

On one occasion, I traveled to an upstate New York town where I had been invited to give a lecture to the local ACS chapter, as I had done elsewhere. During my lecture, I showed a slide that made reference to the new AICR organization. I did not mention my personal association, so the audience was not aware that I was their senior science advisor.

After the lecture, I took questions and my host asked me, "Do you know that AICR is an organization of quacks?"

"No," I said, "I don't." I'm afraid I didn't do such a good job of hiding my skepticism of her comment, because she felt obliged to explain, "That organization is being run by a group of quacks and discredited doctors. Some of them have even served time in prison."

Prison time? This was news to me!

Again, without revealing my association with the AICR, I asked, "How do you know that?" She said she saw a memo that had been circulated to local ACS offices around the country. Before leaving, I arranged for her to send me a copy of the memo she was referring to, and, in a day or so, she did.

The memo had been sent from the office of the national president of the ACS, who also was a senior executive of the prestigious Roswell Park

Memorial Institute for Cancer Research in Buffalo. This memo alleged that the scientific "chair" of the organization, without naming me, was heading up a group of "eight or nine" discredited physicians, several of whom had spent time in prison. It was total fabrication. I didn't even recognize the names of these discredited physicians and had no idea how something so vicious could have gotten started.

After snooping around a little more, I discovered the person in the ACS office in Buffalo who was responsible for the memo. I phoned him. Not surprisingly, he was evasive and only said that he had gotten this information from an unnamed reporter. It was impossible to trace the original source. The one thing I do know for sure was that this memo was distributed by the office of the ACS's president.

I also learned that the National Dairy Council, a powerful industry lobbying group, had obtained a copy of the same memo and proceeded to distribute a notice of its own to its local offices around the country. The smear campaign against the AICR was widespread. The food, pharmaceutical, and medical industries, through and/or parallel to the ACS and the National Dairy Council, were showing their true colors. Prevention of cancer with low-cost, low-profit plant foods was not welcomed by the food and pharmaco-medical industries. With support from a trusting media, their combined power to influence the public was overwhelming.

PERSONAL CONSEQUENCES

The ending of this story, however, is a happy one. Although the AICR's first couple of years were turbulent and difficult for me both personally and professionally, the smear campaigns finally started to wane. No longer considered "on the fringe," the AICR has now expanded to England (the World Cancer Research Fund in London) and elsewhere. For over thirty years now, the AICR has run a program that funds research and education projects on the link between diet and cancer. I initially organized and chaired that grant program, and then continued as the AICR's senior science advisor for several years, in a few different stints, after its initial founding.

One more unfortunate affair, however, bears mention. I was informed by my nutrition society's Board of Directors that two society members (Bob Olson and Alf Harper) had proposed to have me expelled from the society, supposedly because of my association with the AICR. It would have been the first expulsion in the history of the society. I had to go to Washington to be "interviewed" by the president of the society and the director of nutrition at the FDA. Most of their questions concerned the AICR.

The whole ordeal proved stranger than fiction. Expel a prominent society member—shortly after I was nominated to be the organization's president—for being involved with a cancer research organization? Later, I found myself reflecting on the affair with a colleague who knew the inner workings of our society, Professor Sam Tove of North Carolina State University. He, of course, knew all about the investigation, as well as other shenanigans. In our discussion, I told him about AICR being a worthy organization with good intentions. His response has resonated with me ever since. "It's not about AICR," he said. "It's about what you did on the National Academy of Sciences report on diet, nutrition, and cancer."

When the NAS's report concluded in June 1982 that a lower intake of fat and a higher intake of fruits, vegetables, and whole-grain products would make for a healthier diet, I had betrayed, in the eyes of some, the nutrition research community. Supposedly, as one of the two diet and cancer experimental researchers on the panel, it was my duty to protect the reputation of the American diet as it was. After my failure to do so, my subsequent involvement with the AICR and its promotion of the NAS report only made matters worse.

Luckily, reason prevailed in this whole farcical encounter. A board meeting was held to vote on whether I should be expelled from my society, and I handily survived the vote (6–0, with two abstentions).

It was hard not to take all of this personally, but there's a larger point here, and it's not personal. In the world of nutrition and health, scientists are not free to pursue their research wherever it leads. Coming to the "wrong" conclusions, even through first-rate science, can damage your career. Trying to disseminate these "wrong" conclusions to the public, for the sake of public health, can destroy your career. Mine was not destroyed—I was lucky, and some good people stood up for me. But it could have gone much worse.

After all of these numerous ordeals, I have a better understanding of why my society did the things it did. The awards funded by Mead Johnson Nutritionals, Lederle Laboratories, BioServe Biotechnologies, and, previously, Procter & Gamble and the Dannon Institute—all food and drug outfits—represented a strange marriage between industry and my society.[8] Do you believe that these "friends" of the society are interested in pursuing scientific investigation, no matter what the conclusions may be?

CONSEQUENCES FOR THE PUBLIC

Ultimately, the lessons I learned in my career had little to do with specific names or specific institutions and more to do with what goes on behind the scenes of any large institution. What happens behind the scenes during national policy discussions, whether it happens in scientific societies, the government, or industry boardrooms, is supremely important for our health as a nation. The personal experiences I have talked about in this chapter—only a sample of such experiences—have consequences far greater than personal aggravation and damage to my career. They illustrate the dark side of science, the side that harms not just individual researchers who get in the way, but all of society. It does this by systematically attempting to conceal, defeat, and destroy viewpoints that oppose the status quo.

There are some people in very influential government and university positions who operate under the guise of being scientific "experts," whose real jobs are to stifle open and honest scientific debate. Perhaps they receive significant personal compensation for attending to the interests of powerful food and drug companies, or perhaps they merely have an honest personal bias toward a company-friendly viewpoint. Personal bias is stronger than you may think. I know scientists with family members who died from cancer and it angers them to entertain the possibility that personal choices, like diet, could have played a role in the death of their loved ones. Likewise, there are scientists for whom the high-fat, mostly animal-based diet they eat every day is simply what they learned was healthy at a young age; they love the habit, and they don't want to change.

The vast majority of scientists are honorable, intelligent, and dedicated to the search for the common good rather than personal gain. However, a few are willing to sell their souls to the highest bidder. They may not be many in number, but their influence can be vast. They can corrupt the good name of institutions of which they are a part and, most importantly, they can create vast confusion among the public, which often cannot know who is who. You might turn on the TV one day to see an expert praising McDonald's hamburgers, and then read a magazine the same day that says you should eat less high-fat red meat to protect yourself against cancer. Who is to be believed?

Institutions also are part of the dark side of science. Committees like the PNIC and the American Council on Science and Health generate intellectually lopsided panels, committees, and institutions that are far more interested in promoting their point of view than in debating scientific research with an open mind. If a PNIC report says that low-fat diets are fraudulent scams, and an NAS report says the opposite, which one is right?

In addition, this closed-mindedness in science spreads across entire systems. The ACS was not the only health institution that worked to make life difficult for the AICR. The National Cancer Institute's public information office, Harvard Medical School, and a few other universities with medical schools were highly skeptical of the AICR and, in some cases, outright hostile. The hostility of medical schools at first surprised me, but when the ACS, a very traditional medical institution, also pitched in, it became obvious that there really was a "Medical Establishment." The behemoth did not take kindly to the idea of a serious connection between diet and cancer or, for that matter, virtually any other disease. Big Medicine in America is in the business of treating disease with drugs and surgery after symptoms appear. This means that you might turn on the TV to see that the ACS gives almost no credence to the idea that diet is linked to cancer, and then open the paper to see that the AICR says what you eat impacts your risk of getting cancer. Who do you trust?

Only someone familiar with the inside of the system can distinguish between sincere positions based in science and insincere, self-serving positions. I was on the inside for many years, working at the very top levels, and saw enough to be able to say that science is not always the honest search for truth that so many believe it to be. It far too often involves money, power, ego, and protection of personal interests above the common good. Very few, if any, illegal acts need to occur. It doesn't involve large payoffs being delivered to secret bank accounts or to private investigators in smoky hotel lobbies. It's not a Hollywood story; it's just day-to-day government, science, and industry in the United States.

SCIENTIFIC
REDUCTIONISM

14

When our 1982 National Academy of Sciences (NAS) Diet, Nutrition, and Cancer Committee was deciding how to summarize the research on diet and cancer, we included chapters on individual nutrients and nutrient groups. This was the way research had been done, one nutrient at a time. For example, the chapter on vitamins included information on the relationships between cancer and vitamins A, C, E, and some B vitamins. However, in the report summary, we recommended getting these nutrients from foods, not pills or supplements. We explicitly stated that "these recommendations apply only to foods as sources of nutrients—not to dietary supplements of individual nutrients."[1]

The report quickly found its way to the corporate world, which saw a major moneymaking opportunity. They ignored our cautionary message distinguishing foods from pills and began advertising vitamin pills as products that could prevent cancer, arrogantly citing our report as justification. This was a great opening to a vast new market—commercial vitamin supplements.

General Nutrition, Inc., the company with thousands of General Nutrition Centers, started selling a product called "Healthy Greens," a multivitamin supplement of vitamins A, C, and E, beta-carotene, selenium, and a minuscule half-gram of dehydrated vegetables. Then they advertised their product by making the following claims[2]:

[The Diet, Nutrition, and Cancer report] recommended we increase among other things our amounts of specific vegetables to help safeguard our bodies against the risk of certain forms of cancer. These vegetables recommended by the [National Academy of Sciences report] . . . are the ones we should increase[:]

cabbages, Brussels sprouts, cauliflower, broccoli, carrots and
spinach . . . Mom was right!

    Research scientists and technicians at General Nutrition
Labs, realizing the importance of the research, instantly went to
work to harness all of the vegetables and combined all of them
into a natural, easy to take potent tablet.

    [T]he result is Health Greens [sic], a new potent breakthrough
in nutrition that millions of people can now help safeguard their
well-being with . . . the greens that the [National Academy of
Sciences Committee] recommends we eat more of!

GNC was advertising an untested product and improperly using a government document to support its sensational claims. So the Federal Trade Commission went to court to bar the company from making these claims. It was a battle that lasted years, a battle that was rumored to have cost General Nutrition, Inc. about $7 million. The NAS recommended me as their expert witness because of my co-authorship of the report in question and because of my harping on this point during our committee deliberations.

A research associate in my group, Dr. Tom O'Connor, and I spent three intellectually stimulating years working on this project, including my three full days on the witness stand. In 1988, General Nutrition, Inc., settled the false advertising charges relating to Healthy Greens and other food supplements by agreeing to pay $600,000, divided equally, to three different health organizations.[3] This was a small price for the company to pay, considering the ultimate revenues that were generated by the exploding nutrient supplement market.

FOCUS ON FAT

The focus on individual nutrients instead of whole foods has become commonplace in the past three decades, and part of the blame can be put on our 1982 report. As mentioned, our committee organized the scientific information on diet and cancer by nutrient, with a separate chapter for each nutrient or class of nutrients. There were individual chapters for fat, protein, carbohydrate, vitamins, and minerals. I am convinced it was a great mistake on our part. We did not stress enough that our recommendations were concerned with whole foods because many people still regarded the report as cataloging the specific effects of individual nutrients.

The nutrient that our committee focused on the most was fat. The first guideline in the report explicitly stated that high fat consumption is linked to cancer, and recommended reducing our fat intake from 40% to 30% of calories, although this goal of 30% was an arbitrary cutoff point. The accompanying text said, "[T]he data could be used to justify an even greater reduction. However, in the judgment of the committee, the suggested reduction is a moderate and practical target, and is likely to be beneficial." One of the committee members, the director of the United States Department of Agriculture (USDA) Nutrition Laboratory, told us that if we went below 30%, consumers would be required to reduce animal food intake and that would be the death of the report.

At the time of this report, all of the human-based studies showing fat to be related to cancer (mostly breast and large bowel) were actually showing that the populations with more cancer consumed not just more fat, but also more animal-based foods and fewer plant-based foods (see chapter four). This meant that these cancers could just as easily be caused by animal protein, dietary cholesterol, something else exclusively found in animal-based foods, or a lack of plant-based foods (discussed in chapters four and eight). But rather than wagging the finger at animal-based foods in these studies, dietary fat was given as the main culprit. I argued against putting the emphasis on specific nutrients in the committee meetings, but only with modest success. (It was this point of view that landed me the expert witness opportunity at the FTC hearings.)

This mistake of characterizing whole foods by the health effects of specific nutrients is what I call reductionism. For example, the health effect of a hamburger cannot be simply attributed to the effect of a few grams of saturated fat in the meat. Saturated fat is merely one ingredient. Hamburgers also include other types of fat, in addition to cholesterol, protein, and very small amounts of vitamins and minerals. Even if you change the level of saturated fat in the meat, all of the other nutrients are still present and may still have harmful effects on health. It is a case of the whole (the hamburger) being greater than the sum of its parts (the saturated fat, the cholesterol, etc.).

One scientist especially took note[4] of our focused critique of dietary fat, and decided to test the hypothesis that fat causes breast cancer in a large group of American women. He was Dr. Walter Willett of the Harvard School of Public Health, and the study he used is the famous Nurses' Health Study.

Starting in 1976, researchers at the Harvard School of Public Health enrolled over 120,000 nurses from around the country for a study that was intended to investigate the relationship between various diseases and oral contraceptives, postmenopausal hormones, cigarettes, and other factors, such as hair dyes.[5] Beginning in 1980, Professor Willett added a dietary questionnaire to the study; in 1984 he expanded the dietary questionnaire to include more food items. This expanded dietary questionnaire was mailed to nurses again in 1986 and 1990.

Data now have been collected for over three decades. The Nurses' Health Study is widely known as the longest-running, premier study on women's health.[6] It has spawned three satellite studies, altogether costing $4 million to $5 million per year.[6] When I give lectures to health-conscious audiences, upwards of 70% of the people have heard of the Nurses' Health Study.

The scientific community has followed this study closely. The researchers in charge of the study have produced hundreds of scientific articles in the best peer-reviewed journals. The design of the study makes it a prospective cohort study, which means it follows a group of people (a cohort) and records information on diets before disease events are diagnosed, which makes the study "prospective." Many regard a prospective cohort study as the best experimental design for human studies.

The question of whether diets high in fat are linked to breast cancer was a natural outgrowth of the fierce discussion going on in the mid-1970s and the early 1980s. High-fat diets not only were associated with heart disease (the McGovern dietary goals), but also with cancer (the *Diet, Nutrition, and Cancer* report). What better study to answer this question than the Nurses' Health Study? It has a good design, massive numbers of women, top-flight researchers, and a long follow-up period. Sounds perfect, right? Wrong.

The Nurses' Health Study suffers from flaws that seriously doom its results. It is the premier example of how reductionism in science can create massive amounts of confusion and misinformation, even when the scientists involved are honest, well intentioned, and positioned at the top institutions in the world. Hardly any study has done more damage to the nutritional landscape than the Nurses' Health Study, and it should serve as a warning for the rest of science for what not to do.

CARNIVOROUS NURSES

To understand my rather harsh criticism, it is necessary to obtain some perspective on the American diet itself, especially when compared with the international studies that gave impetus to the dietary fat hypothesis.[7] Americans eat a lot of meat and fat compared to developing countries. We eat more total protein, and even more significantly, about 70% or more of our protein comes from animal sources. This fact means only one thing: we are consuming very few fruits and vegetables. To make matters worse, when we eat plant-based foods, we tend to eat a large amount of highly processed products that often have too much added fat, sugar, and salt. For example, the USDA's national school lunch program counts French fried potatoes as a vegetable!

In contrast, people in rural China eat very little animal food; it provides only about 10% of their total protein intake. The striking difference between the two dietary patterns is shown in two ways in Chart 14.1.[8] These distinctions are typical of the dietary differences between Western and traditional cultures. In general, people in Western countries are mostly meat eaters, and people in traditional countries are mostly plant eaters.

So what about the women in the Nurses' Health Study? As you might guess, virtually all of these women consume a diet very rich in animal-based foods, even richer than the average American. Their average protein intake is around 19% of calories, compared with a U.S. average of about 15–16%. To give these figures some perspective, the recommended daily allowance (RDA) for protein is only about 9–10%.

Chart 14.1: Protein Intake in the U.S. and Rural China[8]

Chart 14.2: Percentage of Total Protein that Comes from Animal Food

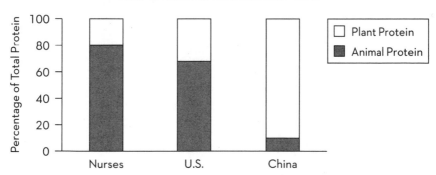

But even more importantly, *of the protein consumed by the nurses in this study, between 78% and 86% comes from animal-based foods*[9], as shown in Chart 14.2.[8,9] Even in the group of nurses that eat the lowest amount of total protein, 79% of it comes from animal-based foods.[9] *In other words, virtually all of these nurses are more carnivorous than an average American woman.* They consume very few whole, plant-based foods.

This is a crucially important point. To get further perspective, we must return to the 1975 international comparison by Ken Carroll shown earlier in Charts 4.7 to 4.9. Chart 4.7 is reproduced here in Chart 14.3.

This chart became one of the most influential observations on diet and chronic disease of the last fifty years. Like other studies, it was a significant part of the reason why the 1982 *Diet, Nutrition, and Cancer* report recommended that Americans cut their fat intake to 30% of total caloric intake to prevent cancer. This report and other consensus reports that followed thereafter eventually set the stage for an explosion of low-fat products in the marketplace ("low-fat" dairy products, lean cuts of meat, "low-fat" sweets and snack foods).

Unfortunately, the emphasis on fat alone was misguided. Carroll's study, like all the other international comparisons, was comparing populations that mostly ate meat and dairy to populations that mostly ate plants. There were many more differences between the diets of these countries than just the fat intake! What Carroll's graph really shows is that the closer a population gets to consuming a plant-based diet, the lower its risk of breast cancer.

Chart 14.3: Fat Intake and Breast Cancer Mortality

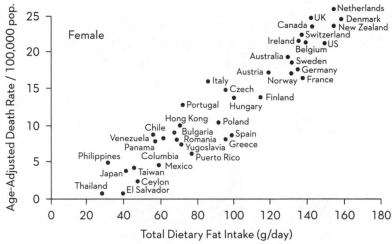

But because the women in the Nurses' Health Study are so far from a plant-based diet, *there is no way to study the diet and breast cancer relation ship originally suggested by the international studies*. Virtually no nurses eat a diet typical of the countries at the bottom of this graph. Make no mistake about it: nearly this entire cohort of nurses is consuming a high-risk diet. Most people who look at the Nurses' Health Study miss this flaw because, as Harvard researchers will point out, there is a wide range of fat intake among the nurses.

The group of nurses who consume the least fat eat 20–25% of their calories as fat, and the group of nurses who consume the most fat eat 50–55% of their calories as fat.[10] At a casual glance, this range appears to indicate substantial differences in the overall nutritional value of their diets, but this is just not true, as almost all women uniformly eat a diet very rich in animal-based foods. That begs the question: How can their fat intake vary dramatically while they all uniformly consume large amounts of animal-based foods?

Ever since "low-fat" became synonymous with "healthy," technology has created many of the same foods that you know and love, without the fat. You can now have all kinds of low-fat or no-fat dairy products, low-fat processed meats, low-fat dressings and sauces, low-fat crackers, low-fat candies, and low-fat "junk food," like chips and cookies. In other words, you can eat mostly the same foods as you did twenty-five years ago, while substantially reducing your fat intake. But you still retain the same proportion of animal- and plant-based food intakes.

In practical terms this means that beef, pork, lamb, and veal consumption is decreasing while lower-fat chicken, turkey, and fish consumption is increasing. In fact, by consuming more poultry and fish, people have been increasing their total meat intake to record-high amounts,[11] while trying (and largely failing[12]) to reduce their fat intake. In addition, whole milk is being consumed less, but low-fat and skim milk are being consumed more. Cheese consumption has increased by 150% in the past thirty years.[13]

Overall, we are as carnivorous now as we were thirty years ago, but we are able to selectively lower our fat intake if we so desire, due to the wonders of food technology.

To illustrate, we need only to look at two typical American meals.[14,15] Meal #1 is served in a health-conscious home, where the main grocery shopper in the family reads the nutrition labels on every food item he or she buys. The result: a low-fat dining experience.

Meal #2 is served in a home where the standard American fare is everyone's favorite. When they cook at home, they make the meal "rich." The result: a high-fat dining experience.

Chart 14.4: Low-Fat and High-Fat American Dinners
(One Person's Dinner)

	Low-Fat Meal #1	High-Fat Meal #2
Dinner	8 oz. roasted turkey	4.5 oz. pan-seared steak
	Low-fat gravy	Green beans almondine
	Golden roasted potatoes	Herb-seasoned potato pockets
Beverage	1 cup skim milk	Water
Dessert	Nonfat yogurt	Apple crisp
	Reduced-fat cheesecake	

Both meals provide roughly 1,000 calories, but are markedly different in their fat content. The low-fat meal (#1) contains about 25 g of fat, and the high-fat meal (#2) contains just over 60 g of fat. In the low-fat meal, 22% of the total calories come from fat, and in the high-fat meal, 54% of the calories come from fat.

The health-conscious home has managed to create a meal that is much lower in fat than the average American dinner, but they've done it without adjusting their proportionate intake of animal- and plant-based foods. Both meals are centered on animal-based foods. In fact, the low-fat meal actually has more animal-based foods than the high-fat meal. In effect, this is how the nurses in the Nurses' Health Study achieved such a wide variation in fat intake. Some nurses simply are more diligent about choosing low-fat animal products.

Many people would consider the low-fat meal to be a triumph of healthy meal planning, but what about the other nutrients in these meals? What about protein and cholesterol? *As it turns out, the low-fat meal contains more than double the protein of the high-fat meal, and almost all of it comes from animal-based foods. In addition, the low-fat meal contains almost twice as much cholesterol* (Chart 14.5).[14,15]

An overwhelming amount of scientific information suggests that diets high in animal-based protein can have unfavorable health consequences, as can diets high in cholesterol. In the low-fat meal, the amount of both of these unhealthy nutrients is significantly *higher*.

Chart 14.5: Nutrient Contents of Two Sample Meals

	Low-Fat Meal #1	High-Fat Meal #2
Fat (percent of total calories)	22%	54%
Protein (percent of total calories)	36%	16%
Percentage of total protein derived from animal-based foods	93%	86%
Cholesterol	307	165

FAT VERSUS ANIMAL FOOD

When women in America, such as those in the Nurses' Health Study and the billion-dollar[4] Women's Health Trial,[16-19] reduce their fat intake, they *do not* do it by reducing their consumption of animal-based foods. Instead, they use low-fat and nonfat animal products, along with less fat during cooking and at the table. Thus, they are not adopting the diets that were shown, in the international correlation studies and in our rural China study, to be associated with low breast cancer rates.

This is a very important discrepancy, and is illustrated by the correlation between the consumption of dietary animal protein and dietary fat for a group of countries (Chart 14.6).[8,9,18,20-22] The most reliable comparison was published in 1975[20]; it showed a highly convincing correlation of more than 90%. This means that as fat intake goes up in various countries, animal protein intake increases in an almost perfectly parallel manner. Likewise, in the China Study, the intakes of fat and animal protein also show a similar correlation of 84%.[8,21]

In the Nurses' Health Study, this is not the case. The correlation between animal protein and total fat intake is only about 16%.[9] In the Women's Health Trial, also including American women, it is even worse, at –17%[18,21,22]; as fat goes down, animal protein goes up. This practice is typical of American women who have been led to believe that, by decreasing their fat intake, they are changing to a healthier diet. A nurse consuming a "low-fat" diet in the Harvard study, like American women everywhere, is likely to continue eating large amounts of animal protein, as shown in meal #1 (Chart 14.4).

Sadly, this evidence on the effects of animal-based food on cancer and other diseases of affluence has been ignored, even maligned, as we continue to focus on fat and other nutrients in isolation. Because of this, the Nurses'

Health Study and virtually every other human epidemiological study published to date have been seriously shortchanged in their investigations of diet and disease associations. Virtually all the subjects under study consume the very diet that causes diseases of affluence. If one kind of animal-based food is substituted for another, then the adverse health effects of both foods, when compared to plant-based food, are easily missed. To make matters worse, these studies often focus on the consumption of just one nutrient, such as fat. Because of these very serious flaws, these studies have been a virtual disaster for discovering the really significant effects of diet on these diseases.

Chart 14.6: Percent Correlations of Total Fat and Animal Protein Consumption

THE $100(+) MILLION RESULTS

So now that you know how I interpret the Nurses' Health Study and its flaws, we should take a look at its conclusions. After more than $100 million and decades of work, there is no shortage of results. So what are they? The logical place to start is, of course, the question of whether fat intake really is linked to breast cancer. Here are some of the findings, cited verbatim:

- "these data provide evidence against both an adverse influence of fat intake and a protective effect of fiber consumption by middle-aged women on breast cancer incidence over eight years."[23] *Translation: The Nurses' Health Study did not detect a relationship between dietary fat and fiber and breast cancer risk.*

- "we found no evidence that lower intake of total fat or specific major types of fat was associated with decreased risk of breast cancer."[10]

Translation: The Nurses' Health Study did not detect a relationship between reducing fat, whether it is total fat or certain kinds of fat, and breast cancer risk.

- "existing data, however, provide little support for the hypothesis that reduction in dietary fat composition, even to 20% of energy during adulthood, will lead to a substantial reduction in breast cancer in Western cultures"[24]
  Translation: The Nurses' Health Study did not detect a breast cancer association with fat even when women reduced their fat consumption all the way down to 20% of calories.

- "relative risks for . . . monounsaturated and polyunsaturated fat . . . were close to unity"[25]
  Translation: The Nurses' Health Study did not detect a relationship between these "good" fats and breast cancer risk.

- "we found no significant associations between intake of meat and dairy products and risk of breast cancer"[26]
  Translation: The Nurses' Heath Study did not detect a relationship between meat and dairy consumption and breast cancer risk.

- "our findings do not support a link between physical activity, in late adolescence or in the recent past, and breast cancer risk among young adult women"[27]
  Translation: The Nurses' Health Study did not detect a relationship between exercise and breast cancer risk.

- "these data are suggestive of only a weak positive association with substitution of saturated fat for carbohydrate consumption; none of the other types of fat examined was significantly associated with breast cancer risk relative to an equivalent reduction in carbohydrate consumption"[28]
  Translation: The Nurses' Health Study detected little or no effect on breast cancer when women substituted fat for carbohydrates.

- "selenium intake later in life is not likely to be an important factor in the etiology of breast cancer"[29]
  Translation: The Nurses' Health Study did not detect a protective effect of selenium on breast cancer risk.

- "these results suggest that fruit and vegetable consumption during adulthood is not significantly associated with reduced breast cancer risk."[30]
Translation: The Nurses' Health Study did not detect a relationship between fruits and vegetables and breast cancer risk.

So there it is, readers. Breast cancer risk does not rise with increased intakes of fat, meat, dairy, or saturated fat. Breast cancer is not prevented by increased intakes of fruits and vegetables, or reduced by exercise (either during the teenage years or during adulthood), dietary fiber, monounsaturated fats, or polyunsaturated fats. Also, the mineral selenium, long considered to be protective against certain cancers, has no effect on breast cancer. *In other words, we might as well conclude that diet is completely unrelated to breast cancer.*

I can understand the frustration of Professor Meir Stampfer, one of the leading researchers in this group, when he was quoted as saying, "This has been our greatest failure and disappointment—that we have not learned more about what people can do to lower their risk."[6] He was making his comment in response to an opinion that "the single biggest challenge for the future [is] sorting out the mess of contradictory findings and lack of information on breast cancer."[6] I applaud Professor Stampfer for his candor, but it's unfortunate that so much money has been spent to learn so little. Perhaps the most rewarding finding, ironically, was the demonstration that tinkering with one nutrient at a time, while maintaining the same overall dietary patterns, does not lead to better health or to better health information.

Despite these challenges, Harvard researchers have been steadily cranking out their findings. Here are some from their slew of studies that I would consider as very troubling contradictions when comparing disease risks for men versus women:

- Men who consume alcohol three or four times a week have a lower heart attack risk.[31]
- Men with Type 2 diabetes who consume a moderate amount of alcohol have a lower risk of coronary heart disease.[32]

And yet . . .

- Alcohol consumption increases breast cancer incidence by 41% for women consuming 30–60 g/day of alcohol compared to non-drinking women.[33]

Apparently alcohol is good for heart disease and bad for breast cancer. The husband can have a drink with dinner but should never share it with his wife. Is this a difference between men and women, or is this a difference in response between heart disease and cancer? Do you feel more informed or more confused?

Then there are those wonderful omega-3 fatty acids. Some types of fish contain relatively large amounts of these fats and have been getting their share of positive press these days. If you've heard anything about omega-3 fatty acids, it's that you need more of them to be healthy. Again, more Harvard findings:

- ". . . contrary to the predominant hypothesis, we found an increased risk of breast cancer associated with omega-3 fat from fish" (This increased risk was statistically significant and was associated with an increase of only 0.1% of the total dietary energy.)[10]
- "our findings suggest that eating fish once per month or more can reduce the risk of ischemic stroke in men"[34]
- "data suggest that consumption of fish at least once per week may reduce the risk of sudden cardiac death in men [but not reduce the] risk of total myocardial infarction, non-sudden cardiac death or total cardiovascular mortality."[35] (In other words, fish may prevent some aspects of heart disease but ultimately has no effect on mortality from heart disease, or even heart attack risk.)

Is this yet another question of deciding which disease you fear the least? Or is this another man versus woman difference?

Here's an even older story: We have been warned for a long time to cut down on our cholesterol intake, and it was largely for this reason that consumption of eggs was brought into question. One egg has a whopping 200 mg or more of cholesterol,[36] which takes up a large proportion of our 300 mg recommended daily limit. So, what do the Harvard studies tell us on this timeworn issue?

> . . . consumption of up to one egg per day is unlikely to have substantial overall impact on the risk of [coronary heart disease] or stroke among healthy men and women[37]

But, for breast cancer,

> Our findings [representing eight prospective studies] suggest a possible modest increase in [breast cancer] risk with egg consumption . . . breast cancer risk was found to increase by 22%

with every 100-g per day increment of egg consumption [about two eggs]. [26] *[There was a 67% increase in risk for the Nurses' Health Study.]*[26]

But earlier, the Harvard researchers took a slightly different position:

. . . among healthy men and women, moderate egg consumption can be part of a nutritious and balanced diet[38]

The Nurses' Health Study then came up with an even more powerful endorsement for eggs. As a news item stated:

Eating eggs during adolescence could protect women against breast cancer . . .[39]

The article goes on to quote a Harvard researcher as saying:

Women who had, during adolescence, a higher consumption of eggs . . . had a lower risk of breast cancer . . .[39]

Most people who read this news article will likely say that eggs are back in favor—even when they don't know how many eggs per day are okay or whether there are exceptions to this generalization. Eggs will only seem to be more healthful when the henhouse industry adds their words of wisdom. But wait a minute—evidence says egg consumption for teenage girls is okay, maybe even good, but evidence also says more egg consumption overall increases breast cancer risk. By the way, here's something else to think about. Multiple studies have rather consistently shown that egg consumption can increase colon cancer risk, more so for women than for men.[40]

What are we to believe? One minute alcohol intake can reduce our disease risks, the next minute it can increase them. One minute fish consumption can help to reduce our disease risks, the next minute it can hurt. One minute eggs are bad, the next minute they can be healthy. It seems to me that what is missing here is the larger context. What you have without that context is just a lot of confusion.

UNRAVELING DIET AND CANCER

In addition to stating that diet and exercise are unrelated to breast cancer, the Harvard researchers have been chipping away at other popular notions regarding diet and cancer. For example, the Harvard studies have not been able to detect any association between colorectal cancer and fiber or fruit and vegetable intake.[4,41,42]

Dietary fiber, of course, only comes from plant-based foods; thus these findings put a dent in the idea that fiber or fruits, vegetables, and cereals prevent large bowel cancer. Keep in mind that the Harvard studies are dealing with uniformly carnivorous populations, almost none of which are using a whole foods, plant-based (WFPB) diet that is naturally low in fat and high in fiber. It is likely that the potential protective effect of fiber or fruits and vegetables does not kick in against colorectal cancer until there is a complete dietary shift away from an animal-based diet.

Between the colon cancer and breast cancer findings, the Nurses' Health Study has done much to confuse, if not discredit, the idea that diet is related to cancer. After these decades of work, Professor Walt Willett says:

> . . . *increasing fruits and vegetables overall appears to be less promising as a way to substantially reduce cancer risk . . . the benefits [of these foods] appear greater for cardiovascular disease than for cancer.*[4]

This statement sounds a bit ominous. Colon cancer, historically one of the first cancers said to be prevented by a plant-based diet,[43–45] now is being described as unrelated to diet? And low-fat diets don't prevent breast cancer? With results like these, it's only a matter of time before the hypothesis of a dietary connection to cancer starts falling apart. In fact, I have already heard people within the scientific community beginning to say that diet may have no effect on cancer.

These are the reasons that I believe that the Nurses' Health Study has done considerable damage to the nutrition landscape. It has virtually nullified many of the advances that have been made over the past fifty years without actually posing a scientifically reliable challenge to earlier findings regarding diet and cancer.

This problem of studying a population that uniformly consumes a high-risk diet and looking at the differences in consumption one nutrient at a time is not unique to the Nurses' Health Study. It is common to virtually all studies using Western subjects. Furthermore, there is little or no value to pooling the results of many large studies for analysis in order to get a more reliable result if all the studies have the same flaw. A pooling strategy is often used for identifying cause-and-effect associations that are more subtle and uncertain within single studies. This is a reliable assumption when each study is properly done, but obviously not when all the studies are similarly flawed. The combined results only give a more reliable picture of the flaw.

The Harvard researchers have done several of these multi-study pooled analyses. One such pooled analysis concerned the question of whether meat and dairy foods had any effect on breast cancer.[26] A previous 1993 pooling of nineteen studies[46] had shown a modest, statistically significant 18% increase in breast cancer risk with increased meat intake and 17% increase with increased milk intake.[46] The Harvard researchers therefore summarized in 2002 a more recent group of studies, this time including eight large prospective studies where dietary information was thought to be more reliable and where a much larger group of women was included. The researchers concluded:

> We found no significant association between intake of meat or dairy products and risk of breast cancer.[26]

Most people would say, "Well, that's it. There is no convincing evidence that meat and dairy foods are associated with breast cancer risk." But let's take another look at this supposedly more sophisticated analysis.

All eight of these studies represented diets that had a high proportion of animal-based foods. In effect, each study in this pool was subject to the same flaw from which the Nurses' Health Study suffered. It makes no sense, and does no good, to combine them. In spite of there being 351,041 women and 7,379 breast cancer cases in this mega-database, these results cannot detect the true effect of diets rich in meat and dairy on breast cancer risk. This would be true even if there were a few million subjects in the study. Like the Nurses' Health Study, these studies all involved typical Western diets highly skewed toward the consumption of animal-based foods, where people are tinkering with the intake of only one nutrient or one food at a time. Every study failed to take into account a broader range of dietary choices—including those that demonstrated positive effects on breast cancer risk in the past.

IGNORING MY CRITIQUE

Once, after reading a publication on animal protein and heart disease in the Nurses' Health Study,[9] I published a critique[47] summarizing some of the same points that I am making in this chapter, including the inability of the Nurses' Health Study to advance our understanding of the original international correlation studies. The lead authors responded, and our exchange is as follows.

First, my comment:

*Within a dietary range [so rich in animal-based foods], it makes
no sense to me that it is possible to reliably detect the so-called
independent associations of the individual constituents of this group
when it can be expected that they share the same disease outcomes
and when there are so many difficult-to-measure and interacting
risk factor exposures. When will it be understood that it is the total
diet and the aggregate and comprehensive effects of large food
groups that make the greatest contribution to the maintenance
of health and prevention of disease? The sort of reductionism
embodied in the interpretation of data from this [Nurses' Health
Study] cohort runs the risk of severely misleading discourse on
meaningful public health and public policy programs.*[47]

Then the response from Dr. Hu and Professor Willett:

*Although we agree that overall dietary patterns are also
important in determining disease risk (ref. cited), we believe
that identification of associations with individual nutrients
should be the first step because it is the specific compounds
or groups of compounds that are fundamentally related to the
[disease process]. Specific components of diet can be modified,
and individuals and the food industry are actively doing so.
Understanding the health effects of specific dietary changes,
which Campbell refers to as "reductionism," is therefore an
important undertaking.*[48]

I agree that studying the independent effects of individual food substances (their identities, functions, mechanisms) is worthwhile, but Willett
and I sharply disagree with how to interpret and use these findings.

I strongly reject the implications in Willett's argument that "specific
components of the diet can be modified" to the benefit of one's health. This
is precisely what is wrong with this area of research. In fact, if the Nurses'
Health Study shows nothing else, it demonstrates that modifying the intake
of one nutrient at a time, without questioning whole dietary patterns, does
not confer significant health benefits. Women who tinker with fat, while
maintaining a near-carnivorous diet, do not have a lower breast cancer risk.

This gets to the heart of reductionism in science. As long as scientists
study highly isolated chemicals and food components, and take the information out of context to make sweeping assumptions about complex diet

and disease relationships, confusion will result. Misleading news headlines about this or that food chemical and this or that disease will be the norm. The more impressive message about the benefits of broad dietary change will be muted as long as we focus on relatively trivial details.

On occasion, when our paths have crossed, Professor Willett and I have had discussions about the findings on fat as they relate to the China Study and the Nurses' Health Study. I have always made the same point: WFPB diets, naturally low in fat, are not included in the Nurses' Health Study cohort, and that it is these types of diets that are the most beneficial for our health. Professor Willett has said to me, in response, on more than one occasion, "You may be right, Colin, but people don't want to go there." This comment has disturbing implications.

Scientists should not be ignoring ideas just because we perceive that the public does not want to hear them. Too often during my career, I have heard comments that seem to be more of an attempt to please the public than to engage in an open, honest debate, wherever it may take us. This is wrong. The role of science in a society is to observe, to ask questions, to form and test hypotheses, and to interpret the findings without bias—not to kowtow to people's perceived desires. Consumers have the ultimate choice of whether to integrate our findings into their lifestyles, but we owe it to them to give them the best information possible with which to make that decision and not decide for them. It is they who paid for this research and it is only they who have the right to decide what to do with it.

The perception in the scientific community that the public only wants magic bullets and simple dietary tinkering is overrated. I have learned in my public lectures that public interest in diet/lifestyle change that really works and is scientifically reliable is greater than some in the academic community are willing to admit.

This method of investigating details out of context, what I call reductionism, and trying to judge complex relationships from the results, is deadly. It is even more damaging than the misbehavior of the small minority of scientists I discussed in chapter thirteen. Unfortunately, this flawed way of investigating nutrition has become the norm. As a consequence, honest, hardworking, well-intentioned scientists around the world are trapped into making judgments about whole-diet effects on the basis of individual nutrient studies—because that is where the funding is. The greatest danger is that reductionism science, standing naked from its larger environment, has come to be the gold standard. Indeed, I know many researchers who would even say that this is what defines "good" science.

These problems are especially egregious in the investigation of vitamin supplements. As I noted at the beginning of the chapter, I spent over three

years during the early history of the nutrient supplement business developing testimony for the Federal Trade Commission and the NAS in their court
case against General Nutrition, Inc. I argued that specific health benefits for
chronic diseases could not be claimed for isolated vitamins and minerals
in supplement form. For this, I took a lot of heat from my colleagues who
believed otherwise. Now, more than twenty-five years later, after hundreds
of millions of dollars of research funding and billions of dollars of consumer
spending, we have this conclusion from a survey of the evidence:

> *The U.S. Preventive Services Task Force . . . concludes that
> the evidence is insufficient to recommend for or against the
> use of supplements of A, C or E; multivitamins with folic acid;
> or antioxidant combinations for the prevention of cancer or
> cardiovascular disease.*[49,50]

How many more billions of dollars must be spent before we understand
the limitations of reductionist research? The endless stream of confusion
generated by the misinterpretation of the findings of reductionist research
undermines not only the entire science of nutrition, but also the health of
America.

AN OPPORTUNITY FOR A TURNING POINT?

This is where this chapter ended in the first edition: with a warning about the
consequences of reductionism in science. While that warning still holds, a
lot has happened in the last decade, including the clarification regarding my
own thinking that led to the writing of *Whole* (as in *wholism*, reductionism's
opposite—the concept of the whole being greater than the sum of its parts),
as well as *The Low-Carb Fraud*, which elaborates on how an emphasis on
reductionism can lead to the idea that carbohydrate is the singular cause of
diseases like heart disease, diabetes, and cancer, thus ignoring the infinite
complexity of nutrition and its effect on the infinitely complex biology of our
bodies. I am increasingly enthusiastic about initiating a conversation on the
conflict between reductionism and wholism because it helps to explain nutrition as a scientific discipline, and to understand the emphasis on drugs in
medical practice and the workings of contemporary scientific research itself.
    I did not personally create the concept of wholism. It has long been used,
by many scholars and laypeople, to describe the content and characteristics
of a wide spectrum of topics. But I now realize that the concept of wholism
was becoming prominent for me even during my time as a member of the

1982 NAS panel that produced the *Diet, Nutrition, and Cancer* report that began this chapter. Two of its messages especially prompted my interest in the singular, reductionist effects of nutrients: the committee's interest in the reported effect of dietary fat (especially saturated fat) on cancer, and the inferences on the effects of *individual* nutrients (e.g., vitamins) on cancer. Both presumed the importance of single-nutrient effects on one's health, such as the subtraction of dietary fat or the addition of micronutrients. These messages, one intended by our committee (reduction of dietary fat) and the other not (nutrient supplementation), offered me unusual insight into how we establish our research priorities and how this information is provided to, and used by, the public in the marketplace.

Ten years later, I remain ambivalent both about our NAS report and many of the reductionism-oriented studies its findings led to, including the Nurses' Health Study—which continues to this day, now in its third generation of nurses. Without question, this study has been the most productive diet and health study ever conducted, with a vast collection of well-written professional reports. My original concern, however, remains. To my knowledge, all of these nurses (238,000+, depending on which individual records are selected for analysis) still consume typical American diets,[51] high in total fat, higher than average in protein, low in fruit and vegetable consumption, and high in animal products. Virtually none of these nurses appear to consume a WFPB diet like that described here, nor are they made aware of its benefits.

In 2015 researchers involved in the Nurses' Health Study published a review[52] of the advantages and disadvantages of varied epidemiological study designs. Although it is an excellent summary, it still refuses to even acknowledge the existence of a WFPB diet despite the recent growth in its prominence, leading me to still conclude, as Professor Willett previously suggested to me, "people don't want to go there." Interestingly, much of the evidence in this Harvard summary may even support the benefits of the WFPB diet, but because individual nutrient associations mostly exist as fragments that are not merged into a larger dietary perspective, this support is hard to discern.

The evidence against supplement use has also continued to grow during this past decade.[53] According to *The Economist*, in 2015 there were 85,000 kinds of "pills, powders and elixirs in America alone."[53] It is difficult to know the size of the market, depending on who reports the estimate; the industry estimate is $37 billion[54] but this has been challenged as inflated,[55] and a much more conservative estimate says $12 billion.[55] *The Economist* says supplement sales were $88 billion worldwide in 2014. Part of this disparity depends on which dietary supplement group is included in the estimate. Regardless of what is the best estimate, it is a huge industry that has grown continuously since the first edition of this book.[53] Yet, during this same period, still more studies have found varied nutrient supplements to have no effect or even increase disease risk. A meta-analysis of 89 studies found that "omega 3 fats [found in fish oil] do not have a clear effect on total mortality, combined cardiovascular events, or cancer."[56] Although not statistically significant, "clinically important harm [cancer risk] could not be excluded." And in a study of 195,000 individuals followed for 14–18 years that resulted in 9,380 Type 2 diabetes cases, higher consumption of long-chain omega-3 fat supplements was highly significantly associated with *increased* risk of disease. (Interestingly, even fish as a source of long-chain omega-3 fats was significantly associated with *increased* disease risk.)

The researchers for the women-based Nurses' Health Study and the men-based Physicians' Health Study published a series of papers in 2009 on the health effects of nutrient supplements on their subjects that mostly showed the same lack of benefit, except for some cases where there was *increased* disease risk. Vitamin E and C supplementation did not reduce the risk of prostate or total cancer,[57] and had no beneficial effect on the risk of cataracts[58]; multivitamin supplementation barely reduced cataracts and had no effect on macular degeneration,[59] cardiovascular events, and total mortality,[60] or total cancer;[61] and vitamins C and E had no effects on total cancers, prostate cancer, or other site-specific cancers.[62] (The reasons for these studies mostly arose from associations observed for consuming these vitamins in whole food, but isolating them from their food context does not give the same effects.) I also am not impressed with any findings so far regarding vitamin D supplementation for the prevention or treatment of chronic disease, including a study on its effects on breast cancer.[63] The only benefit that might be significant in the recent series of vitamin D supplement studies is the minimal (only 14%) reduction of colorectal adenoma.[64]

These research findings, along with other, similar findings during the last ten years, tell us two important things: First, a huge amount of research money has been spent seeking the hoped-for benefits of nutrient supplements over a relatively short period of time. And second, few if any benefits have been demonstrated—some supplements even *increased* disease risk.

In a way, I'm glad this research was done. It means we now have clear evidence that the hoped-for health benefits of nutrient supplements are not forthcoming. But what a waste of money, spent on selling nonsense! It is abundantly clear to me that the vitamin supplement industry has nothing to do with science and everything to do with marketing—nothing to do with the health for the many and everything to do with wealth for the few. And in the process, this focus on supplemental nutrition has detracted from efforts to develop sound whole-food nutrition information for the public, which would have taken far less cost and had far greater improvements in health.

THE "SCIENCE"
OF INDUSTRY

15

W hat does every American spend money on several times a day? Eating. After a lifetime of eating, what do we all do? Die—a process that usually involves large costs as we try to postpone it for as long as possible. We're all customers of hunger and death, so there's a lot of money to be spent and made.

Because of this, the food and health industries in America are among the most influential organizations in the world. The revenue they generate is staggering; many individual food companies have over $10 billion in annual revenues. Kraft has revenues of roughly $18 billion a year. The Danone Group, an international dairy company based in France, operates the Dannon brand and has revenues of almost $25 billion a year. And of course, there are the large fast-food companies. McDonald's has revenues in excess of $25 billion a year, and Wendy's International generates almost $4 billion a year. *Total food expenditures, including food bought by individuals, government, and business, were $1.24 trillion in 2010.*[1]

The massive drug company Pfizer had $48 billion in revenue in 2015, while Eli Lilly & Co. chalked up over $23 billion. Johnson and Johnson collected over $70 billion from selling their products. As of 2010, over $1 *trillion* has been riding on what we choose to eat and how we choose to treat sickness and promote health. That's a lot of money.

Powerful players are competing for your food and health dollars. Individual companies, of course, do what they can to sell more of their products, but there are also industry groups that work to increase general demand for their products. The National Dairy Council, National Dairy Promotion and Research Board, National Fluid Milk Processor Promotion Board, International Sprout Growers Association, American Meat Institute, Florida Citrus

Processors Association, and United Egg Producers are examples of such industry groups. These organizations, operating independently of any single company, wield significant influence—the most powerful among them have yearly budgets in the hundreds of millions of dollars.

These food companies and associations use whatever methods they can to enhance their products' appeal and grow their market. One way to accomplish this is to claim nutritional benefits for the food products they sell. At the same time, these companies and associations must protect their products from being considered unhealthy. If a product is linked to cancer or some other disease, profits and revenue will evaporate. Food business interests need to claim that their product is good for you, or, at least, that it's not bad for you. In this process, the "science" of nutrition becomes the "business" of marketing.

THE AIRPORT CLUB

While I was getting the China Project off the ground, I learned of a committee of seven prominent research scientists who had been retained by the animal-based foods industry (the National Dairy Council and the American Meat Institute) to keep tabs on any research projects in the U.S. likely to cause harm to their industry. I knew six of the seven members, four of them quite well. A graduate student of mine was visiting with one of these scientists and was given a file on the committee activity. I have never learned exactly why the file passed hands. Perhaps the scientist's conscience was getting the better of him. In any case, the file was ultimately given to me.

The file contained minutes of committee meetings, the latest being held at Chicago's O'Hare Airport. From then on, I have called this group of scientists "The Airport Club." It was run by Professors E. M. Foster and Michael Pariza, faculty members of the University of Wisconsin (where Alf Harper was located), and was funded by the meat and dairy industry. This committee's main objective was to have members observe projects that might do "harm" to their industry. With such surveillance, the industry could more effectively respond to unexpected discoveries from researchers that might make otherwise unanticipated news. I had learned well that, when the stakes are high, industry was not averse to putting its own spin on a story.

They listed about nine potentially damaging projects, and I had the dubious distinction of being the only researcher responsible for two of them. I was named once for the China Project, which one of the members was assigned to watch over, and once for my association with the American Institute for Cancer Research (AICR), especially my chairing of the review panel that decided which research applications on diet and cancer got funded. Another panel member had the task of keeping an eye on the AICR activity.

After learning of The Airport Club, and of the individual assigned to watch over me at the AICR grant meetings, I was in a position to see how his spying was going to unfold. I went into the first AICR review panel meeting after learning of the Club with an eye on the spy who was keeping an eye on me!

One might argue that this industry-funded "spying" was not illegal, and that it is prudent for a business to keep tabs on potentially damaging information that might affect its future. I agree completely, even if it was disconcerting to find myself on the list of those being spied on. But industry does more than just keep tabs on "dangerous" research. It actively markets its version, regardless of potentially disastrous health effects, and corrupts the integrity of the science to do so. This is especially troubling when academic scientists do the spying and hide their intentions.

POWERFUL GROUPS

The dairy industry, one of the sponsors of The Airport Club, is particularly powerful in this country. Founded in 1915, the well-organized, well-funded National Dairy Council has been promoting milk for over a hundred years.[2] In 1995, two major milk industry groups put a new face on their old establishment, renaming it Dairy Management, Inc. The purpose of this new group was "to do one thing: increase demand for U.S.-produced dairy products," to quote their website.[3] They had a 2003 marketing budget of more than $165 million to do it.[4] In comparison, the National Watermelon Promotion Board has a budget of $1.6 million.[5] A Dairy Management, Inc., press release includes the following items[4]:

> Rosemont, Illinois—National, state and regional dairy producer directors have approved a budget of $165.7 million for a 2003 Unified Marketing Plan (UMP) designed to help increase dairy demand....
> ... Major program areas include:
> Fluid Milk: In addition to key ongoing activities in advertising, promotion and public relations efforts targeted to children ages six to twelve and their mothers, 2003 dairy checkoff efforts will focus on developing and extending partnerships with major food marketers, including Kellogg's*, Kraft foods* and McDonald's*...

. . . School Marketing: As part of an effort to guide school-age children to become life-long consumers of dairy products, 2003 activities will target students, parents, educators and school food-service professionals. Programs are underway in both the classroom and the lunchroom, where dairy checkoff organizations look to widen the success of last year's School Milk Pilot Test . . .

. . . Dairy Image/Confidence: This ongoing program area aims to protect and enhance consumer confidence in dairy products and the dairy industry. A major component involves conducting and communicating the results of dairy nutrition research showing the healthfulness of dairy products, as well as issues and crisis management . . .

If I may paraphrase the dairy industry's efforts: their goals are to 1) market to young children and their mothers; 2) use schools as a channel to young customers; 3) conduct and publicize research favorable to the industry.

Many people are not aware of the dairy industry's presence in our schools. But make no mistake: on nutrition information, the dairy industry reaches young children more effectively than any other industry. It has enlisted the public education system as the primary vehicle for increasing demand for its products. The 2001 Dairy Management, Inc., annual report stated[6]:

As the best avenue to increase fluid milk consumption long-term, children are without a doubt the future of dairy consumption. That's why the dairy checkoff continues to implement school milk marketing programs as one way to help increase kids' fluid milk consumption.

Dairy producers . . . launched two groundbreaking initiatives in 2001. A yearlong school milk research program that began in the fall of 2001 examines how improved packaging, additional flavors, coolers with merchandising and better temperature regulation can affect fluid milk consumption and kids' attitudes toward milk both in and out of school. The study concludes at the end of the 2001–02 school year. Also, dairy producers and processors worked together to conduct a five-month vending study in middle and high schools in five major U.S. markets. The study revealed that many students would choose milk over competitive beverages if it were available when, where and how they wanted.

Many other successful school programs continue to encourage children to drink milk. Nutrition education programs, such as "Pyramid Explorations" and "Pyramid Café," teach students that dairy products are a key part of a healthy diet; the "Cold Is Cool" program teaches school cafeteria managers how to keep milk cold, just how kids like it; and the checkoff is helping expand dairy-friendly school breakfast programs. In addition, the popular "Got Milk?" campaign continues to reach children at school and through such kid-focused media outlets as Nickelodeon and the Cartoon Network.

These activities are far from small-scale; in 1999, "Chef Combo's Fantastic Adventures," an "educational" (marketing) set of lesson plans produced by the dairy industry, "was placed in 76% of preschool kindergarten sites nationally."[7] According to a dairy industry report to Congress,[8] the dairy industry's "nutrition education" programs are doing quite well:

> "Pyramid Cafe®" and "Pyramid Explorations™," targeted to second and fourth grades, reach over 12 million students with messages that milk and dairy products are a key part of a healthy diet. Survey results continue to show a very high utilization rate for these two programs, currently at over 70% of the instructors that have the programs.

America is entrusting the important task of educating our children about nutrition and health to the dairy industry. In addition to ubiquitous nutrition lesson plans and "educational" kits, the industry supplies high schools with videos, posters, and teaching guides regarding nutrition; it runs special promotions in cafeterias to increase milk consumption in thousands of schools; it distributes information to principals at national conferences; it runs back-to-school promotions with over 20,000 schools; and it runs sports promotions targeted toward youth.

Should we be worried? In a word, yes. If you are curious as to what kind of "education" is being taught by the dairy industry, take a look at their website.[9] When I visited the site in July 2003, one of the first bits of information to greet me was, "July is National Ice Cream Month." Upon clicking for more information on National Ice Cream Month, I read, "If you're wondering if you can have your ice cream and good nutrition too, the answer is 'yes'!"[9] Great. So much for combating childhood obesity and diabetes!

The website is divided into three sections, one for educators, one for parents, and one for food service professionals. When I looked at the site in July 2003 (it regularly changes its content), in the educator portion of the site, teachers could download lesson plans to teach nutrition to their classrooms. Lesson plans included making hand puppets of cows and dairy foods and doing a finger play. Once the puppets are made, the teacher should "[t]ell the students they're going to meet five special friends, and these friends want boys and girls to grow up to be strong and healthy."[9] Another lesson was "Dairy Treat Day," where each child gets to taste cheese, pudding, yogurt, cottage cheese, and ice cream.[9] Or teachers could lead their classes in making "Moo Masks."[9] For the more advanced fourth grader, teachers could do a lesson plan from Pyramid Explorations in which students explore the five food groups, and their health benefits, as follows[9]:

Milk Group (Build strong bones and teeth.)
Meat Group (Build strong muscles.)
Vegetable Group (Help you see in the dark.)
Fruit Group (Help heal cuts and bruises.)
Grain Group (Give us energy.)

Based on the evidence presented in the previous chapters, you know that if this is what our children are learning about nutrition and health, then we are in for a painful journey, courtesy of Dairy Management, Inc. Obviously neither kids nor their parents are learning about how milk has been linked to Type 1 diabetes, prostate cancer, osteoporosis, multiple sclerosis, or other autoimmune diseases, and how casein, the main protein in dairy foods, has been shown to experimentally promote cancer and increase blood cholesterol and atherosclerotic plaque.

In 2002, this marketing website delivered over 70,000 lesson plans to educators.[8] The dairy industry truly is teaching its version of nutrition to the next generation of Americans.

The industry has been doing this for decades, and it has been successful. I have encountered many people who, when they hear about the potential adverse effects of dairy foods, immediately say, "Milk can't be bad." Usually these people don't have any evidence to support their position; they just have a feeling that milk is good. They've always known it to be that way, and they like it that way. You can trace some of their opinions back to their school days, when they learned that there are seven continents, two plus two equals four, and milk is healthy. If you think about it this way, you will understand why the dairy industry has had such exceptional influence in this country by using education for its marketing purposes.

If this marketing program weren't such a widespread threat to our children's health, it would be downright laughable that an industry group would try to peddle its food product under such a thinly veiled "education" plan. Don't people wonder what's going on when almost every single children's book advertised in the "Nutrition Bookshelf" portion of this website revolved around either milk, cheese, or ice cream, with such titles as *Ice Cream: Great Moments in Ice Cream History*?[9] After all, during July 2003, there were no vegetable books anywhere to be found on this "Nutrition Bookshelf"! Aren't they healthy?

At least when the dairy industry describes all of these school-related activities in the official reports to Congress and in industry press releases, it rightly refers to them as "marketing" activities.

CONJUGATED LINOLEIC ACID

The dairy industry doesn't stop with kids. For adults, the industry puts a heavy emphasis on "science" and the communication of research results that might be construed as showing health benefits from eating dairy foods. The dairy industry spends $4 to $5 million a year to fund research toward the goal of finding something healthy to talk about.[7,10] In addition, the dairy industry promoters employ a Medical Advisory Board made up of doctors, academics, and other health professionals. These scientists are the ones who appear as medical professionals in the media, providing science-based statements supporting the health benefits of milk.

The Airport Club was a good example of industry efforts to maintain favorable product image and "confidence." In addition to keeping an eye on potentially damaging projects, the Club was trying to generate research that might show that cancer could be prevented by drinking cow's milk. What a coup that would be! At that time, the industry was getting quite edgy about the growing evidence showing that the consumption of animal-based foods is associated with cancer and related ailments.

Their hook for this research was an unusual group of fatty acids produced by bacteria in the cow's rumen (the biggest of the four stomachs). These fatty acids were collectively called conjugated linoleic acid (CLA), which is produced from the linoleic acid commonly found in corn that the cow eats. From the cow's rumen, CLA is then absorbed and gets stored in the meat and milk of the animal, eventually to be consumed by humans.

The big payday for The Airport Club was when initial tests on experimental mice suggested that CLA might help to block the formation of stomach tumors produced by a weak chemical carcinogen called benzo(a) pyrene.[11,12] But there was a catch in this research: researchers gave CLA to the mice first, and then gave the carcinogen benzo(a)pyrene. The ordering of these chemical feedings was backwards. In the body there is an enzyme system that works to minimize the amount of cancer caused by a carcinogen. When a chemical such as CLA is initially consumed, it "excites" that enzyme system so that it has increased activity. So the trick was to administer CLA first, to excite the enzyme system, and then administer the carcinogen. In this order, the enzyme system excited by CLA would be more effective at getting rid of the carcinogen. As a result, CLA could be called an anticarcinogen.

Let me give you an analogous situation. Let's say you have a bag of a potent pesticide in your garage. The pesticide bag says, "Do not swallow! In case of ingestion, contact your local poison control health authorities," or some such warning. But let's say you're hungry and you eat a handful of pesticide anyway. That pesticide in your body will "rev up" the enzyme systems in all of your cells that are responsible for eliminating nasty things. If you then go inside and eat a handful of peanuts dripping with aflatoxin, your body's enzyme systems will be primed to deal with the aflatoxin, and you'll end up with fewer aflatoxin-induced tumors. So, the pesticide, which will ultimately do all sorts of nasty things in your body, is an anticarcinogen! This scenario is obviously absurd, and the research on mice that initially showed CLA to be an anticarcinogen was similarly absurd. However, the end results of the mice research sounded pretty good to people who don't know this methodology (including most scientists).

Airport Club member Michael Pariza headed the research that studied CLA in some detail.[13–15] Later, at Roswell Park Memorial Institute for Cancer Research in Buffalo, a very good researcher and his group extended the research still further and demonstrated that it did more than merely block the first step in the formation of tumors. CLA also appeared to slow down subsequent tumor growth[16,17] when fed after the carcinogen. This was a more convincing finding of the anticancer properties of CLA than the initial studies,[11,12] which showed only an inhibition of tumor initiation.

Regardless of how promising these mouse and cow studies were becoming, this research remained two major steps removed from human cancer. First, it had not been shown that cow's milk containing CLA, as a whole food (as opposed to the isolated chemical CLA), prevents cancer in mice. Second, even if such an effect existed in mice, it would need to be confirmed in humans. In fact, as has been discussed earlier in this book, if cow's milk has any effect at all, it has been shown to increase, not decrease, cancer. The far more significant nutrient in milk is protein, whose potent cancer-promoting properties are consistent with the human data.

In other words, to make any health claims regarding CLA in milk and its effect on human cancer would require unreasonably large leaps of faith. But never doubt the tenacity (i.e., money) of those who would like to have the public believe that cow's milk prevents cancer. Lo and behold, a front-page headline in our local newspaper, the *Ithaca Journal*, stated "Changing Cows' Diets Elevates Milk's Cancer-Fighting."[18] This article concerned the studies of a Cornell professor who was instrumental in the development of bovine growth hormone now fed to cows. He showed that he could increase CLA in cow's milk by feeding the animals more corn oil (i.e., linoleic acid, the parent of CLA).

The *Ithaca Journal* article, although only in a local, hometown newspaper, really was a dream come true for the sponsors of The Airport Club. The headline delivers a powerful but very simple message to the public: drinking milk reduces cancer risk. I know that media people like punchy statements so, initially, I suspected that the reporter had made claims beyond what the researchers had said. But in the article the enthusiasm expressed by Professor Bauman for the implications for this research equaled that of the headline. The study cited in this article only showed that CLA is higher in the milk of cows fed corn oil. That's a long way from having any relevance to human cancer. No studies had yet shown that humans or even mice drinking cow's milk had a lower risk of cancer—of any kind. Yet Bauman, who is a technically competent researcher, was quoted as saying that these findings have "good potential because CLA happens to be [a] very potent [anticarcinogen]." The journalist went on to say "CLA has been shown to suppress carcinogens and inhibit the spread of colon, prostate, ovarian and breast cancers and leukemia," and concluded that "all indications are that CLA is effective in humans even in low concentrations." According to the article, Bauman says that this "research represents the new focus on designing foods to enhance their nutritional and health qualities." These claims could not be more dramatic, considering the absence of the necessary human research.

Bauman, Pariza, and their many other colleagues[19] have vigorously pursued this line of research for about fifteen years and have published a large number of research papers. Although additional beneficial effects of CLA are said to exist, the key research still has not been done: namely, testing whether the consumption of milk from cows fed high-corn-oil diets really will reduce human cancer risk.

In addition, Bauman and his colleagues have attempted to take a step toward finding this essential connection. They have shown that the milk fat of cows fed high amounts of natural CLA in corn oil, like synthetic CLA, was able to decrease tumors in rats treated with a carcinogen.[20] But again, they used the tricky experimental method. They administered the milk fat before, not after, the carcinogen. Yet their claims will be as dramatic as ever, because this is the first time that CLA, as present in food (i.e., the fat), is shown to be as anticarcinogenic as the isolated chemical. Translated: eat butter from cows fed corn oil—it prevents cancer!

THE SCIENCE OF INDUSTRY

The CLA story is a good example of how industry uses science to increase demand for its product to make more money. At the very least, industry science often leads to public confusion (Are eggs good? Are they bad?), and at its worst, industry science leads unsuspecting consumers to foods that are actually bad for them, all in the name of better health.

Conflicts of interest abound in this science of industry. The CLA research was created with special-interest money and has grown and been sustained with special-interest money. The National Dairy Council,[20–22] Kraft Foods, Inc.,[20] the Northeast Dairy Foods Research Center,[20,21] the Cattlemen's Beef Board,[23] and the Cattlemen's Beef Association[23] have frequently funded these studies.

Corporate influence in the academic research world can take many forms, ranging from flagrant abuses of personal power to conflicts of interest, all hidden from public view. This influence does not need to be a crass payoff to researchers to fabricate data. That sort of behavior is rare. The more significant way for corporate interests to influence academic research is much more sophisticated and effective. As illustrated by the CLA example, scientists investigate a detail out of context that can be construed as a favorable message and industry exploits it for all it's worth. Almost no one knows where the CLA hypothesis started and who originally funded it.

Few people really question such research if it is published in the best journals. Very few people, especially among the public, know which studies are "benefiting" from direct corporate funding. Very few people are able to sort out the technical details and recognize the missing information that would otherwise establish context. Almost everyone, however, understands that headline in my local newspaper.

I could play this game, too. If I wanted to hurt the dairy industry and be a little wild in my interpretation of study results, I could produce another headline to say, "New birth control chemical discovered in cow's milk." Research has shown, for example, that CLA dramatically kills chick embryos.[13] Also, CLA increases the tissue level of saturated fats that could (using our dramatic method of interpretation) exacerbate heart disease risk. Of course, I have taken these two unrelated effects grossly out of context in my example. I don't really know whether these CLA effects actually translate into less fertility and more heart disease for humans, but if I were playing the game the way industry enthusiasts do, I wouldn't mind. It would make a great headline, and that can go a long way.

I subsequently met with one of the members of The Airport Club, a scientist who has been involved in the CLA effort, and he confessed that the

CLA effect will never be anything more than a drug effect. However, you can bet that what is known in private will not be told in public.

INDUSTRY'S LOVE OF TINKERING

The Airport Club and CLA stories mostly tell a story about the "dark side" of science, which I detailed in chapter thirteen. But the CLA story is also about the dangers of reductionism, of taking details out of context and making claims about diet and health, which I discussed in the previous chapter. Like academia, industry is also an essential player in the system of scientific reductionism that undermines the knowledge we have about dietary patterns and disease. Industry, you see, loves to tinker. Securing patents based on details leads to marketing claims and, ultimately, to greater revenues.

In a 1999 paper[20] by several CLA researchers (including Professor Dale Bauman, a long-time friend of the animal foods industry), the following sentence appeared, revealing much about how some industry enthusiasts feel as we "tinker" our way to health:

The concept of CLA-enriched foods could be particularly appealing to people who desire a diet-based approach to cancer prevention without making radical changes in their eating habits.[20]

I know that, for Bauman and others, "making radical changes in . . . eating habits" means consuming a diet rich in plant-based foods. Rather than avoiding bad foods altogether, these researchers are suggesting that we tinker with the existing, but problematic, foods to correct the problem. Instead of working with nature to maintain health, they want us to rely on technology—their technology.

This faith in technological tinkering, in humans over nature, is ever-present. It is not limited to the dairy industry, or the meat industry, or the processed foods industry. It has become part of every single food and health industry in the country, from oranges to tomatoes, from cereals to vitamin supplements.

The plant food industry got carried away in the early 2000s when another carotenoid was "discovered." You've probably heard of it. It is called lycopene, and it provides the red color in tomatoes. In 1995, it was reported that people who ate more tomatoes, including whole tomatoes and tomato-containing foods like pasta sauces, had a lower risk for prostate cancer,[24] which supported an earlier report.[25]

For those companies that make foods with tomato products, this was a gift from above. Marketing people in the corporate world quickly got the message. But what they zeroed in on was lycopene, not tomatoes. The media, willing to oblige, rose to the occasion. It was lycopene time! Suddenly lycopene became widely known as something to eat more of if you don't want prostate cancer. The scientific world, investigating details, escalated its efforts to decipher the "lycopene magic." As of 2015, the National Library of Medicine listed 3,653 (!) scientific publications on lycopene.[26] A major market is under way, with trade names like Lycopene 10 Cold Water Dispersion and LycoVit 10% to be used as food supplements.[27] If you only listened to their health claims, we might be on the way to bringing prostate cancer, a leading cancer among men, under control.

There are, though, a couple of disquieting thoughts. First, after spending millions of research and development dollars, there is some doubt whether lycopene, as an isolated chemical, can prevent prostate cancer. According to one review publication, six studies now have shown a statistically significant decrease in prostate cancer risk with increased lycopene intake; three nonstatistically significant studies agree; and seven studies show no association.[28] But these studies measured lycopene intake from *whole foods*, namely tomatoes. So, while these studies certainly indicate that the tomato is a healthy food,[28] does that mean we can assume that lycopene, by itself, reduces prostate cancer risk? There are hundreds, even thousands, of chemicals in tomatoes. Do we have evidence that a lycopene pill will do what tomatoes do, especially for those who don't like tomatoes? The answer is no.[29]

Nonetheless, the lycopene business is up and running. In-depth studies are under way to determine the most effective dose of lycopene and whether commercial lycopene preparations are safe (when tested in rats and rabbits, that is).[27] Also, the industry is considering genetically modifying plants for higher levels of lycopene and other carotenoids.[30] It is a real stretch to call this series of lycopene reports legitimate science. In my book, this is what I call technological tinkering and marketing, not science.

Five years before the latest "discovery" of lycopene, a graduate student of mine, Youping He, compared four different carotenoids (beta-carotene, lycopene from tomatoes, canthaxanthin from carrots, and cryptoxanthin from oranges) for their ability to prevent cancer in experimental animals.[31,32] Depending on what we were testing and how we did the test, single carotenoids could have widely ranging potencies. While one carotenoid is potent in one reaction, the same carotenoid is far less potent in another. This variation manifests itself in countless ways involving hundreds of antioxidants and thousands of different reactions, forming a nearly indecipherable network. Consuming one carotenoid at a time in the form of a pill will never be the same as eating the whole food, which provides the natural network of health-supporting nutrients.

And in fact, the most recent research on lycopene has borne this out. According to a May 2016 review of the lycopene research literature (as part of a review of the use of phytochemicals to prevent cancer[33]), there is no convincing evidence that lycopene, in supplemental form, has any significant benefit over just eating a tomato. Indeed, "high doses of lycopene . . . [were] associated with a higher incidence of prostate cancer," and readers were warned that "the use of these supplements should be avoided."[34]

FRUIT CLAIMS

The fruit industry plays this game just like everyone else. For example, when you think of vitamin C, what food product comes to mind? If you don't think of oranges and orange juice, you are unusual. Most of us have heard ad nauseam that oranges are a good source of vitamin C.

This belief, however, is just another result of good marketing. How much do you know, for example, about vitamin C's relationship to diet and disease? Let's start with the basics. Although you probably know that oranges are a good source of vitamin C, you may be surprised to know that many other plant foods have considerably more. One cup of peppers, strawberries, broccoli, or peas all have more. One papaya has as much as four times more vitamin C than one orange.[35]

Beyond the fact that many other foods are better sources of vitamin C, what can we say about the vitamin C that is in oranges? This concerns the ability of the vitamin to act as an antioxidant. How much of the total antioxidant activity in an orange is actually contributed by its vitamin C? Probably not more than 1–2%.[36] Furthermore, measuring antioxidant activity by using "test tube" studies does not represent the same vitamin C activity that takes place in our bodies.

Most of our impressions about vitamin C and oranges are a mixture of conjectures and assumptions about out-of-context evidence. Who first established these assumptions? Orange merchants. Did they justify their assumptions on the basis of careful research? Of course not. Did these assumptions (presented as fact) sound good to the marketing people? Of course they did. Would I eat an orange to get my vitamin C? No. Would I eat an orange because it is a healthy plant food with a complex network of chemicals that almost certainly offer health benefits? Absolutely.

I played a small role in this story a couple of decades ago. In the 1970s and 1980s, I appeared in a television ad for citrus fruits. A New York public relations firm for the Florida Citrus Commission had earlier interviewed me about fruit, nutrition, and health. This interview, unknown to me at the time, was the source of my presence in the ad. I had not seen the ad and I did not get paid for it, but, nonetheless, I was one of the talking heads that helped the Florida Citrus Commission build its case for the vitamin C content of oranges. Why did I do the interview? At that point in my career, I probably thought that the vitamin C in oranges was important, and, regardless of vitamin C, oranges were very healthy foods to eat.

It is very easy for scientists to get caught in the reductionism web of thinking, even if they have other intentions. Not until recently, after a lifetime of research, did I come to realize how damaging it is to take details out of context and to make subsequent claims about diet and health. Industry uses these details extremely well, and the result is public confusion. Every year, it seems, some new product is being touted as the key to good health. The situation is so bad that "health" sections of grocery stores are often stocked more with supplements and special preparations of seemingly magic ingredients than they are with real food. Don't be tricked: the healthiest section of any store is the place where they sell whole fruits and vegetables—the produce section.

Perhaps worst of all, industry corrupts scientific evidence even when its product has been linked to serious health problems. Our kids are often the most coveted targets of their marketing. The American government has passed legislation preventing cigarette and alcohol companies from marketing their products to children. Why have we ignored food? Even though it is accepted that food plays a major role in many chronic diseases, we allow food industries not only to market directly to children, but also to use our publicly funded school systems to do it. The long-term burden of our shortsighted indiscretion is incalculable.

THE MISUSE OF SCIENCE CONTINUES UNABATED

As I return to the topic of science's relationship with industry for this second edition, ten years later, I do not believe it is necessary to regale you with still more stories like those told here, although there is no shortage of them.

The biggest question is not why there are so many of these stories, but why these stories are such a surprise to so many people. Industry has a mandate, first and foremost, to meet the needs of its investors. Almost every industry leader is beholden to their shareholders to make a profitable business. If they fail to reach expectations, there are others ready and willing to take their place. This is Business 101.

But when it comes to the business of health products and their marketing, what sells can't be the most important driver—accuracy and reliability of industry food-health claims is. Industry leaders and their scientists should be ready to answer vital questions about the health benefits of the products they tout: Should side effects be required alongside benefit claims? How serious must a side effect be for it to be listed on a label alongside a health claim? Should the chances of experiencing the side effect be stated? (When the chances of a chemical causing cancer are less than one in a million, for example, we do not have to label it as a carcinogen.) It's difficult, if not impossible, to give definitive answers to these questions. Yet the public tends to want reasonably definite answers—and so marketing offers them, even when they shouldn't.

There is financial pressure to push health claims to their limits—to use science to sell. And as a result, we have a contest between the marketing manager, who is driven to sell, and the scientist, who must be mindful of their reputation. As a scientist, I know this tension all too well, especially from my time as a witness in Federal Trade Commission hearings. The "science" of the marketing manager is seldom my science.

GOVERNMENT: IS IT FOR THE PEOPLE?

16

D uring the past two to three decades, we have acquired substantial evidence that most chronic diseases in America can be partially attributed to bad nutrition. Expert government panels have said it, the surgeon general has said it, and academic scientists have said it. More people die because of the way they eat than from tobacco use, accidents, or any other lifestyle or environmental factor. We know that the incidence of obesity and diabetes is skyrocketing and that Americans' health is slipping away, and we know what to blame: diet. So shouldn't the government be leading us to better nutrition? The government can take no greater action to prevent pain and suffering in this country than to tell Americans unequivocally to eat fewer animal products, fewer highly refined plant products, and more whole, plant-based foods. It is a message soundly based on the breadth and depth of scientific evidence, and the government could make this clear, as it did with cigarettes. Cigarettes kill, and so do these bad foods. *But instead of doing this, the government is saying that animal products—dairy and meat—refined sugar, and fat in your diet are good for you!* The government is turning a blind eye to the evidence as well as to the millions of Americans who suffer from nutrition-related illnesses. The covenant of trust between the U.S. government and the American citizen has been broken. It is not only failing to put out our fires—it is actively fanning the flames.

DIETARY RANGES: THE LATEST ASSAULT

The Food and Nutrition Board (FNB), as part of the Institute of Medicine (IOM) of the National Academy of Sciences, has the responsibility every five years or so to review and update the recommended consumption of individual nutrients. The FNB has been making nutrient recommendations since 1943 when it established a plan for the U.S. Armed Forces that included recommended daily allowances (RDAs) for each individual nutrient.

In the 2002 FNB report,[1] nutrient recommendations were presented as ranges instead of single numbers, as had been the practice. For good health, we are now advised to consume from 45% to 65% of our calories as carbohydrates. There are ranges for fat and protein as well.

A few quotes from the news release announcing this massive 900-plus-page report say it all. Here is the first sentence[2]:

To meet the body's daily energy and nutritional needs while minimizing risk for chronic disease, adults should get 45% to 65% of their calories from carbohydrates, 20% to 35% from fat and 10% to 35% from protein . . .

Further, we find:

. . . added sugars should comprise no more than 25% of total calories consumed. . . . added sugars are those incorporated into foods and beverages during production [and] major sources include candy, soft drinks, fruit drinks, pastries and other sweets.[2]

Let's take a closer look. What are these recommendations really saying? Remember, the news release starts off by stating the report's objective of "minimizing risk for chronic disease."[2] This report says that we can consume a diet containing up to 35% of calories as fat; this is up from the 30% limit of previous reports. It also recommends that we can consume up to 35% of calories as protein; this number is far higher than the suggestion of any other responsible authority.

The last recommendation puts the frosting on the cake, so to speak. We can consume up to 25% of calories as added sugars. Remember, sugars are the most refined type of carbohydrates. In effect, although the report advises that we need a minimum of 45% of calories as carbohydrates, more than half of this amount (i.e., 25%) can be the sugars present in candies, soft drinks, and pastries. The critical assumption of this report is this: the American diet is not only the best there is, but you should now feel free to eat an even richer diet and still be confident that you are "minimizing risk for chronic disease." Forget any words of caution you may find in this report—with such a range of possibilities, virtually any diet can be advocated as minimizing disease risk.

You may have trouble getting your mind around what these figures mean in everyday terms, so I have prepared the following menu plan that supplies nutrients in accordance with these guidelines (Chart 16.1).[3,4]

Chart 16.1: Sample Menu That Fits into the Acceptable Nutrient Ranges

Meal	Foods
Breakfast	1 cup Froot Loops 1 cup skim milk 1 package M&M milk chocolate candies Fiber and vitamin supplements
Lunch	Grilled cheddar cheeseburger
Dinner	3 slices pepperoni pizza, 1 16-oz. soda 1 serving Archway sugar cookies

Charts 16.2: Nutrient Profile of Sample Menu Plan and Report Recommendations

Nutrient	Sample Menu Content	Recommended Ranges
Total Calories	~1,800	Varies by height/weight
Protein (% of total calories)	~18%	10–35%
Fat (% of total calories)	~31%	20–35%
Carbohydrates (% of total calories)	~51%	45–65%
Sugars in Sweets, or Added Sugars (% of total calories)	~23%	Up to 25%

Folks, I'm not kidding. This disastrous menu plan fits the recommendations of the report and is supposedly consistent with "minimizing chronic disease."

What's amazing is that I could put together a variety of menus, all drenched in animal foods and added sugars, that conform to these recommended daily allowances. At this point in the book, I don't need to tell you that when we eat a diet like this day in and day out, we will be not just marching, but *sprinting* into the arms of chronic disease. In sad fact, this is what a large proportion of our population already does.

PROTEIN

Perhaps the most shocking figure is the upper limit on protein intake. Relative to total calorie intake, only 5–6% dietary protein is required to replace the protein regularly excreted by the body (as amino acids). About 9–10% protein, however, is the amount that has been recommended for the past fifty years to be assured that most people at least get their 5–6% "requirement." This 9–10% recommendation is equivalent to the well-known RDA.[5]

Almost all Americans exceed this 9–10% recommendation; we consume protein within the range of about 11–21%, with an average of about 15–16%.[6] The relatively few people consuming more than 21% protein mostly are those who "pump iron," joined by those on high-protein diets.

It is extremely puzzling that these government-sponsored 2002 FNB recommendations now say that we should be able to consume protein up to the extraordinary level of 35% as a means of minimizing chronic illnesses like cancer and heart disease. This is an unbelievable travesty, considering the scientific evidence. The evidence presented in this book shows that increasing dietary protein within the range of about 10–20% is associated with a broad array of health problems, especially when most of the protein is from animal sources.

As reviewed earlier in this book, diets with more animal-based protein will create higher blood cholesterol levels and higher risk of atherosclerosis, cancer, osteoporosis, Alzheimer's disease, and kidney stones, to name just a few chronic diseases that the FNB committee mysteriously chose to ignore.

Furthermore, the FNB panel had the audacity to say that this 10–35% recommendation range is the same as previous reports. Their press release clearly states, "Protein intake recommendations are the same [as previous reports]." *I know of no report that has even remotely suggested a level as high as this.*

When I initially saw this protein recommendation, I honestly thought that it was a printing error. But, no, it was correct. I know several of the people on the panel who wrote this report and decided to give them a ring. The first panel member, a long-time acquaintance, said this was the first time he had even heard about the 35% protein limit! He suggested that this protein recommendation might have been drafted in the last days of preparing the report. He also told me that there was little discussion of the evidence on protein, for or against a high consumption level, although he recollected there being some pro-Atkins sympathy on the committee. He had not worked in the protein area, so he did not know the literature. In any event, this important recommendation slipped through the panel without much notice and made the first sentence of the FNB news release!

The second panel member, a long-time friend and colleague, was a sub-committee chair during the latter part of the panel's existence. He is not a nutritional scientist and also was surprised to hear my concerns about the upper limit for protein. He did not recall much discussion on the topic, either. When I reminded him of some of the evidence linking diets high in animal protein to chronic disease, he initially was somewhat defensive. But with a little more persistence on my part about the evidence, he finally said, "Colin, you know that I really don't know anything about nutrition." How, then, was he a member—let alone the chair—of this important subcommittee? *And it gets worse.* The chair of the standing committee on the evaluation of these recommendations left the panel shortly before its completion for a senior executive position in a very large food company—a company that will salivate over these new recommendations.

A SUGARCOATED REPORT

The recommendation on added sugar is as outrageous as the one for protein. At about the time this FNB report was being released, an expert panel put together by the WHO (World Health Organization) and the FAO (Food and Agriculture Organization) was completing a new report on diet, nutrition, and preventing chronic diseases. Professor Phillip James, another friend of mine, was a member of this panel and a panel spokesperson on the added sugar recommendation. Early rumors of the report's findings indicated that the WHO/FAO was on the verge of recommending an upper safe limit of 10% for added sugar, far lower than the 25% established by the American FNB group.

Politics, however, had entered the discussion early, as it had done in earlier reports on added sugars.[7] According to a news release from the director-general's office at the WHO, the U.S.-based Sugar Association and the World Sugar Research Organization, who "represent the interests of the sugar growers and refiners, had mounted a strong lobbying campaign in an attempt to discredit the [WHO] report and suppress its release."[8] They did not like setting the upper safe limit so low. According to the *Guardian* newspaper of London,[7] the U.S. sugar industry was threatening "to bring the World Health Organization to its knees" unless it abandoned these guidelines on added sugar. WHO people were describing the threat "as tantamount to blackmail and worse than any pressure exerted by the tobacco industry."[7] The U.S.-based group even publicly threatened to lobby the U.S. Congress to reduce the $406 million U.S. funding of the WHO if it persisted in keeping the upper limit so low at 10%! There were reports, after a letter was sent by the industry to Secretary of Health and Human Services Tommy Thompson, that the Bush administration was inclined to side with the sugar industry. I, and many other scientists, were being encouraged at that time to contact our congressional representatives to stop this outrageous strong-armed tactic by the U.S. sugar companies.

So, for added sugars, we now have two different upper "safe" limits: a 10% limit for the international community and a 25% limit for the U.S. Why such a huge difference? Did the sugar industry succeed in controlling the U.S.-based FNB report but fail with the WHO/FAO report? What does this say about the FNB scientists who also devised the new protein recommendation? These wildly different estimates are not a matter of scientific interpretation. This is nothing more than naked political muscle. Professor James and his colleagues at the WHO stood up to the pressure; the FNB group appears to have caved in. The U.S. panel received funding from the M&M Mars candy company and a consortium of soft drink companies. Is it possible that the U.S. group felt an obligation to these sugar companies? Incidentally, the sugar industry, in their fight against the WHO conclusion, has relied heavily[7] on the FNB report with its 25% limit. In other words, the FNB committee produces a friendly recommendation for the sugar industry, which then turns around and uses this finding to support its claim against the WHO report.

It's true that when government leaders need advice on policy development, they often turn to expert panels, most composed of academics. But having served on several of these panels, it is clear to me that the government leaders responsible for funding these panels exercise considerable control over their recommendations. Aside from providing the funding, they write the panels' remits and are generally active in choosing each panel's chair. The chair, whose views on the topic are often (though not always) known to be acceptable to the government agency, often helps to select the remaining members. Because of this, these panels do not often stray too far from government interests. Keep in mind, also, that panel recommendations are almost always, in my experience, advisory only—meaning that the government staff can select what they like from the report. There are several ways that government and industry can work for a common purpose but, from my firsthand experience, I believe that this linkage is one of the subtlest but nonetheless most powerful collaborations. The policy that flows from such bodies can be far reaching.

THE INFLUENCE OF INDUSTRY

This discussion still leaves unanswered the question of how industry develops such extraordinary influence. Industry mostly develops consultancies with a few publicly visible figures in academia, who then take leadership in policy positions outside of academia. However, these industry consultants continue to wear their academic hats. They organize symposia and workshops, write commissioned reviews, chair expert policy groups, and/or become officers of key professional societies. They gravitate toward the leadership positions in science-based organizations that develop significant policy and publicity.

Once in these positions, these people then have the opportunity to assemble teams to their liking by choosing committee members, symposia speakers, management staff, and so forth. The kinds of people most helpful to the team are either colleagues with similar prejudices and/or colleagues who are oblivious to who is "calling the shots." It's called "stacking the deck," and it really works.

In the case of the FNB, its panel was organized while being chaired by an academic with strong personal ties with the dairy industry. He helped in selecting the "right" people and setting the agenda for the report, the most significant roles that anyone could have played. Is it surprising that the dairy industry, which must have been ecstatic with the panel's findings, also helped to finance the report? You might be surprised to learn that academic scientists can receive personal compensation from industry while simultaneously undertaking government-sponsored activities of considerable public importance. Ironically, they can even help set the agenda for the same government authorities who have long been restricted from such corporate associations. It is a huge conflict of interest loophole that allows industries to exercise their influence through the side door of academia. In effect, the entire system is essentially under the control of industry. The government and academic communities, playing their respective roles, mostly do as they are expected to do.

In addition to the M&M Mars company, the corporate sponsors of the FNB report also included major food and drug companies that would benefit from higher protein and sugar allowances.[2] The Dannon Institute, a leading dairy-industry consortium promoting its own brand of nutrition information, and the International Life Sciences Institute (ILSI), a front group for about fifty food, supplement, and drug companies, both contributed fund-ing for the FNB report. Corporate members include Coca-Cola, Taco Bell, Burger King, Nestlé, Pfizer, and Roche Vitamins.[9] Some drug companies sponsored the report directly, in addition to their support through ILSI. I don't recall private corporations providing financial support for the NAS expert panels that I served on.

It seems as if there is no end to this story. The chair of the FNB has been an important consultant to several major dairy-related companies (e.g., National Dairy Council; Mead Johnson Nutritionals, a major seller of dairy-based products; Nestlé Company; and a Dannon yogurt affiliate).[10] While chairing FNB, he was also chair of the Dietary Guidelines Commit-tee, which establishes the Food Guide Pyramid and sets national nutrition policy affecting the National School Lunch and Breakfast programs, the Food Stamp Program, and the Women, Infants, and Children (WIC) Supple-mental Feeding Program.[1,10] As chair of this latter committee, his personal financial associations with the food industry were not publicly revealed as required by federal law.[11] Eventually a court order, initiated by the Physi-cian's Committee for Responsible Medicine,[12] was required to force him and his fellow colleagues to reveal their relationships with the food indus-try. Although the chair's industry associations were more substantial, *six of the eleven committee members also were shown to have ties to the dairy industry*.[10,11]

The entire system of developing public nutrition information, as I orig-inally saw with the Public Nutrition Information Committee that I once chaired (see chapter thirteen), has been invaded and co-opted by industry sources that have the interest and resources to do so. They run the show. They buy a few academic hacks who have gained positions of power and who exercise considerable influence, both within academia and government.

It seems curious that while government scientists are not allowed to receive personal compensation from the private sector, their colleagues in academia can receive all that they can get. In turn, these conflicted individu-als then run the show in collaboration with their government counterparts. However, restricting academics from receiving corporate consultancies is not the answer. That would only drive it underground. Rather, the situation would be best handled by making one's industry connections a matter of public disclosure. Everyone needs to know the full extent of each academ-ic's associations with the private sector. Disclosure and full transparency is in everyone's interest. These associations should not be something we have to go to court to discover.

SETTING US BACK FOR YEARS

Lest you think that this Food and Nutrition Board report is merely a five-second news bite that then gets filed into a dusty old cabinet somewhere in Washington, let me assure you that this panel's findings directly affect tens of millions of people. According to the summary of the report itself,[13] the recommended levels of nutrient consumption that are set by this panel are

> *the basis for nutrition labeling of foods, for the Food Guide Pyramid and for other nutrition education programs . . . [They are] used to determine the types and amounts of food:*
>
> - *provided in the WIC . . . Supplemental Feeding Program and the Child Nutrition Programs such as School Lunch,*
> - *served in hospitals and nursing homes for Medicare reimbursement,*
> - *found in the food supply that should be fortified with specific nutrients,*
> - *used in a host of other important federal and state programs and activities [such as establishing reference values used in food labeling]*[13]

The School Lunch Program fed 29.5 million children every day in May 2015.[14] With officially recommended consumption patterns like these, we are at liberty to put any agricultural commodity we want into the hungry mouths of children already suffering from unprecedented levels of obesity and diabetes. By the way, the 2002 FNB report does make one special exception for children: it says that they can consume up to 40% of calories as fat, up from 35% for the rest of us, while minimizing the risk of chronic disease. The WIC Program affects the diets of another 8.3 million Americans,[15] and the Medicare hospital programs feed millions of people every year. It is safe to say that the food provided by these government programs directly feeds at least 39 million Americans a month.

For people who are not directly fed by the government, this nutrient information still has significant consequences. From September 2002 onwards, nutrition education programs around the country have incorporated these new guidelines. This includes education in primary schools, universities, health professional programs, and other community-based programs. Food labels also will be affected by these changes, as will the nutrition information that seeps into our lives via advertising.

Almost all of the wide-ranging effects of this 2002 FNB report will be profoundly harmful. In school, our children can be fed more fat, more meat, more milk, more animal protein, and more sugar. They will also learn that this food is consistent with good health. The ramifications of this are serious, as a whole generation will walk the path of obesity, diabetes, and other chronic illnesses, all the while believing that they are doing the right thing. Meanwhile, our government and its academic hacks can feel free to unload more meat, more fat, more animal protein, and more sugar onto the neediest among us (e.g., WIC participants). I consider this to be an irresponsible and callous disregard for American citizens. Of course, these women and infants are not in a position to pay for research, donate to politicians, give academics special favors, or fund government panels! For others concerned about nutrition, every time they see a dietitian, every time they see their doctor, every time they see a nutritionist, and every time they go to a community health center, they may be told that a diet high in fat, animal protein, meat, and dairy is consistent with good health, and they needn't worry about eating too many sweets. Posters that deck the bulletin boards of public institutions will now feature these new government guidelines as well.

In short, this 2002 FNB report, which represents the most sweeping, regressive nutrition policy statement I have ever seen, will either indirectly or directly promote sickness among Americans for many years to come. Having been a member of several diet- and health-policy-making expert panels over a twenty-year period, I harbored the view that these panels were dedicated to the promotion of consumer health. I no longer believe this to be true.

UNFUNDED NUTRITION

Not only is the government failing to promote health through its recommendations and reports, it is squandering an opportunity to promote public health through scientific research. The U.S. National Institutes of Health (NIH) is responsible for funding at least 80–90% of all biomedical and nutrition-related research that is published in the scientific literature. To address a range of health topics, the NIH comprises twenty-seven separate institutes and centers, including its two largest, the National Cancer Institute (NCI) and the National Heart, Lung, and Blood Institute.[16] With a 2015 budget of $30.55 billion,[17] the NIH is the center of the government's gigantic medical research efforts.

In terms of nutrition research, however, something is amiss. None of these twenty-seven institutes and centers at the NIH is devoted to nutrition, despite the pivotal nature of nutrition in health, and despite the public interest in the subject. One of the arguments against having a separate institute for nutrition is that the existing institutes already concern themselves with nutrition. But this does not happen. Chart 16.3 shows the funding priorities for various health topics at the NIH.[18]

Of the $30.55 billion NIH budget for 2015, only about 5% is designated for projects that are related in some way to nutrition[19] and 23% for projects that are related to prevention. That may not sound too bad. But these figures are seriously misleading.

Chart 16.3: NIH 2015 Estimated Funding for Different Health Topics[18]

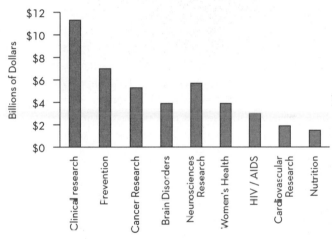

Most of the prevention and nutrition budgets have absolutely nothing to do with prevention and nutrition, as I have written in this book. We won't be hearing about exciting research on dietary patterns, nor will there be serious efforts to tell the public how diet affects health. Instead, the prevention and nutrition budgets will be designated for developing drugs and nutrient supplements. Several years ago, the director of the NCI, the oldest of the NIH institutes, described prevention as "efforts to directly prevent and/or inhibit malignant transformation, to identify, characterize and manipulate factors that might be effective in achieving that inhibition and attempts to promote preventative measures."[20] This so-called prevention is all about manipulation of isolated chemicals. To "identify, characterize and manipulate factors" is a not-so-secret code for drug discovery.

Considered from another perspective, the NCI (of the NIH), in 1999, had a budget of $2.93 billion.[21] In a "major" 5-A-Day dietary program, it was spending $500,000 to $1 million to educate the public to consume five or more servings of fruits and vegetables per day.[20] This is only *three-hundredths of one percent* (0.0256%) of its budget. That's $2.56 for every $10,000! If it calls this a major campaign, I pity its minor campaigns.

The NCI also has been funding a couple of multi-year large studies, including the Nurses' Health Study at Harvard (discussed in chapter fourteen) and the Women's Health Initiative, which is mostly devoted to the testing of hormone replacement therapy, vitamin D and calcium supplementation, and the effect of a moderately low-fat diet on prevention of breast and colon cancer. These rare nutrition-related studies unfortunately suffer from the same experimental flaws described in chapter fourteen. Almost always, these studies are designed to tinker with one nutrient at a time, among an experimental population that uniformly consumes a high-risk, animal-based diet. These studies have a very high probability of creating some very unnecessary—and very expensive—confusion.

If very few of our tax dollars are used to fund nutrition research, what do they fund? Almost all of the billions of dollars of taxpayer money the NIH spends annually funds projects to develop drugs, supplements, and mechanical devices. In essence, the vast bulk of biomedical research funded by you and me is basic research to discover products that the pharmaceutical industry can develop and market. In 2000, Dr. Marcia Angell, a former editor of the *New England Journal of Medicine*, summarized it well when she wrote:

> . . . the pharmaceutical industry enjoys extraordinary government protections and subsidies. Much of the early basic research that may lead to drug development is funded by the National Institutes of Health (ref. cited). It is usually only later, when the research shows practical promise, that the drug companies become involved. The industry also enjoys great tax advantages. Not only are its research and development costs deductible, but so are its massive marketing expenses. The average tax rate of major U.S. industries from 1993 to 1996 was 27.3% of revenues. During the same period the pharmaceutical industry was reportedly taxed at a rate of only 16.2% (ref. cited). Most important, the drug companies enjoy seventeen-year government-granted monopolies on their new drugs—that is, patent protection. Once a drug is patented, no one else may sell it, and the drug company is free to charge whatever the traffic will bear.[22]

Our tax dollars are used to make the pharmaceutical industry more profitable. One could argue that this is justified by gains in public health, but the alarming fact is that this tide of money into drugs, genes, devices, and technology research *will never cure our chronic diseases*. Our chronic diseases are largely the result of infinitely complex assaults on our bodies resulting from eating bad food. No single chemical intervention will ever equal the power of consuming the healthiest food. In addition, isolated chemicals in drug form can be very dangerous. The National Cancer Institute itself states, "What is clear is that most of our current treatments will produce some measure of adversity."[23] There is no danger to eating a healthy diet, and there are far more benefits, including massive cost savings both on the front end of preventing disease and on the back end of treating disease. So why is our government ignoring the abundant scientific research supporting a dietary approach in favor of largely ineffective, potentially dangerous drug and device interventions?

PERSONAL ACCOUNTS

In terms of public nutrition policy, I want to leave you with one short story that says so much about the government's priorities. One of my former graduate students at Cornell, Dr. Antonia Demas, did her doctoral research in education by teaching a healthy food-and-nutrition-based curriculum[24] to elementary school kids and then integrating those healthy foods into the school lunch program. She had been doing this work as a volunteer mother in her children's schools for seventeen years prior to her graduate studies. I was her advisor for the nutrition part of her dissertation research.

The U.S. Department of Agriculture administers the school lunch program to 29.5 million children, largely relying on an inventory of government-subsidized foods. The government program, as it now stands, uses mostly animal-based products and even requires that participating schools make available cow's milk. At the local level, this usually means that consumption of milk is mandatory.

Dr. Demas's innovative research on the school lunch program was a great success; children loved the learning style and were excited to eat the healthy foods when they went through the lunch line. The children then convinced their parents to eat the healthy food at home. Dr. Demas's program won national awards for the "most creative implementation of the dietary guidelines" and "excellence in nutrition education." The program proved to be of interest to more than 300 school lunch and behavioral rehabilitation programs around the U.S., including schools in areas as widely dispersed as Hawaii, Florida, Indiana, New England, California, and New Mexico. In this effort, Dr. Demas has organized a nonprofit foundation (Food Studies Institute, Trumansburg, New York) and written a curriculum ("Food is Elementary"). And here's the kicker: Dr. Demas's program is entirely plant-based.

I had the opportunity to go to Washington and talk with Dr. Eileen Kennedy, who was then the director of the Center for Nutrition Policy and Promotion at the USDA. Dr. Kennedy was deeply involved both in the school lunch program and the dietary guidelines committee, on which it was revealed that she had ties to the dairy industry. The topic of our discussion was Dr. Demas's innovative school lunch program and how it was garnering national attention. At the end of this discussion, I said to her, "You know, that program is entirely plant-based." She looked at me, wagged her finger as if I were being a bad boy, and said, "*We can't have that.*"

Here's an even more recent story: After publication of the first edition of this book in 2005, I was afforded the opportunity to call on some of my political and government friends who were expressing interest in the book's contents. On a couple of my visits to Washington, I invited my colleague Dr. Caldwell Esselstyn to join me. Together we talked with some senior officials, especially at the USDA, about our views and books. We received courteous, warm receptions by government administrators of food and health programs.

At the time, I was tentatively hopeful of our making some progress, because I once thought that getting support from government program leaders would be an effective way to inform the public. I mostly learned that I was wrong. Nothing came of all those visits. To give one example, we met five of the six top USDA administrators, a couple of whom I had had prior personal acquaintance with and who were familiar with my interests and my work in days gone by, when I was less problematic. Although, as professionals, they acknowledged our achievements without question, it also quickly became clear to me that they were merely being courteous in meeting with us. These program leaders do not have to stand for elections, but they still answer to superiors who do—and we now know how elections are won, especially since the *Citizens United* case was decided by the Supreme Court in a way that gave much more power to the corporate sector. That is, elected officials and their subordinates are now even more subservient to corporate interests.

It is also worth mentioning the 2015 Dietary Guidelines Advisory Committee, which generated a lot of controversy and news. This is the scientific advisory group that writes the Scientific Report of the Dietary Guidelines Advisory Committee, which should form the basis of the final dietary guidelines. In 2015, in the executive summary of their report, the scientific panel stated, "The overall body of evidence examined by the 2015 [Dietary Guidelines Advisory Committee] identifies that a healthy dietary pattern is higher in vegetables, fruits, whole grains, low- or non-fat dairy, seafood, legumes, and nuts; moderate in alcohol (among adults); lower in red and processed meat; and low in sugar-sweetened foods and drinks and refined grains."[25] They also considered environmental sustainability, given the importance of food choices in our environment: "The major findings regarding sustainable diets were that a diet higher in plant-based foods, such as vegetables, fruits, whole grains, legumes, nuts, and seeds, and lower in calories and animal-based foods is more health promoting and is associated with less environmental impact than is the current U.S. diet."[25]

Despite not embracing a whole-foods, plant-based diet, these exceptionally conservative, easily justified statements certainly are more progressive than the government reports we discussed in the first part of this chapter, written for the first edition.

The 2015 Scientific Report met with tremendous resistance, unsurprisingly. Detractors claimed that environmental sustainability is not relevant to guidelines on food and nutrition—an odd complaint, seeing as no one seemed to have a problem with including physical activity guidance and commentary, a completely non-food issue, as part of the nutrition guidelines.

But the idea that got these critics riled was that the government might recommend eating less red and processed meat in favor of plants. Thirty senators (all Republican) drafted a letter critical of the Scientific Report. They wrote:

> Not only do we represent farmers and ranchers who raise animals to provide healthy meat products, but we also represent consumers who enjoy lean meat as an important food in their diet. The inconsistencies brought forward in the Dietary Guidelines Advisory Committee's report are significant. We encourage you to carefully consider the most relevant nutrition scientific literature and reject the Dietary Guidelines Advisory Committee's inconsistent conclusions regarding the role of meat in Americans' diets as you finalize the Dietary Guidelines.[26]

Seventy-one representatives in the House (all of whom were Republican) signed a similarly critical letter as well.[27] They wrote, "The Dietary Guidelines Advisory Committee's recommendation on lean red meat directly contradicts years of peer reviewed scientific research on the benefits of lean red meat as a high quality source of protein in a healthy diet."

What's going on here? I never knew we had such a well-versed cadre of nutrition science enthusiasts among our elected officials! Could major portions of the Senate and House of Representatives have been quietly reading abundant primary research on nutrition and health? And could the scientific body failed to have considered some large body of nutrition research that these apparent nutrition enthusiasts read in their spare time?

Or is it something else? One analysis showed that the senators had received over $1 million from the food industry in the previous year, about half of which was from the beef industry.[28] The House signers received at least $2 million from food and agricultural interests during the previous year.

In our opinion, their agendas could not be more plain.

Of course, in the end, the scientists were only advisors. Never a group to let scientists dictate scientific recommendations, government administrators formulating the final report gutted the executive summary in a blatant effort to bury any anti-industry themes. Any anti-animal food sentiment was replaced or eliminated. When discussing what people might consider cutting back on, they focused on nutrients and not foods—a common tactic to make recommendations harder to understand. After the administrators were done, the main guidelines, as stated in the executive summary, were:

1. Follow a healthy eating pattern across the lifespan.
2. Focus on variety, nutrient density, and amount. (. . . choose a variety of nutrient-dense foods across and within all food groups . . .)
3. Limit calories from added sugars and saturated fats and reduce sodium intake.
4. Shift to healthier food and beverage choices. (Choose nutrient-dense foods and beverages across and within all food groups in place of less healthy choices. Consider cultural personal preferences to make these shifts easier to accomplish and maintain.)
5. Support healthy eating patterns for all.[29]

What meaningless drivel! Industry couldn't have written the executive summary any differently if they themselves had drafted it. Only the sugar industry remained targeted. The focus on sugar in some ways has been a more politically palatable, even welcome, distraction from the evidence against red meat and milk.

During the 2015 guidelines battle, the House of Representatives wrote a section of a bill to appropriate a million dollars to fund a formal review of how the Dietary Guidelines are drafted. They wanted to ensure that there are broad viewpoints among panel members and that they follow rigid scientific standards (whose, I wonder?) to make recommendations. I can only interpret this to mean that those friendly to industry wanted to take steps to fundamentally change the guidelines process so industry never again has to publicly deny science and flex their political muscle. The whole episode could not have been good PR. It is much better for industry (and elected officials) if industry can pull the strings of government outside public view.

I have concluded that when it comes to health, government is not for the people; it is for the food industry and the pharmaceutical industry at the expense of the people. It is a systemic problem where industry, academia, and government combine to determine the health of this country. Industry funds public health reports, and academic leaders with industry ties play key roles in developing them. A revolving door exists between government jobs and industry jobs, and government research funding goes to develop drugs and devices instead of healthy nutrition. It is a system built by people who play their isolated parts, often unaware of the top decision makers and their ulterior motivations. In the rare cases when this system doesn't work, industry can rely on elected officials to directly intervene in any recommendations or determinations that do not favor their bottom line. The system is a waste of taxpayer money and is profoundly damaging to our health.

BIG MEDICINE: WHOSE HEALTH ARE THEY PROTECTING?

17

When was the last time you went to the doctor and he or she told you what to eat or what not to eat? You've probably never had that experience. But the vast majority of Americans will fall prey to one of the chronic diseases of affluence discussed in Part II, and, as you have seen, there is a wealth of published research that suggests these diseases are a result of poor nutrition, not poor genes or bad luck. So why doesn't the medical system take nutrition seriously?

Four words: money, ego, power, and control. While it is unfair to generalize about individual doctors, it is safe to say that the system they work in, the system that currently takes responsibility for promoting the health of Americans, is failing us. No one knows this better than the tiny minority of doctors who treat their patients from a nutritional perspective. Two of the most prominent doctors in this minority have spent many years emphasizing diet and health, both in public within their profession and in private with their patients. They have had exceptionally impressive results protecting their patients' health. These two doctors are Caldwell B. Esselstyn, Jr., whose work we discussed in chapter five, and John McDougall, an internist. My son Tom and I sat down with these men to discuss their experience advocating a whole foods, plant-based (WFPB) diet in the medical setting.

DR. SPROUTS

Long before our country was founded, Dutch pioneers had settled in the Hudson Valley north of New York City. One of these settler families were the Esselstyns. They started farming a plot of land in 1675. Nine generations later, that farm still belongs to the Esselstyn family. Dr. Esselstyn and his wife, Ann, own the several-hundred-acre Hudson Valley farm, just over two hours north of New York City. They spent the summer of 2003 living in the country, working the farm, growing a garden, hosting their kids and grandkids, and enjoying a more relaxed life than what they're used to in Cleveland, Ohio.

Ess and Ann have a modest house: a large, rectangular, converted storage building. The simplicity of it belies the fact that this is one of the oldest family farms in America. Only upon closer inspection does it become apparent that there is something unusual about this place. Hanging on the wall is a framed certificate from New York State given to the Esselstyn family in recognition of their family farm, one that has now seen parts of five different centuries. Nearby an oar hangs on the wall. It is the oar Ess used in 1955 as an oarsman at Yale, when Yale beat Harvard by five seconds. Ess explains he has three other oars: two from beating Harvard in other years, and one for winning the gold medal in the Olympics with the Yale crew in 1956.

Downstairs, there is an exceptionally old photograph of Ess's great-great-grandfather on the farm. Around the corner there's an impressive-looking museum-style schematic of the Esselstyn family tree, and at the other end of the hall, there's a large black-and-white picture of Ess's father standing in front of a microphone, exchanging comments with John F. Kennedy during a White House address. Despite its humble appearance, it is very clear that this is a place with a distinguished history.

After touring the farm on a tractor, we sat down with Ess and asked him about his past. After graduating from Yale, he was trained as a surgeon at the Cleveland Clinic and at St. George's Hospital in London. He remembers fondly some of his most influential mentors: Dr. George Crile, Jr., Dr. Turnbull, and Dr. Brook. Dr. Crile, a giant at the Cleveland Clinic, eventually became Ess's father-in-law upon Ess's marriage to Ann. Dr. Crile was a man of exceptional accomplishment, playing a courageous leading role in questioning the macabre surgery called "radical mastectomy."[1] Dr. Turnbull and Dr. Brook were also renowned surgeons. In addition, Ess's own father was a distinguished physician with a national reputation. But, as Ess remembers, despite being "health experts," all four of these men were "ravaged by cardiovascular disease." His own father had a heart attack at age forty-two and Dr. Brook had a heart attack at age fifty-two.

These were the men he looked up to, and when it came to cardiovascular disease, all of them were helpless. Shaking his head, Ess said, "You can't escape this disease. These people, who were giants in the prime of their years, just *withered*." As he took a moment to remember his father, he said, "It was the last year or two of my dad's life, and we were just strolling along one day. He was saying, 'We are going to have to show people how to lead healthier lives.' *He was right on it.* He was intensely interested in preventive medicine, but he didn't have any information." His father's interest has been a driving influence in Ess's life.

Following in these men's footsteps, Ess went on to amass an extraordinarily impressive list of awards and credentials: an Olympic gold medal in rowing; a Bronze Star for military service in Vietnam; President of the Staff, member of the Board of Governors, chairman of the Breast Cancer Task Force, and head of the Section of Thyroid and Parathyroid Surgery at the Cleveland Clinic, one of the top-ranked medical institutions in the world; president of the American Association of Endocrine Surgeons; over 100 professional scientific articles; and inclusion on a list in 1994–95 of the best doctors in America.[2] He remembers, "For about a ten- to fifteen-year period I was the top earner in the department of general surgery. As Dr. Crile's son-in-law, I was panicked about not pulling my weight. I didn't get home until late at night, but I had a position that was secure." When the then-president of the American Medical Association needed thyroid surgery, he wanted Ess to be the one to operate.

But despite the accolades, the titles, and the awards, something was not right. *So often, Ess's patients did not regain their health, even after his best efforts.* As Ess described it, he had "this haunting feeling that was really beginning to bother me. I kept looking at how the patients were doing after these operations." Slightly exasperated, he said, "What is the survival rate for cancer of the colon? It's not so great!" He recounted the operation for colon cancer on one of his best friends. During surgery, they saw that the cancer had spread throughout the intestines. Ess lowered his voice ever so slightly in remembering this, saying, "You get there after the horse has left the barn." In thinking about all the breast surgery he had done, the lumpectomies and mastectomies, he expressed disgust at the idea of "disfiguring somebody when you know that you haven't changed their chances for recovery."

He began to do some soul searching. "What is my epitaph going to be? Five thousand mastectomies! You've disfigured more women than anybody else in Ohio!" Dropping the sarcasm, he said with sincerity, "I think everybody likes to leave the planet thinking that maybe . . . maybe you've helped a little."

Dr. Esselstyn began studying the literature on the diseases he commonly treated. He read some of the popular work of Dr. John McDougall, who had just written a best-selling diet and health book called *The McDougall Plan*.[3] He read the scientific literature that compared international disease rates and lifestyle choices, and a study by a University of Chicago pathologist showing that a low-fat, low-cholesterol diet fed to nonhuman primates could reverse atherosclerosis. He came to the realization that the diseases that so often plagued his patients were due to a diet rich in meat, fat, and highly refined foods.

As mentioned in chapter five, he got the idea to treat heart patients with a low-fat, plant-based diet, and in 1985 went to the head of the Cleveland Clinic to discuss his study. She said that nobody had ever shown that heart disease in humans could be reversed by using dietary treatment. Still, Ess knew he was on the right track and went about quietly conducting his study over the next several years. The study he published, of eighteen patients with heart disease, demonstrated the most dramatic reversal of heart disease in the history of medicine, simply by using a low-fat, plant-based diet and a minimal amount of cholesterol-reducing medication.

Esselstyn has become a champion of dietary treatment of disease, and he has the data to prove his case. But it hasn't been easy. Rather than recognizing him as a hero, some in the medical establishment would rather he disappear. Somewhere in this transition from top-ranked, self-described "macho, hard-ass surgeon" to dietary advocate, he has become known, behind his back, as Dr. Sprouts.

A DAUNTING TASK

What's interesting about this story is that a man who had reached the pinnacle of a highly respected profession dared to try something different, succeeded, and then quickly found himself on the outside of the establishment looking in. He had threatened the status quo by circumventing standard treatments.

Some of Ess's colleagues have disparaged his treatment as being too "extreme." Some doctors have dismissed it by saying, "I think the research in this area is pretty soft," which is an absurd comment considering the breadth and depth of the international studies, the animal studies, and the intervention studies. Some doctors have said to Ess, "Yeah, okay, but nobody is going to eat like that. I can't even get my patients to stop smoking." Ess's response was, "Well, you really have no training in this. This requires just as much expertise as doing a bypass. It takes three hours for me to counsel a patient," not to mention the diligence required for the constant follow-up and monitoring of the patient's health. One patient told his cardiologist that he wanted to see Ess and commit to a dietary program to reverse his heart disease. The cardiologist responded, "Now you listen to me. There is no way to reverse this disease." You'd think that doctors would be more excited about healing their patients!

In talking about doctors and their unwillingness to embrace a WFPB diet, Ess says, "You can't get frustrated. These aren't evil people. There are sixty cardiologists [at the Cleveland Clinic], any number of whom are closet believers in what I do, but they're a little afraid because of the power structure."

For Ess, however, it has been impossible to avoid his share of frustration. Early on, when he was first suggesting dietary treatment of heart disease, colleagues greeted the idea with caution. Ess figured that their attitude was born out of the fact that scientific research showing effective dietary intervention of heart disease in humans wasn't yet strong enough. But later, scientific results of unparalleled success, including Esselstyn's, were published. The data have been strong, consistent, and deep, yet Ess still encountered reluctance to embrace this idea:

> You take a cardiologist and he's learned all about beta blockers, he's learned about calcium antagonists, he's learned about how to run this catheter up into your heart and blow up balloons or laser it or stent it without killing you and it's very sophisticated. And there's all these nurses and there's lights out and there's drama. I mean it's just, oh my god, the doctor blows up the balloon in his head. The ego of these people is enormous. And then someone comes along and says, "You know, I think we can cure this with Brussels sprouts and broccoli." The doctor's response is, "WHAT? I learned all this crap, I'm making a freakin' fortune, and you want to take it all away?"

Then when that person comes along and actually cures patients with Brussels sprouts and broccoli, as Esselstyn did, and gets better results than any other pill or procedure known, you've suddenly announced that something works, hands down, better than what 99% of the profession is doing. Summarizing his point, Ess says:

> Cardiologists are supposed to be experts in diseases of the heart—and yet they have no expertise in treating heart disease, and when that awareness strikes them, they get very defensive. They can treat the symptoms, they can take care of arrhythmias, they can

*get you interventions, but they don't know how to treat the disease,
which is a nutritional treatment . . . Imagine a dietitian training a
heart surgeon!*

Esselstyn has found that merely saying that patients can have control over their own health is a challenge to many. These experts, after all, are built up to be the dispensers of health and healing. "Intellectually it's very challenging to think that the patient can do this with greater alacrity, dispatch, safety, and it's something that's going to endure." With all of the doctor's gadgets, technologies, training, and knowledge, nothing is more effective than guiding the patient to make the right lifestyle choices.

But Ess is quick to point out that doctors are not malicious people engaged in a conspiracy:

*The only person that likes change is a newborn, and it's natural,
it's human nature. Anywhere you go, 99% of the people are eating
incorrectly. The numbers are against you, and it's very hard for
those 99% to look at you in the 1% and say, "Yes, he's right, we are
all wrong."*

Another obstacle: lack of nutrition knowledge among physicians. Ess has had his share of interaction with ignorant doctors, and his impression is that "it's absolutely daunting, the lack of physician knowledge that there is about the fact that disease can be reversed. You wonder, what is the literature that these guys read?"

Physician knowledge often involves only the standard treatments: pills and procedures. "What does the twentieth century of medicine have to offer? We have pills and we have procedures. Right?" Esselstyn leans forward and, with a slight grin, as if he's about to tell us the emperor has no clothes, he says, "*But who ever says, 'Maybe we ought to stop disease'?*" In Dr. Esselstyn's experience, stopping disease does not figure prominently into the status quo.

LACK OF TRAINING

The medical status quo relies heavily on medication and surgery, to the exclusion of nutrition and lifestyle. Doctors have virtually *no training in nutrition and how it relates to health*. In 1985 the United States National Research Council funded an expert panel report that investigated the quantity and quality of nutrition education in U.S. medical schools.[4] The committee's findings were clear: "The committee concluded that nutrition education programs in U.S. medical schools are largely inadequate to meet the present and future demands of the medical profession."[4] But this finding was nothing new. The committee noted that in 1961 the "American Medical Association Council on Foods and Nutrition reported that nutrition in the U.S. medical schools received 'inadequate recognition, support and attention.'"[4,5] In other words, over forty years ago, the doctors themselves said that their nutrition training was inadequate. Nothing had changed by 1985, and up to the present time, articles continue to be written documenting the lack of nutrition training in medical schools.[6,7]

This situation is dangerous. Nutrition training of doctors is not merely inadequate; it is practically nonexistent. The 1985 National Research Council report found that physicians receive, on average, only twenty-one classroom hours (about two credits) of nutrition training during their four years of medical school.[4] The majority of the schools surveyed actually taught less than twenty contact hours of nutrition, or one to two credit hours. By comparison, an undergraduate nutrition major at Cornell will receive twenty-five to forty credit hours of instruction, or about 250–500 contact hours; registered dietitians will have more than 500 contact hours.

It gets worse. The bulk of these nutrition hours are taught in the first year of medical school, as part of other basic science courses. Topics covered in a basic biochemistry course may include nutrient metabolism and/or biochemical reactions involving certain vitamins or minerals. *In other words, nutrition is often not taught in relation to public health problems, like obesity, cancer, diabetes, etc.* In conjunction with the 1985 government report, the president of the American Medical Students Association, William Kassler, writes[8]:

> *Most nutrition in the formal curriculum is incorporated into other courses. Biochemistry, physiology, and pharmacology are the courses most often alleged to contain some nutrition instruction. Too often in such courses, nutrition is touched on briefly, with the primary emphasis on the major discipline.* It is quite possible to finish such a course and not even realize that nutrition was covered *[our emphasis]. Nutrition taught by those whose interest and expertise lie elsewhere simply doesn't work.*

It gets even worse! When nutrition education is provided in relation to public health problems, guess who is supplying the "educational" material? The Dannon Institute, Egg Nutrition Board, National Cattlemen's Beef Association, National Dairy Council, Nestlé Clinical Nutrition, Wyeth-Ayerst

Laboratories, Bristol-Myers Squibb Company, Baxter Healthcare Corporation, and others have all joined forces to produce a Nutrition in Medicine program and the Medical Nutrition Curriculum Initiative.[9,10] Do you think that this all-star team of animal foods and drug industries representatives is going to objectively judge and promote optimal nutrition, which science has shown to be a WFPB diet that minimizes the need for drugs? Or might they try to protect the meat-centered, Western diet where everyone expects to pop a pill for every sickness? This organization is creating nutrition curricula on CD-ROMs and giving them away to medical schools for free. As of late 2003, 112 medical schools were using the curriculum[11]; according to their website at the time, "Plans are underway for developing versions for undergraduate nutrition students, continuing medical education and other health professions audiences."

The dairy industry has also funded research investigations into nutrition education in medical schools[12] and has funded "prestigious" awards.[13,14] These efforts show that industry is well prepared to promote its monetary interests whenever the opportunity presents itself.

You should not assume that your doctor has any more knowledge about food and its relation to health than your neighbors and coworkers. It's a situation in which nutritionally untrained doctors prescribe milk- and sugar-based meal-replacement shakes for overweight diabetics, high-meat, high-fat diets for patients who ask how to lose weight, and extra milk for patients who have osteoporosis. *The health damage that results from doctors' ignorance of nutrition is astounding.*

Apparently, there aren't enough "nutrition-oriented physician role models" in medical education. One survey found "a shortage of nutrition-oriented physician role models is probably the major constraint in teaching nutrition to residents."[12] It may be that these medical programs lack nutrition-oriented physicians simply because they do not make it a priority to hire them. Nobody knows this better than Dr. John McDougall.

DR. MCDOUGALL'S CHALLENGE

Dr. John McDougall has been advocating a WFPB approach to health longer than any practitioner we know. He has written ten books, including several that have sold over half a million copies each. His nutrition and health knowledge is phenomenal, greater than any other doctor we've met and greater than any of our nutrition colleagues in academia. Colin met John in his Northern California home, and one of the first things he showed Colin was his bank of four or five full-size metal file cabinets lined up along the back of his study. There can't be many people in the country with a collection of scientific literature on diet and disease that could rival John McDougall's, and, most importantly, John maintains a high level of familiarity with all of it. It is not unusual for him to spend a couple of hours a day on the internet reviewing the latest journal articles. If anybody would be a perfect "nutrition-oriented physician role model" in an educational setting, it would be Dr. John McDougall.

Growing up, John ate a rich, Western diet. As he says, he had four feasts a day: Easter during breakfast, Thanksgiving at lunch, Christmas at dinner, and a birthday party for dessert. It caught up to him, and at the age of eighteen, a few months into college, John had a stroke. After recovering with a new appreciation for life, he became a straight-A student as an undergraduate and then completed medical school in Michigan and an internship in Hawaii. He chose to practice on the Big Island of Hawaii, where he cared for thousands of patients, some of whom had recently migrated from China or the Philippines, and some who were fourth-generation Chinese or Filipino Americans.

It was there that John became an unhappy doctor. Many of his patients' health problems were a result of chronic illnesses, such as obesity, diabetes, cancer, heart disease, and arthritis. John would treat them as he was taught, with the standard sets of pills and procedures, but very few of them became healthy. Their chronic diseases didn't go away, and John quickly realized that he had severe limitations as a doctor. He also started to learn something else from his patients: the first- and second-generation Americans from Asia, the ones who ate more traditional, Asian staple diets of rice and vegetables, were trim, fit, and not afflicted with the chronic diseases that plagued John's other patients. The third- and fourth-generation Asian Americans, however, had fully adopted America's eating habits and suffered from obesity, diabetes, and the whole host of other chronic diseases. It was from these people that John began to notice how important diet was for health.

Because John wasn't healing people, and the pills and procedures weren't working, he decided he needed more education and entered a graduate medical program (residency) at the Queens Medical Center in Honolulu. It was there that he began to understand the boundaries that the medical establishment had set and the way that medical education molds the way doctors are supposed to think.

John went into the program hoping to find out how to perfect the pills and procedures so that he could become a better doctor. But after observing experienced doctors treating their patients with pills and procedures, he realized *that these authoritative doctors didn't do any better than he did.* Their patients didn't just stay sick—they got worse. John realized something was wrong with the system, not him, so he began to read the scientific literature. Like Dr. Esselstyn, once he did so, John became convinced that a WFPB diet had the potential not only to prevent these diseases that were plaguing patients, but also the potential to treat them. This idea, he was to find out, was not received kindly by his teachers and colleagues.

In this environment, diet was considered quackery. John would ask, "Doesn't diet have something to do with heart disease?" and his colleagues would tell him that the science was controversial. John continued to read the scientific research and to talk to his colleagues but only became even more baffled: "When I looked at the literature, I couldn't find the controversy. It was absolutely clear what the literature said." Through those years, John came to understand why so many physicians claimed diet was controversial: "The scientist is sitting down at the breakfast table and in the one hand he has a paper that says that cholesterol will rot your arteries and kill you, and in the other hand he has a fork shoveling bacon and eggs into his mouth, and he says, 'There's something confusing here. I'm confused.' And that's the controversy. That's all it is."

John tells a story about seeing a thirty-eight-year-old man and his wife after the man had suffered a second heart attack. As the resident physician (not their primary attending physician), he asked the patient what he was going to do to prevent a third, fatal heart attack. "You're thirty-eight years old with a beautiful young wife, five kids. What are you going to do to keep your wife from being a widow and your kids from becoming fatherless?" The man was despondent, frustrated, and said, "There's nothing I can do. I don't drink. I don't smoke. I exercise, I follow the same diet the dietitian gave me after my last heart attack. There's nothing more I can do."

John told the couple what he had been learning about diet. He suggested that the man might reverse his disease if he ate the right way. The patient and his wife received the news with enthusiasm. John talked with them for quite a long time, left the room, and felt great. He had finally helped someone; he had finally done his job.

That lasted for about two hours. He was called into the Chief of Medicine's office. The Chief of Medicine wields absolute authority over the residents. If he fires a resident, not only is that person out of his or her job, that person is out of his or her career. The excited couple had told their attending physician what they had just learned. The doctor replied that what they had been told wasn't true, and promptly reported John to the Chief of Medicine.

The Chief of Medicine had a serious conversation with John, who remembers being told that "I was stepping far beyond my duties as a resident. I should get serious about medicine and give up all this nonsense about food having anything to do with disease." The Chief of Medicine made it clear that on this point, John's job, and his subsequent career, was on the line. So John bit his tongue for the rest of his education.

On the day of John's graduation, he and the Chief of Medicine had a final talk. John remembers the man as being smart, with a good heart, but he was too entrenched in the status quo. The Chief of Medicine sat him down and said, "John, I think you're a good doctor. I want you to know that. I want you to know that I like your family. That's why I'm going to tell you this. I'm concerned that you're going to starve to death with all your crazy ideas about food. All you're going to do is collect a bunch of bums and hippies."

John paused to gather his thoughts, and then said, "That may be the case. Then I'll have to starve. I can't put people on drugs or surgeries that don't work. Besides, I think you're wrong. I don't think it will be bums and hippies. I think it will be successful people who have done well in life. They'll ask themselves, 'I'm such a big success, so how come I'm so fat?'" With that, John looked at the Chief's generous belly, and continued, "They'll ask, 'If I'm such a big success, why are my health and my future out of control?' They'll look at what I have to say, and they're going to buy it."

John finished his formal medical education having had only one hour of nutrition instruction, which involved learning which infant formulas to use. His experience confirms every study that has found nutrition training among physicians to be sorely inadequate.

HOOKED ON DRUGS

John touched on another important area where the medical profession has lost credibility: its ties to the drug industry. Medical education and drug companies are in bed together, and have been for quite some time. John talked some about the depth of the problem and how the educational system has been corrupted. He said:

> The problem with doctors starts with our education. The whole
> system is paid for by the drug industry, from education to research.
> The drug industry has bought the minds of the medical profession.
> It starts the day you enter medical school. All the way through
> medical school everything is supported by the drug industry.

John is not alone in criticizing the way in which the medical establishment has partnered with the drug industry. Many prominent scientists have published scathing observations showing how corrupt the system has become. Among the common observations are:

- The drug industry ingratiates itself with medical students with free gifts, including meals, entertainment, and travel; educational events, including lectures, which are little more than drug advertisements; and conferences, which include speakers who are little more than drug spokespeople.[15–17]
- Graduate medical students (physician residents) and other physicians actually change their prescribing habits because of information provided by drug salespeople,[18–20] even though this information is known to be "overly positive and prescribing habits are less appropriate as a result."[17, 21, 22]
- Research and academic medicine merely carry out the pharmaceutical industry's bidding. This can happen because the drug companies, and not researchers, may design the research, which allows the company to "rig" the study[23,24]; the researchers may have a direct financial stake in the drug company whose product they are studying[15,25]; the drug company may be responsible for collecting and collating the raw data, and then only selectively allow researchers to view the data[23,26]; the drug company may retain veto power over whether the findings are published, and may retain editorial rights over any scientific publications resulting from the research[23,25,27]; the drug company may hire a communications firm to write the scientific article, and then find researchers willing to attach their names as authors of the paper after it has already been written.[26]
- The major scientific journals have turned into little more than marketing vehicles for drug companies. The leading medical journals derive their primary income from drug advertising. This advertising is not adequately reviewed by the journal, and companies often present misleading claims about drugs. Perhaps more disconcerting, the majority of clinical trial research reported in the journals is funded by drug company money, and the financial interests of the researchers involved are not fully acknowledged.[24]

In the past couple of years there have been well-publicized scandals at major medical centers that confirm these charges. In one instance, a scientist's integrity was maligned in a variety of ways by both a drug company and her university administration after she found that a drug under study had strong side effects and lost its effectiveness.[27] In another case, a scientist speaking out about the possible side effects of antidepressants lost a job opportunity at the University of Toronto.[26] The examples go on and on.

Dr. Marcia Angell, an ex-editor of the *New England Journal of Medicine*, wrote a scathing editorial called "Is Academic Medicine for Sale?"[15]:

> *The ties between clinical researchers and industry include not only grant support, but also a host of other financial arrangements. Researchers serve as consultants to companies whose products they are studying, join advisory boards and speakers' bureaus, enter into patent and royalty arrangements, agree to be the listed authors of articles ghostwritten by interested companies, promote drugs and devices at company-sponsored symposiums and allow themselves to be plied with expensive gifts and trips to luxurious settings. Many also have equity interest in the companies.*

Dr. Angell goes on to say that these financial associations often significantly "bias research, both the kind of work that is done and the way it is reported."

Even more dangerous than the threat of fraudulent findings is the fact that the only type of research that is funded and recognized is research on drugs. Research on the causes of disease and non-drug interventions simply doesn't occur in medical education settings. For example, academic researchers may be furiously trying to find a pill that will treat the symptoms of obesity, but not be devoting any time or money to teaching people how to live a healthier life. Dr. Angell writes[15]:

> *In terms of education, medical students and house officers, under the constant tutelage of industry representatives,* learn to rely on drugs and devices more than they probably should *[our emphasis]. As the critics of medicine so often charge,* young physicians learn that for every problem, there is a pill (and a drug company representative to explain it) *[our emphasis]. They also become accustomed to receiving gifts and favors from an industry that uses these courtesies to influence their continuing education. The academic medical centers, in allowing themselves to become research outposts for industry, contribute to the overemphasis on drugs and devices.*

In this environment, is it possible for nutrition to be given fair and honest consideration? Despite the fact that our leading killers can be prevented and even reversed using good nutrition, will you ever hear about it from your doctor? Not as long as this environment persists in our medical schools and hospitals. Not unless your doctor has decided that standard medical practice as it is taught does not work, and decides to spend a significant amount of time educating himself or herself about good nutrition. This takes a rare individual.

The situation has gotten so bad that Dr. John McDougall said, "I don't know what to believe anymore. When I read a paper that says I should be giving my heart patients beta blockers and ACE inhibitors, two classes of heart drugs, *I don't know whether it's true. I honestly don't know if it's true because* [drug research] *is so tainted*."

Do you think the following headlines are related?

> *"Schools report research interest conflicts" (between drug companies and researchers)*[28]
> *"Prescription use by children multiplying, study says"*[29]
> *"Survey: Many guidelines written by doctors with ties to companies"*[30]
> *"Correctly Prescribed Drugs Take Heavy Toll; Millions Affected by Toxic Reactions"*[31]

We pay a high price for allowing these medical biases. A *Journal of the American Medical Association* study found that one in five new drugs will either get a "black box warning," indicating a previously unknown serious adverse reaction that may result in death or serious injury, or will be withdrawn from the market within twenty-five years.[32] Twenty percent of all new drugs have serious unknown side effects, and more than 100,000 Americans die every year from *correctly* taking their properly *prescribed medication*.[33] This is one of the leading causes of death in America!

DR. MCDOUGALL'S FATE

When Dr. John McDougall finished his formal medical education, he set up a practice on the Hawaiian island of Oahu. He began writing books about nutrition and health and established a national reputation. In the mid-1980s John was contacted by St. Helena Hospital in Napa Valley, California, and asked if he would accept a position running its health center. The hospital was a Seventh-day Adventist hospital; if you recall from chapter seven, the Seventh-day Adventists encourage followers to eat a vegetarian diet (even though they consume higher-than-average amounts of dairy products). It was an opportunity too good to pass up, and John left Hawaii for California.

John had a good home at St. Helena for a number of years. He taught nutrition and used nutrition to treat sick patients, which he did with fantastic success. He treated over 2,000 very sick patients, and over the course of sixteen years, he has never been sued or even had a letter of complaint. Perhaps more importantly, John saw these patients get well. Throughout this time, he continued his publishing activity, maintaining a national reputation. But as time passed, he realized that things weren't quite the same as when he first arrived. His discontent was growing. Of those later years he says, "I just didn't think I was going anyplace. The program had 150 or 170 people a year and that was it. Never grew. Wasn't getting any support from the hospital and we had gone through a lot of administrators."

He had small clashes with the other doctors at the hospital. At one point, the heart department objected to what John was doing with heart patients. John told them, "I'll tell you what, I'll send every one of my heart patients to you for a second opinion if you'll send yours to me." It was quite an offer, but they didn't accept it. On another occasion, John had referred a patient to a cardiologist and the cardiologist incorrectly told the patient that he needed to have bypass surgery. After a couple of these incidents, John had reached the limit of his patience. Finally, after the cardiologist recommended surgery for another one of John's patients, John called him and said, "I want to talk with you and the patient about this. I would like to discuss the scientific literature that causes you to make this recommendation." The cardiologist said that he wouldn't do that, to which John responded, "Why not? You just recommended that this guy have his heart opened! And you're going to charge him 50,000 or 100,000 bucks for it. Why don't we discuss it? Don't you think that's fair to the patient?" The cardiologist declined, saying that it would just confuse the patient. That was the last time he recommended heart surgery for one of John's patients.

Meanwhile, none of the other physicians in the hospital had ever referred a patient to John. Not once. Other physicians would send their own wives and children to see him but they would never refer a patient. The reason, according to John:

> They were worried [about what would happen when] their
> patients would come to see me, and it happened all the time when
> patients would come on their own. They'd come to me with heart
> disease or high blood pressure or diabetes. I'd put them on the
> diet and they'd go back off all their pills and soon their numbers
> would be normal. They'd go to their doctor and say, "Why the hell
> didn't you tell me about this before? Why did you let me suffer,
> spend all this money, almost die, when all I had to do was eat
> oatmeal?" The doctors didn't want to hear this.

There were other moments of friction between John and the hospital, but the last straw involved Dr. Roy Swank's multiple sclerosis program mentioned in chapter nine.

John had contacted Dr. Swank when he learned that Swank was about to retire. John had known and respected Dr. Roy Swank for a long time, and he offered to take over the Swank MS program and merge it with his health clinic at St. Helena Hospital, preserving it in honor of Dr. Swank. Dr. Swank agreed, much to John's excitement. As John said, there were four reasons that this would be a perfect fit for St. Helena's:

- it fit in with the philosophy of the Adventists: dietary treatment of disease
- they would be helping people who desperately needed their help
- it would double their patient census, helping to grow the program
- it would cost almost nothing

In thinking back on it, John said, "Could you think of any reason not to do this? It [was] obvious!" So he took the proposal to the head of his department. After listening, she said that she didn't think the hospital wanted to do this. She said, "Well, I don't think we really want to introduce any new programs right now." John, dumbfounded, asked her, "Please tell me why. What does it mean to be a hospital? Why are we here? I thought we were here to take care of sick people."

Her response was a doozy: "Well, you know we are, but you know, MS patients are not really desirable patients. You told me yourself that most neurologists don't like to take care of MS patients." John could not believe what he had just heard. In a very tense moment, he said:

Wait a minute. I'm a doctor. This is a hospital. As far as I know our job is to relieve the suffering of the sick. These are sick people. Just because other doctors can't help them in their suffering doesn't mean that we can't. Here's the evidence that says we can. I have an effective treatment for people who need my care and this is a hospital. Will you explain to me why we don't want to take care of those kinds of patients?

He continued:

I want to talk to the head of the hospital. I want to explain to her why I need this program and why the hospital needs this program

and why the patients need this program. I want you to get me an
appointment.

Ultimately, though, the head of the hospital proved to be just as difficult. John reflected on the situation with his wife. He was supposed to renew his contract with the hospital in a couple of weeks, and he decided not to do it. He left on cordial terms, and to this day he does not hold personal grudges. He just explains it by saying that their directions in life were different. John would prefer to remember St. Helena for what it was: a good home to him for sixteen years, but a place nonetheless that was "just into that whole drug money thing."

Now, John runs a highly successful "lifestyle medicine" program with his family's help, writes a popular newsletter that he makes freely available (http://www.drmcdougall.com), organizes group trips with past patients and new friends, and has more time to go windsurfing when the wind picks up on Bodega Bay. This is a man with a wealth of knowledge and qualifications, who could benefit the health of millions of Americans. He has never been challenged by any of his colleagues for physician "misbehavior," and yet the medical establishment does not want his services. He is reminded of this fact all the time:

Patients will come in with rheumatoid arthritis. They'll be in
wheelchairs, they can't even turn the key on their car. And I'll take
care of them and three or four weeks later, they'll go back to see
their doctor. They'll walk up to their doctor, grab their hand, and
shake it hard. Doctor will say, "Wonderful." The patient, all excited,
will say, "Well, I want to tell you what I did. I went to see this Dr.
McDougall, I changed my diet, and now my arthritis is gone." Their
doctor simply responds, "Oh my goodness. That's great. Whatever
you're doing, just keep doing it. I'll see you later." That's always the
response. It's not, "Please, my god, tell me what you did so I can
tell the next patient." It's, "Whatever you're doing, that's just great."
If the patient starts to tell them they changed to a vegetarian diet,
the doctor will cut in with, "Yeah okay, fine, you're really a strong
person. Thanks a lot. See you later." Get them out of the office as
quickly as they can. It's very threatening . . . very threatening.

ESSELSTYN'S REWARD

Back in Ohio, Dr. Esselstyn retired from active surgery in June of 2000 and assumed the position of preventive cardiology consultant in the department of general surgery at the Cleveland Clinic. He has continued to do research and to visit with patients. He holds three-hour counseling sessions in his home with new heart disease patients, gives them research evidence, and provides a delicious "heart-safe" meal. In addition, he gives talks around the country and abroad.

In March of 2002, Ess and his wife, Ann, whose grandfather founded the Cleveland Clinic, drafted a letter to the head of the cardiology department and the head of the hospital at the Clinic. The letter started off by saying how proud they were of the reputation and excellence of the Clinic and the innovation of the surgical procedures, but that everyone recognized that surgery was never going to be the answer to this epidemic of heart disease. Ess formally proposed the idea that he could help set up an arrest-and-reversal dietary program in the department of preventive cardiology at the Cleveland Clinic. The program would mirror his own and could be administered by nurse clinicians and physician assistants. Ideally, a young physician with passion for the idea would head the program. Ultimately, every patient with heart disease at the Clinic would be offered the option of arrest-and-reversal therapy using dietary means, which costs very little, harbors no risks, and puts the control back into the patients' hands.

You'd think that if an opportunity arose to profoundly heal sick people, and one of the most reputable people in the country was going to help you, a hospital would jump at the opportunity. But after being one of the star surgeons at the Cleveland Clinic for decades, after initiating a heart-disease reversal study that had greater success than anything ever done at the Clinic, and after graciously offering a plan to help heal even more people, Ess wasn't even contacted. Neither the head of the hospital nor the department head had the respect to even acknowledge that he had written to them. They didn't call. They didn't write. They completely ignored him.

Seven weeks passed, and finally Ess called the department head and the hospital head, and neither of them would take his call. Finally, after seven calls, the head of the hospital got on the phone. This man had praised Ess for years for his research and seemed excited by his results, but now he was singing a different tune. He obviously knew exactly what Ess was calling about, and told Ess that the head of the cardiology department didn't want to do it. In other words, he just passed the buck. If the head of the hospital wanted it to be done, it would be done, regardless of what the head of cardiology wanted. So Ess called the head of cardiology, who finally took his call. The man was abrasive and rude. He made it clear he had no interest in what Ess was trying to do.

Ess hasn't talked to either of these doctors since, but he still has hope that he can change their minds as more and more research supports what he has been saying. Meanwhile, many people at the Clinic are still excited about Ess's work. Many of them want to see a wider application of his program, but the powers that be will not let it happen. They get frustrated, and Ess is likewise frustrated because the current program in preventive cardiology is a disaster:

> They still eat meat, they still eat dairy, and they don't have any cholesterol goal. It's all just so vague. Preventive cardiology takes great pride when they are able to slow the rate of progression of this disease. This isn't cancer for God's sake!

An interesting situation is now developing: just as with Dr. McDougall, many of the Clinic "bigwigs" with heart disease have themselves gone to Esselstyn for treatment and lifestyle counseling. They know it works, and they seek out the program on their own. As Ess says, this could be developing into a very interesting crisis:

> I have now treated a number of senior staff with coronary disease at the Clinic—senior staff physicians. I have also treated a number of senior staff trustees. One of the trustees knows about the frustrations that we've had trying to get this into the Clinic, and he says, "I think, if the word gets out that Esselstyn has this treatment that arrests and reverses this disease at the Cleveland Clinic, and it's been used by senior staff and he's treated senior trustees, but he's not permitted to treat the common herd, we could be open for a lawsuit."

For the time being, Ess, with his wife's help, will continue to run counseling sessions out of his own home because the institution to which he gave the greater part of his life does not want to endorse a dietary approach that competes with its standard menu of pills and procedures. This past summer Ess spent much more time than usual at his upstate New York farm, making hay. As much as Ess likes a more relaxed life, he would also love to continue to help diseased people get better with the aid of the Cleveland Clinic. But they won't allow him to. This is nothing short of criminal. We, the public, turn to doctors and hospitals in times of great need. For them to provide care that is knowingly less than optimal, that doesn't protect our health, doesn't heal our disease, and costs us tens of thousands of dollars is morally inexcusable. Ess sums up the situation:

The Clinic is now injecting stem cells to try to make new heart vessels grow. Wouldn't it be easier to stop the disease? It's appalling, isn't it? It's just so grippingly unbelievable to think that we're being led around by people who refuse to believe the obvious!

Both Esselstyn and McDougall have now been denied reentry into the establishment, after headline-making success at healing people with a nutritional approach. You can focus on the money—according to John and Ess, 80% of St. Helena's and 65% of the Cleveland Clinic's respective incomes were generated by traditional heart disease treatments, surgical interventions—but it's something more than just money. It may also be the intellectual threat that the patient should be in control, and not the doctor; that something as simple as food could be more powerful than all the knowledge of pills and high-tech procedures; it may be the lack of credible nutrition education in medical school; it may be the influence of the drug industry. Whatever it is, it has become clear that the medical industry in this country is not protecting our health as it should. As McDougall reaches his arms out, palms up, and scrunches his shoulders up, he simply says, "It's beyond comprehension."

SINCE THE FIRST EDITION— FROM THOMAS M. CAMPBELL, MD

After co-authoring the first edition of *The China Study* with my dad, I had a new passion for nutrition and health and decided to pursue a medical degree. The four years I spent working closely with my dad on this book were a sort of apprenticeship in nutrition literature review and communication. I had spent time with thousands of abstracts, reading hundreds of nutrition science publications, and discussing and arguing and learning with one of the top nutritional biochemists of the past fifty years. I knew how powerful a WFPB diet could be in preventing and reversing some of our more common chronic diseases, and I knew well that my medical education would be a time largely devoid of diet and lifestyle information.

Since the first edition of this book, the amount of nutrition education in medical school remains scandalous. Survey results published in 2010 show that, on average, medical students get a total of about twenty hours of nutrition education during their four-year education—essentially nothing.[34] My own training experience reinforced the notion that nutrition is ignored. The small number of hours present were focused almost entirely on biochemistry and metabolism and had almost no bearing on using nutrition to prevent and treat the illnesses that all doctors see every day.

What I believe has improved since the first edition of this book is the extent of the direct marketing relationship between industry and medical education. In the mid- to late 2000s, when I was in medical school, I was at clinics that sometimes had lunches provided by drug representatives, who in turn were able to attend and share promotional materials for their products. My impression is that this type of direct marketing has been seriously subsiding over the past ten years, at least among academic medical centers. As a resident doctor and then as a board-certified family physician at a major academic medical center, I did not benefit from any industry-branded gifts (free lunches, pens, drug samples, etc.) during my training. That is true generally of students, residents, and practitioners at the University of Rochester. The University of Rochester Medical Center has a strict policy that regulates interactions between pharmaceutical and device industries and practitioners. Industry continues to play a major role in medical research, and this core relationship has far-reaching implications in setting the paradigms of how we identify and treat disease, perpetuating the status quo. But in a growing percentage of academic medical centers, industry no longer has a direct line to market their products directly to trainees and practitioners.

I was prepared for the terrible gap in education that leaves nutrition out of the picture, but I could not be fully prepared for the individual suffering that results. Countless individuals are suffering terribly, right now, with illnesses caused or strongly exacerbated by poor nutrition. These patients have often interacted with dozens of health professionals, most of whom are, without a doubt, extraordinarily hardworking, intelligent, caring, and kind, and these patients have never been told about the potential of nutrition to prevent and reverse illness. Through my journey they have been a stark reminder of how poorly our medical system sometimes functions.

Since the original publication of *The China Study*, though, there has been great reason for hope and optimism. The Cleveland Clinic Wellness Institute now offers a six-hour group counseling seminar with Dr. Esselstyn. Montefiore Hospital offers a similar program. Continuing medical education conferences on plant-based nutrition draw hundreds of health practitioners annually. A preventive medicine training program at Maine Medical Center will incorporate plant-based nutrition training. Kaiser Permanente, one of the largest health systems in the country, published a paper in its journal suggesting that physicians recommend plant-based diets to all their patients. Other hospital systems from Lee County, Florida, to Midland, Texas, have been incorporating plant-based nutrition into their patient care (with the help of PlantPure Wellness, my brother Nelson Campbell's organization), as have a growing variety of private medical practices, like the Barnard Medical Center. Thousands of laypeople and hundreds of health care practitioners are getting educated in plant-based nutrition through the T. Colin Campbell Center for Nutrition Studies, which offers an online certificate program in conjunction with eCornell.

As part of the primary care network at my own institution, I and my wife, Erin Campbell, who is a board-certified preventive medicine physician, have been supported to start a small program that offers plant-based nutrition as an option for patients interested in preventing or reversing disease: the University of Rochester Program for Nutrition in Medicine (URNutritionInMedicine.com). We're proud to offer one of the more comprehensive offerings using plant-based nutrition at an academic medical center that I know of in the country. Our services include individual consultations, community education, and a variety of group patient programs, including immersion programs for people from around the country. In addition, we have had a small number of trainees work with us to learn about plant-based nutrition in clinical practice and have opportunities to do further research on plant-based nutrition. Remarkably, this is all under the umbrella of a major academic medical center at the University of Rochester. This is a testament to the groundswell of interest and support in plant-based nutrition for prevention and also *treatment* of disease.

Yet we stand with great work ahead of us. Humans are strongly social creatures, and those who currently eat a WFPB diet remain a tiny minority of the population. I believe that a great many of our behavioral choices are made with a strong, mostly subconscious deference to social norms, and many people, including patients and health care providers, remain uninterested in trying a plant-based diet. Nutrition training in medical school remains woefully absent, and we live in a paradigm that regards pills and procedures as the only legitimate treatment for our common diseases. While industry's direct, in-person marketing to health providers may be less active, the device and pharmaceutical industries continue to strongly shape the medical paradigm by providing funding for research, in turn helping the careers of those researchers and educators who shape important medical guidelines. As long as this is the case, nutrition education and behavior change will not be seriously considered as the powerful treatment that it can be.

And perhaps most difficult, reimbursement systems do not pay for patients to undergo most comprehensive nutrition programs. For an uninsured patient, the average cost of a coronary artery bypass procedure in the U.S. in 2015 was about $150,000, with great variation between different locations[35]—some hospitals charge over $400,000. Those with insurance can easily get this service covered, even at astronomical prices (though insurance companies may work out deals to pay substantially less than what the hospital officially charges). Yet there are no, or very few, satisfactory mechanisms to get insurance to pay adequately for most patients to participate in physician-led group nutrition programs at a tiny fraction of this cost. This is a fundamental barrier to the widespread practice of nutrition as medicine. Until this changes, there will be very limited movement toward the systemic changes needed to help patients lead healthier lives by addressing diet and lifestyle as the leading causes of death and disability in the U.S.

One of the great sources of physician burnout is the feeling that what we do isn't helping our patients in the way we'd hope. It's a loss of meaning in our work. I have frequently seen tragic illness fought impressively by patients and their health care providers using pills and procedures, while simultaneously ignoring diet and lifestyle's role as cause, or promoter, of their illness. There is inevitable frustration in a medical system trying to fight chronic disease while unknowingly withholding their greatest weapon: diet and lifestyle change. And the surveys bear this out: Over 50% of physicians in the U.S. are experiencing burnout,[36] something I believe to be worsened under the current standard of care by seeing our work fail to yield significant benefits in many cases.

Our present situation is unsustainable and largely unsatisfying for a great many people on both sides of the stethoscope (patients and doctors). Not only in spite of these challenges, but also because of these challenges, many people are now looking for an improved approach, yielding the innovative changes and programs I previously mentioned. Given all the positive examples of change around the country, I believe medicine is on its way to seriously helping people lead healthier lives though addressing lifestyle choices, even though we have many barriers to overcome. This movement is finally gaining traction—a remarkable change from eleven years ago, when the first edition of *The China Study* was published.

I have had the mother of an eleven-year-old child cry in my office when she got the cholesterol results showing that her child wouldn't need to start lifelong statins and instead could just focus on eating a healthy plant-based diet. I have delighted in taking patients off medications when they received dramatic health benefits by enjoying new, delicious breakfast, lunch, and dinner habits. Patients in our group programs have called them "life-changing" and are grateful for an alternative option to maintaining and regaining health. The tagline for University of Rochester Medicine is "Medicine of the Highest Order." The most heartwarming compliment we've had so far, as we've worked so incredibly hard to build a plant-based program at a major medical institution, is from a patient at the end of one of our eight-week group lifestyle programs who referred to her experience by saying, "THIS . . . THIS is medicine of the highest order."

ACADEMIA

18

cademia is the societal sector I know best. As I write this chapter for *The China Study*'s second edition, it's been my professional home for sixty years and two days. Yet in the first edition of this book, except for some comments on the "dark side" of science, we did not discuss how academia as an *institution* relates to this book's message.

We provided some discussion in the first edition on how industry, government, and medical practice create confusing and misleading diet and health information. But that discussion mostly focused on conflicts that arise from the way research is designed and data are interpreted by each of these sectors. It did not go deeply enough into our fundamental assumptions and definitions of nutrition, health, medical practice, and the discipline of science itself. These ideas were further fleshed out in *Whole*. However, in that book, too, we omitted what role the institution of academia might be playing.

It is tempting to lay the blame for public confusion about health and nutrition at the feet of any of the institutions discussed here. As we've seen, each has played a role. However, I prefer not to blame industry for this problem because I understand (even though I often disagree with) their main purpose: to produce products and services that will sell. Shareholder interests, jobs, and revenue matter; otherwise, there is no business. Unfortunately, however, companies often act extremely irresponsibly when interpreting science for their own selfish interests.

Neither do I hold responsible medical practitioners and administrators, because they mostly rely on the highly reductionist scientific evidence that is provided to them. Practitioners also suffer from an almost total lack of training in nutrition, a wholistic science with its own set of principles and criteria. When all of one's training has been highly reductionist, it can be difficult to fully grasp the paradigm of wholism as a basis for their understanding of nutrition.

We might also blame institutions not mentioned here—the media, for example, who are responsible for disseminating this information. For the most part, however, media communicate what they are told by those who create information. Most journalists do not have the educational background necessary to assess the reliability of the information given to them—and are under pressure to present "balanced" reports—so they run a very high risk of selecting unqualified people to present the opposing side of stories where only one side has merit. And as in industry, media publications are companies, beholden to advertisers and other outside interests that affect their continued existence.

On the question of the government sector, it is my experience that although most government personnel concerned with human health research do their best to provide reliable facts to the public, their interpretation of these facts into regulations and public policy may become quite subjective. It is during this interpretation phase of evaluating scientific evidence that outside corporate interests can best exert their influence. I have seen this interplay between industry and government sectors becoming so significant in so many ways that it is fair to say that government and industry now act, in effect, as one mega-institution.

Each of these sectors—industry, medical practice, the media, government—has specific interests and responsibilities, but these also overlap. Although I once thought it reasonable to ask which sector was most responsible for the public's confusion about diet and health, I now realize that it makes little or no sense to estimate who is most responsible. Each sector depends, more or less, on the same fundamental information provided to them. Each sector will use it to its best advantage.

And who has the responsibility to create this knowledge and to determine its validity? In one way or another, it is academia.

The impact of academia on society goes well beyond the ivory tower; its reach into the intellectual, social, and corporate fabric of our society is overwhelming. Academia, aside from educating, in the fall of 2016, twenty-one million college-age young people,[1] conducts or oversees most of our basic research in the health sciences. The National Institutes of Health (NIH) alone send most of its annual $30 billion in medical research to "300,000 researchers at more than 2,500 universities, medical schools, and other institutions in every state and around the world."[2]

When we speak of academia, however, we do not refer only to the university campuses where most of this information is produced. Significant amounts of work by academics occurs outside of their institutions, and these activities are related to and strongly influenced by their academic reputation and continued "membership" and responsibilities within academia.

One of the more prominent of these activities is helping to develop public health policies, projects, and services, usually by sitting on committees of experts (which I discussed further in chapter 13).

Academia also takes a lead role in managing a vast proportion of agricultural outreach activities. Through a government program more than a century old, universities and colleges administer "cooperative extension" outreach programs that, according to the United States Department of Agriculture, "bring evidence-based science and modern technologies to farmers, consumers and families."[3]

In other words, academia is the sector of our society best positioned, at least theoretically, to gather the kind and quality of information that is fundamental to how we think about diet and health. But this can happen only if academia promotes and ensures the necessary freedom for its professionals to practice their art, and then ensures that these ideas are regularly exposed to the fresh air of public and professional scrutiny. Academia should be expanding the boundaries of knowledge through original research, then sharing this information not only with professional peers but also with various public communities: classroom students, independent study students, and the community. A free society cannot exist without a venue and an environment for honest research and discourse.

Regrettably, in my experience, academia is falling far short of this standard.

THE CHALLENGE TO ACADEMIC FREEDOM: CORNELL AS CASE STUDY

The importance of academia to any society aspiring to be free and progressive can hardly be overemphasized. But to truly benefit society, academics must be free to think, to investigate, and to share ideas in an environment where integrity and honesty flourish. Unfortunately, I have come to see academia as a victim of the steady erosion of free speech once granted them.

I have spent virtually my entire career in the academy: three years at MIT, ten years at Virginia Tech, and forty years at Cornell (counting four years of graduate studies and sixteen years as professor emeritus), with one-year sabbaticals at Oxford University and the headquarters of our professional biomedical societies in Bethesda, Maryland. I was recruited back to Cornell in 1975 as a full professor with tenure at the unusually young age of forty, fourteen years after finishing my doctoral studies there. My principal faculty appointment was in the Division of Nutritional Sciences, newly enlarged and renamed but long ranked as the number one nutrition science department in the country. But I was also invited to become a member of two other graduate fields of study (biochemistry and international agriculture), which also qualified me to chair graduate students' research dissertations in each of these disciplines. I then co-founded a new graduate field of toxicology, thus providing me four graduate fields in which to work and mentor students.

During my time at Cornell, my research group hosted about twenty-five visiting professors and scholars from six different countries (Japan, England, France, China, Canada, and Nigeria) for periods of about one year each to work in my laboratory. (To all these people, I am grateful; without their participation, I would not have written this book or *Whole*.) Many of these young people went on to have distinguished careers in science. My research program was, for many years, the largest, best-funded, and most published in the entire Division of Nutritional Sciences.

My long career at Cornell also has been especially rewarding for me off campus. Cornell's name and reputation certainly opened doors, including the opportunity for me to stay very busy for about twenty years as a member of, and contributor to, several highly recognized expert panels responsible for developing or contributing to national and international policies on diet and health. These activities provided unusually broad experiences and perspectives that shaped a critically important vision for our society, indeed our planet.

In short, academia has given me, as it has many others, exceptionally rich opportunities for career development. Unless we academics brush too close to the edge of well-established and cherished beliefs and practices, we can create and share our own perspectives on knowledge within the classroom with our students, we can choose our own colleagues, and we can imagine and test our own research questions—provided that we are able to compete for funding. We have a lot of room to create our reality.

However, I have seen what happens when an academic's work *does* brush too close to—indeed, outright challenges—those established beliefs and practices.

Prior to 1990, my research group's extensively published findings had often been featured in the media, thanks to the assistance of Cornell's communications department. But in 1990, our project in China added a substantial new dimension to our research that further ratcheted up national and international attention. Lead stories on the China project appeared in *USA Today*, the *New York Times,* and the *Saturday Evening Post*, among other popular media outlets. The news surrounding this research in China was considerable, undoubtedly enhanced by this project's being the first joint research collaboration between our two countries.

I became quite interested in the massive new data from China. The combination of laboratory and human research findings hinted at a story that had great potential to fundamentally reshape the way we thought about nutrition. From that time onwards, events began to expand in many different directions: a first-of-its kind university course on "Vegetarian Nutrition" was taught at Cornell (until it was moved to an online offering); this book was published in 2005; at least fifteen videos and movie documentaries have been made that included, even featured, our work; and I've been offered an increasing number of speaking engagements, beyond my capacity to fulfill. A "movement" about plant-based nutrition was beginning to emerge.

If I were to select a singular event that became a turning point, it would be the *New York Times* story on our China project findings in their Science section in 1990. It signaled a new path, one that made my academic pursuits much more public. The years that followed gradually provided an opportunity for me to reconsider the meanings of nutrition, health, and science itself, although I did not appreciate how much of a departure from traditional science these new meanings would eventually be. I had experienced the difficulties of challenging dogma in earlier years, as already told elsewhere in this book, but these new developments begun in the early 1990s presented fresh challenges.

As all these events were unfolding, certain Cornell administrators were taking interest, but not in the way I would have hoped. Their interest might be better described as uncertain curiosity, rather than constructive interest, and I began to face what often felt like a concerted effort to prevent my work from reaching not only the public, but also others, including students, within the university.

At around that same time, the director of our Division of Nutritional Sciences at Cornell (long the number one nutritional sciences program in the country), Dr. Cutberto Garza, was serving as vice president of the powerful multinational food-products and dairy company the Danone Group (in Europe) or the Dannon Company (in the U.S.). In 1995, he also became chair of the USDA Dietary Guidelines Committee (the source of the government's Food Pyramid). During his tenure, he and his committee were successfully sued for their suppression of information regarding their conflicts of interest with the dairy industry. Six of the eleven members of the committee had financial ties to the industry that had not been revealed. That lawsuit also uncovered that Garza had failed to declare personal compensation in excess of the amount that required declaration.[4]

In the midst of this period, I organized a course in our division titled "Vegetarian Nutrition"—a title that I did not particularly like but that our director thought appropriate. I was more interested in challenging some of the fundamental practices of nutritional science. Although an elective course, it soon became quite popular.

However, when I chose, six years into the class's offering, to skip a year in order to present some lectures off campus that were arising because of the release of first edition of this book, the director deleted the course from the course catalog with no consultation with me, shortly before leaving campus to take a provost position at Boston University. I was told by a staffer of the student newspaper that between 3,000 and 5,000 students signed a petition to have it reinstated but, in spite of my appeal through channels all the way to the university president (who himself was a vegetarian), the course remained cancelled. The last year of its offering was hosted by another department on campus, when I was piloting a teaching model to allow students elsewhere in the U.S. to take the course and transfer credits from Cornell to their institution. But this, too, hit a snag. Garza's successor, geneticist Patrick Stover, wrote a letter to the director of the host department to say that his department could not sponsor the course because it was no longer approved by our department, a fabrication. Both the university ombudsman and the dean of faculty offered to help and suggested that I seek re-approval of the course from our department committee, who originally approved the course. But Stover nixed that idea as well by writing a letter to the committee that even if they reapproved it, he would block its offering.

(It's worth noting, also, that Garza's challenges to the concept of academic freedom were not limited to Cornell. After leaving our campus for Boston University, he denied a request of 88% of the faculty there to establish a faculty senate shortly before his stepping down from that position.)

Stover continued his unexplained interference in my work by cancelling (through one of his staff), a mere three days before the lecture date, a previously scheduled room for dual lectures by visiting lecturer Dr. Caldwell Esselstyn and myself (the room remained unused during that time slot). When I asked for the staffer's assistance at that late date in locating another lecture hall, I was told, "Dr. Campbell, you will never have another room for lectures on this campus!"

I also learned from a colleague that the retiring director of our large and influential communications department had been instructed by a high university official that his staff was not to give me "any more ink." I had been the beneficiary of these university communication services for all the years I'd been with Cornell (national news releases, articles in Cornell's publications), and was once shown a tracking report by this office that more than 200 state and national media reports on our work came from their news releases. However reliable my colleague's comment, that office did terminate communications about our work with off-campus media sources. And so, for the next three or so years—silence.

Back when my nutrition course was cancelled, the final "solution" suggested by the dean of our college was to bring it to Cornell's then-new online program, eCornell, which was struggling to survive. Although it was like going down to the minors in baseball and seemed to me like another way of making the course disappear, I was willing to give it a try. I had started a nonprofit organization to fund the work of a couple graduate students of mine and, with the help of some enterprising former students who had previously put my courses online (in those days not a very easy thing to do), especially Meghan Murphy, and a donor, who paid to staff the reenergized nonprofit, we organized and began offering the course online. By 2014, the course, now qualified as a certificate program and offering thirty Category 1 continuing medical education credits for physicians, was ranked number one out of the hundred or so courses hosted by eCornell. Learning of our success, a senior writer at Cornell's communications office composed an article about the course for their *Cornell Chronicle* (Cornell's primary news source).

The article's author had been at Cornell for thirty-two years and was planning her retirement that October. Many years before, her first article upon her employment at Cornell concerned my co-authorship of the 1982 *Diet, Nutrition, and Cancer* report of the National Academy of Sciences[5] and the unusual national publicity that arose with that report, so it seemed fitting that she began and concluded her career with articles on my research work.

But when a draft of the proposed news item was shared with Cornell's president, he in turn shared it with a few administrators, including the dean of the College of Agriculture and Life Sciences, the director of the Division of Nutritional Sciences, and the dean of the College of Human Ecology, and they refused to allow its publication. According to the journalist, they did so because they did not "endorse" my views. *Cornell Chronicle* staff countered that blocking its publication for that reason was contrary to academic freedom and offered them an opportunity to publish their own interpretation of this information alongside the article. But this, too, was denied.

Incidentally, when the *Cornell Chronicle* journalist was initially interviewing me for her article, I reminded her that her office had been forbidden three years before to write "any more ink" on my work, but she assured me that this was no longer true because that director had recently retired. However, something had clearly changed since she had first interviewed me for the article. Someone higher up in the administration was calling the shots, regardless of who occupied the director's chair.

I really dislike sharing with the public this "dirty laundry" of a university for which I have had so much respect and which is still so enriched with so many brilliant scholars and teachers. I would not hesitate to advise students to attend Cornell. But it is important to me to share enough of this information to demonstrate how academia has the power to modify science to its liking and discredit scientific information not to their liking. This story, although based on my own experiences, is not one intended to focus on me personally, either favorably or unfavorably. It simply is the version I know best of a story that has been repeated too many times elsewhere with serious societal consequences.

THE CONTINUING EROSION OF ACADEMIC FREEDOM

I wish I could follow up these stories with something hopeful about the future, but recent trends show that the conditions that encourage the loss of academic freedom are getting worse. More and more of the lecturers and researchers in our universities are non-tenure-track employees whose jobs are vulnerable to the wishes and control of their employers. In effect, they are contractors carrying out their employers' propaganda. Without tenure, they can be released from their positions at any time when their opinions and findings run afoul of gutless authorities. In 1980, 68% of academics held tenure or tenure-track positions.[6] Now this number is only 32%.[7] This means 68% are non-tenure-track, when the American Association of University Professors recommends that the number of non-tenure-track academics on staff should not exceed 15%.[6]

The higher-level bureaucrats who control these non-tenure and tenure-track faculty positions are also more and more beholden to corporate interests, because corporations are paying more and more of the institution's bill. In 1965, when I assumed my first faculty position at Virginia Tech, the private sector funded less than 40% of scientific research and development; by 2006, that number had increased to 65%.[8]

I know well the protection that tenure affords. When I first returned to Cornell as a tenured full professor in 1975, I was invited to join two other faculty on a lecture tour around the state led by our dean of the College of Agriculture. I had already started to question the consumption of animal-based protein based on my research findings, and this prompted a letter from the New York State Egg Board, an industry advocacy group, who urged the dean and the university president to fire me. The dean, although very much a livestock industry enthusiast in his personal life, was a man of personal character. He replied that he could not and would not do this. My tenure was working for me and it continues—at least in principle—to do so until the present day. Despite my research having led me further and further astray from the conventional positions backed by corporate interests, I have kept both my position and my ability to speak what I believe to be the truth. While the proportion of faculty who enjoy the privilege of tenure continues to decline, its further erosion is catalyzed by a few individual faculty who sell their souls to the highest bidder by accepting personal consultancies for personal gain. In this system, unfortunately, these are also the people who get the most media attention as scientific, university-based authorities, especially when also publicized and supported by their corporate associates.

THE IDEALS OF THE ACADEMY

The Board of Directors of the Association of American Colleges & Universities[9] provides the following guidelines on academic conduct and freedom—guidelines that should be obvious and that are assumed by most people.

> *Students do have a right to hear and examine diverse opinions . . .*
> *. . . scholars require the freedom to pursue their ideas wherever they lead, unconstrained by political, religious, or other dictums.*
> *. . . the academy ensures that no proposal stands without alternatives or arrogates to itself the claim of possessing the sole truth [as the claim of administrators that they know best].*
> *Academic freedom is protected by society so that faculty and students can use that freedom to promote the larger good.*

But these high-minded ideals become a fairy tale when institutions are beholden to corporate sponsors.

I am confident that the vast majority of academics are honorable, socially conscious scholars who are willing to participate in honest discourse. What so many of us in academia don't realize, however, is that we live within intellectual silos, generally unaware—even unconscious—of the limits that are imposed on our speech and the direction of our research. Too many of us working on narrow topics of diet, health, and medicine never get to see those limits, because when working in an environment of scientific reductionism, there are countless well-focused ideas to study that do not challenge the boundaries of big paradigms and big practices. As well, our continual search for external sources of research funding prevents us from straying too far outside of conventional lines, lest we be unable to find the funding necessary for promotion and tenure. The idea of "publish or perish" is alive and well. I've been on tenure review committees and have watched highly qualified and promising young scholars be released because they failed to get the research funding to pursue their interests. In many ways, our system favors the status quo.

Academia is no longer what it once was. I am now convinced that among the sectors of industry, government, and health care discussed in the first edition of this book, academia is more to blame for the public confusion and distortion of health information than any other sector. However, it is critically important to know that this is *not* the fault of the vast majority of academic researchers and teachers. Rather, the blame lies with those few academics, however few they may be, who are happy to oblige corporate interests for their own self-serving reasons. If they gain an administrative position, it affords them even more leverage. And those who are intellectually capable of offering an opposing opinion are becoming fewer and fewer as academic freedom diminishes.

To illustrate my concern about how academia has become too enmeshed with corporate interests, here are a few pictures worth more than proverbial words can tell. The picture on the left is the front of Stocking Hall at Cornell University, the dairy science building on its "ag" (agriculture) campus. This building housed my graduate student office where my desk was that of the recently passed professor who was the first Nobel Laureate from Cornell, James Sumner (the desk is now in a campus museum with his name rightfully on it, not mine).

A couple of years ago, Stocking Hall was massively renovated, at an estimated cost of $105 million. This meant gutting out the innards of the building (including my old office) and replacing it with what is, both inside and out, an impressive, very modern building, as seen on the right.. The side of the building that faces the road is all glass so that people can see within some marvelous machinery used for creating dairy products.

Just outside the entrance of this new cow castle is a "monument" of a milk bottle 15- to 20-feet tall, shown in the picture on the left. What a piece of art!

On the inside is the entranceway to a beautiful new Pepsico auditorium, as seen on the right, that replaces the old auditorium where I attended several classes.

I know well that I am being unusually harsh in this chapter on the institution that has been my professional home longer, I suspect, than almost anyone else at Cornell. I also know that Cornell University provided for me an incredible opportunity to do many mutually rewarding things, especially including the opportunities to work with so many outstanding students, faculty, and administrators. These individuals are people whom I am more than happy to call personal colleagues and friends. However, I also know the oftentimes subtle but powerful ability of institutions and paradigms to exercise control of what we do and think. The journey I took in following my research and lecturing led me to cross boundaries, sometimes unknowingly, that have been etched into our collective consciousness. Our research findings challenged the nutritional supremacy of animal-based protein, the reductionist bias that underlies biomedical research, the supposed irreversibility of cancer, the key mechanism concept that underlies drug development, the inadequacy of nutrient supplementation, and the chemical carcinogen causation of cancer, among others. I had no choice. And it is there, on the other side of those boundaries, that I have seen a new world and where I have acquired many new friends and colleagues who know and cherish this information. I can only hope that more of my colleagues will someday say, "Tell me more."

My research was funded for thirty-five years by taxpayer money, at least 90% of which was NIH funding that I competed for on the basis of rigorous review by peers (the rest mostly being my yearly salary, provided by the U.S. State Department for six years of my work in the Philippines). Restricting my research funding to the public sector was my intent from the beginning of my career, as I did not want to use funding from self-serving, for-profit organizations, and I am more than grateful for that funding.

I did not start my research journey with any preconceived agenda—not ideological, not corporate. I simply wanted to investigate how diet relates to human health, and to do so by using public, neutral funding. My father's advice when we were young was, "Always tell the truth and nothing but the truth." His words have been my shield, no matter how inconvenient and treacherous this path has become. Research findings that initially seemed inconceivable were no exceptions. Such findings must be either confirmed or rejected; they cannot be ignored. That's science—to the best of my knowledge.

Professionally, I have had everything—professional position and reputation, generous research funding, student access, collegial interchange, genuine support from a few Cornell greats, excellent facilities, a generous amount of personal awards, and more. Equipped with such largesse, I naïvely thought I was relatively immune to the tyranny of incompetent second- and third-level administrators. But I confess: my path has been steeper and more challenging than I had thought. Searching for truths, whatever the path, seems not to be part of the calculus of administrators personally beholden to corporate interests.

I have known, over the years, a few faculty and (especially) students who sought truth as they saw it but who were defenseless against administrative misbehavior because they did not have enough professional credentials to defend themselves. These victims were sincere, competent people with an unusual sense of personal honor. I had credentials and those victims did not. Thus, in their name and nameless others, I will stubbornly pursue what I set out to do and what others were not able to do. My main interest now becomes furthering the cause of academic freedom.

Tom Riner, long-time representative in the Kentucky Legislature, says it best in the film *Plant Pure Nation*: "Truth is a stubborn thing. It just won't go away."

REPEATING
HISTORIES

19

I n 1985, when I was on sabbatical in Oxford, England, I had the opportunity
to study the history of diet and disease at some of the great medical history
libraries in the Western world. I made use of the famous Bodleian Library
in Oxford and the London libraries of the Royal College of Surgeons and the
Imperial Cancer Research Fund. In the quiet recesses of these marble-lined
sanctuaries, I was thrilled to find authors who wrote eloquently on the topic
of diet and cancer, among other diseases, over 150 years ago.

One such author was George Macilwain, who wrote fourteen books on
medicine and health. Macilwain was born and raised in Northern Ireland.
He later moved to London where he became a prominent surgeon in the
early 1800s. He was to become a member, and later, an honorary fellow,
of the Royal College of Surgeons. He became vegetarian at the age of forty,
after identifying "grease, fat, and alcohol" as the chief causes of cancer.[1]
Macilwain also popularized the theory of the "constitutional nature of disease," mostly in reference to the origins and treatment of cancer.

The constitutional nature of disease concept meant that disease is not
the result of one organ, one cell, or one reaction gone awry, or the result of
one external cause acting independently. It is the result of *multiple systems
throughout the body breaking down*. Opposing this view was the local theory of disease, which said that disease is caused by a single external agent
acting at a specific site in the body. At that time, a fierce fight was under
way between those who believed in diet and those who supported surgery
and the emerging use of drugs. The "local disease" proponents argued that
disease could be cut out or treated in isolation with chemicals. In contrast,
those who favored diet and lifestyle believed that disease was a symptom
resulting from the "constitutional" characteristics of the whole body.

I was impressed that these old books contained the same ideas about diet and disease that had resurfaced in the health battles of the 1980s. As I learned more about Macilwain, I came to realize that he was a relative of mine. My paternal grandmother's maiden name was Macilwain, and that "branch" of the family had lived in the same part of Northern Ireland that George Macilwain had come from. Furthermore, there were family stories about a famous Macilwain who had left the family farm in Ireland to become a very well-known doctor in London in the early 1800s. My father, who had emigrated from Northern Ireland, had referred to an Uncle George when I was young, but I never knew who this man was.

Two years ago, my wife, Karen, and I traveled to England and Ireland to look further into my relation to Macilwain. We learned he was buried in Messing, England, after having lived for most of his adult life in that country. Unfortunately we have not been able to find his death certificate, and when we traveled to the graveyard in Messing, we found the unusually soft head-stones marking the graves of people who died before about 1900 had mostly worn away—and Macilwain died in 1883. Through this and further genea-logical research, I have come to the near certain conclusion that George Macilwain was either my great-great uncle or my great-great grandfather.

This discovery has been one of the more remarkable stories of my life. Karen says, "If there's such a thing as reincarnation . . ." I agree: if I ever lived a past life, it was as George Macilwain. He and I had similar careers; both of us became acutely aware of the importance of diet in disease, and both of us became vegetarian (to use this term loosely). Some of his ideas, written over 150 years ago, were so close to what I believed that I felt they could have come from my own mouth.

Since the first edition of this book, I've retrieved eleven of Macilwain's books and have read many of them. Like so many of the medical texts of that day, they are wordy and sometimes difficult to understand. But one thing is clear: his writing during the 1800s weaves a story of wholism—although he called it "constitutionalism"—that fits very nicely into my own thoughts regarding wholism as the best way to describe nutrition and what the guiding principle of medical practice ought to be.

I discovered more than my family history while reading in these august, history-laden libraries. I found out that scholars have been arguing over the nature of health for millennia. Almost 2,500 years ago, Plato wrote a dialogue between two characters, Socrates and Glaucon, in which they discuss the future of their cities. Socrates says cities should be simple, and the citizens should subsist on barley and wheat, with "relishes" of salt, olives, cheese, and "country fare of boiled onions and cabbage," and desserts of "figs, pease, beans," roasted myrtle-berries and beechnuts, and wine in moderation.[2] Socrates says, "And thus, passing their days in tranquility and sound health, they will, in all probability, live to an advanced age."

But Glaucon replies that such a diet would only be appropriate for "a community of swine," and that the citizens should live "in a civilized manner." He continues, "They ought to recline on couches . . . and have the usual dishes and dessert of a modern dinner." In other words, the citizens should have the "luxury" of eating meat. Socrates replies, "If you wish us also to contemplate a city that is suffering from inflammation . . . We shall also need great quantities of all kinds of cattle for those who may wish to eat them, shall we not?" Glaucon says, "Of course we shall."

Socrates then says, "Then shall we not experience the need of medical men also to a much greater extent under this than under the former régime?" Glaucon can't deny it: "Yes, indeed."

Socrates goes on to say that this luxurious city will be short of land because of the extra acreage required to raise animals for food. This shortage will lead the citizens to take land from others, which could precipitate violence and war, and thus a need for justice. Socrates further says, "When dissoluteness and diseases abound in a city, are not law courts and surgeries opened in abundance, and do not Law and Physic begin to hold their heads high, when numbers even of well-born persons devote themselves with eagerness to these professions?" In other words, in this luxurious city of sickness and disease, lawyers and doctors will become the norm.[2]

Though it is indeed remarkable that one of the greatest intellectuals in the history of the Western world condemned meat eating almost 2,500 years ago, I find it even more remarkable that few know about this history. Hardly anybody knows, for example, that the father of Western medicine, Hippocrates, advocated diet as the chief way to prevent and treat disease, or that George Macilwain knew that diet was the way to prevent and treat disease, or that the man instrumental in founding the American Cancer Society, Frederick L. Hoffman, knew that diet was the way to prevent and treat disease.

How did Plato predict the future so accurately? He knew that consuming animal foods would not lead to true health and prosperity. Instead, the false sense of rich luxury granted by being able to eat animals would only lead to a culture of sickness, disease, land disputes, lawyers, and doctors. This is a pretty good description of some of the challenges faced by modern America!

How did Seneca, one of the great scholars 2,000 years ago, a tutor and advisor to Roman Emperor Nero, know with such certainty the trouble with consuming animals when he wrote[2]:

An Ox is satisfied with the pasture of an acre or two: one wood suffices for several Elephants. Man alone supports himself by the pillage of the whole earth and sea. What! Has Nature indeed given us so insatiable a stomach, while she has given us so insignificant bodies? . . . The slaves of the belly (as says Sallust) are to be counted in the number of the lower animals, not of men. Nay, not of them, but rather of the dead . . . You might inscribe on their doors, "These have anticipated death."

How did George Macilwain predict the future when he said that the local theory of disease would not lead to health? Even today, we don't have any pills or procedures that effectively prevent, eliminate, or even treat the causes of any chronic diseases. The most promising preventions and treatments have now been shown to be diet and lifestyle changes, a constitutional approach to health.

How did we forget these lessons from the past? How did we go from knowing that the best athletes in the ancient Greek Olympics must have consumed a plant-based diet to fearing that vegetarians don't get enough protein? How did we get to a place where the healers of our society, our doctors, know little, if anything, about nutrition; where our medical institutions denigrate the subject; where using prescription drugs and going to hospitals is the third leading cause of death? How did we get to a place where advocating a plant-based diet can jeopardize a professional career, where scientists spend more time overcoming and mastering nature than respecting it? How did we get to a place where the companies that profit from our sickness are the ones telling us how to be healthy; where the companies that profit from our food choices are the ones telling us what to eat; where the public's hard-earned money is being spent by the government to boost the drug industry's profits; and where there is more distrust than trust of our government's policies on foods, drugs, and health? How did we get to a place where Americans are so confused about what is healthy that they no longer care?

Our country's population, which numbers over 300 million people,[3] is sick.

- 82% of American adults have at least one risk factor for heart disease[4]
- 81% of Americans take at least one medication during any given week[5]
- 50% of Americans take at least one prescription drug during any given week[5]

- 65% of American adults are overweight[6]
- 31% of American adults are obese[6]
- Roughly one in three youths in America (ages six to nineteen) is already overweight or at risk of becoming overweight
- About 105 million American adults have dangerously high cholesterol levels[7] (defined as 200 mg/dL or higher—heart-safe cholesterol level is under 150 mg/dL)
- About 50 million Americans have high blood pressure[8]
- Over 63 million American adults have pain in the lower back (considerably related to circulation and excess body weight, both influenced by diet and aggravated by physical inactivity) during any given three-month period[9]
- Over 33 million American adults have a migraine or severe headache during any given three-month period[9]
- 23 million Americans had heart disease in 2001[9]
- At least 16 million Americans have diabetes
- Over 700,000 Americans died from heart disease in 2000
- Over 550,000 Americans died from cancer in 2000
- Over 280,000 Americans died from cerebrovascular diseases (stroke), diabetes, or Alzheimer's in 2000

At the great peril of ignoring the warnings of Plato and others, America has, in the words of Seneca, "anticipated death." Starvation, poor sanitation, and communicable diseases—symbols of impoverishment—have been largely minimized in the Western world. Now we have an urgency of excess, and some of the previously less developed countries are racing to get where we are. Never before have such large percentages of the population died from diseases of "affluence." Is this the affluence that Socrates predicted 2,500 years ago—a society full of doctors and lawyers wrestling with the problems caused by people living luxuriously and eating cattle? Never before have so many people suffered such high levels of obesity and diabetes. Never before has the financial strain of health care distressed every sector of our society, from business to education to government to everyday families with inadequate insurance. If we have to decide between health insurance for our teachers and textbooks for our kids, which will we choose?

Never before have we affected the natural environment to such an extent that we are losing our topsoil, our massive North American aquifers, and our world's rain forests.[10] We are changing our climate so rapidly that many of the world's best-informed scientists fear the future. Never before have we been eliminating plant and animal species from the face of the earth as we are doing now. Never before have we introduced, on such a large scale, genetically altered varieties of plants into the environment without knowing what the repercussions will be. All of these changes in our environment are strongly affected by what we choose to eat.[11]

As billions of people in the developing world accumulate more wealth and adopt Western diets and lifestyles, problems created by nutritional excess are becoming exponentially more urgent with each passing year. In 1997, the director-general of the World Health Organization, Dr. Hiroshi Nakajima, referred to the future chronic disease burden in developing countries as "a crisis of suffering on a global scale."[12]

We've fumbled around for the past 2,500 years, building up the unsustainable behemoth that we now call modern society. We certainly won't have another 2,500 years to remember the teachings of Plato, Socrates, Pythagoras, Seneca, and Macilwain; we won't even have 250 years. From this urgency arises great opportunity, and because of that I am filled with hope. People are beginning to sense the need for change and to question some of the most basic assumptions that we have about food and health. People are beginning to understand the conclusions of scientific literature and are changing their lives for the better.

Never before has there been such a mountain of empirical research supporting a whole foods, plant-based (WFPB) diet. Now, for example, we can obtain images of the arteries in the heart, and then show conclusively, as Drs. Dean Ornish and Caldwell Esselstyn, Jr., have done, that a WFPB diet reverses heart disease.[13] We now have the knowledge to understand how this actually works. Animal protein, even more than saturated fat and dietary cholesterol, raises blood cholesterol levels in experimental animals, individual humans, and entire populations. International comparisons between countries show that populations subsisting on traditional plant-based diets have far less heart disease, and studies of individuals within single populations show that those who eat more whole, plant-based foods not only have lower cholesterol levels, but less heart disease. *We now have a deep and broad range of evidence showing that a WFPB diet is best for the heart.*

Never before have we had such a depth of understanding of how diet affects cancer both on a cellular level as well as a population level. Published data show that animal protein promotes the growth of tumors. Animal protein increases the levels of a hormone, IGF-1, which is a risk factor for cancer, and high-casein (the main protein of cow's milk) diets allow more carcinogens into cells, which allow more dangerous carcinogen products to bind to DNA, which allow more mutagenic reactions that give rise to cancer cells, which allow more rapid growth of tumors once they are initially formed. Data show that a diet based on animal-based foods increases a woman's production of reproductive hormones over her lifetime, which may lead to breast cancer. *We now have a deep and broad range of evidence showing that a WFPB diet is best for preventing, and possibly also for treating, cancer.*

Never before have we had technology to measure the biomarkers associated with diabetes, and the evidence to show that blood sugar, blood cholesterol, and insulin levels improve more with a WFPB diet than with any other treatment. Intervention studies show that Type 2 diabetics treated with a WFPB diet may reverse their disease and go off their medications. A broad range of international studies shows that Type 1 diabetes, a serious autoimmune disease, is related to cow's milk consumption and premature weaning. We now know how our autoimmune system can attack our own bodies through a process of molecular mimicry induced by animal proteins that find their way into our bloodstream. We also have tantalizing evidence linking multiple sclerosis with animal food consumption, and especially dairy consumption. Dietary intervention studies have shown that diet may help slow, and perhaps even halt, multiple sclerosis. *We now have a deep and broad range of evidence showing that a WFPB diet is best for diabetes and autoimmune diseases.*

Never before have we had such a broad range of evidence showing that diets containing excess animal protein can destroy our kidneys. Kidney stones arise because the consumption of animal protein creates excessive calcium and oxalate in the kidney. We now know that cataracts and age-related macular degeneration might be prevented by foods containing large amounts of antioxidants. In addition, research has shown that cognitive dysfunction, vascular dementia caused by small strokes, and Alzheimer's are all related to the food we eat. Investigations of human populations show that our risk of hip fracture and osteoporosis is made worse by diets high in animal-based foods. Animal protein leeches calcium from the bones by creating an acidic environment in the blood. *We now have a deep and broad range of evidence showing that a WFPB diet is best for our kidneys, bones, eyes, and brains.*

More research can and should be done, but the idea that WFPB diets can protect against and even treat a wide variety of chronic diseases can no longer be denied. No longer are there just a few people making claims about a plant-based diet based on their personal experience, philosophy, or the occasional supporting scientific study. Now there are hundreds of detailed, comprehensive, well-done research studies that point in the same direction.

Furthermore, I have hope for the future because of our new ability to exchange information across the country and around the world. A much greater proportion of the world population is literate, and a much greater proportion of that population has the luxury of choosing what they eat from a wide variety of readily accessible foods. People can make a WFPB diet varied, interesting, tasty, and convenient. I have hope because people in small towns and in previously isolated parts of the country can now readily access cutting-edge health information and put it into practice.

All of these things together create an atmosphere unlike any other, an atmosphere that demands change. Contrary to the situation in 1982, when a few colleagues tried to destroy the reputations of scientists who suggested that diet had anything to do with cancer, it is now more commonly accepted that what you eat can determine your risk of multiple cancers. I have also seen the public image of vegetarianism emerge from being considered a dangerous, passing fad to a healthful, enduring lifestyle choice. The popularity of plant-based diets has been increasing, and both the variety and availability of convenient vegetarian foods have been skyrocketing.[14] Restaurants around the country now regularly offer meat-free and dairy-free options.[15] Scientists are publishing more articles about vegetarianism and writing more about the health potential of a plant-based diet.[16] Now, over 150 years after my ancestor George Macilwain wrote books about diet and disease, I am writing a book about diet and disease with the help of my youngest son, Tom. Tom's middle name is McIlwain (the family changed the spelling over the past couple of generations), which means that not only am I writing about many of the same ideas Macilwain wrote about, but a relative bearing his name is the co-author. History can repeat itself. This time, however, instead of the message being forgotten and confined to library stacks, I believe that the world is finally ready to accept it. More than that, I believe the world is finally ready to change. We have reached a point in our history where our bad habits can no longer be tolerated. We, as a society, are on the edge of a great precipice: we can fall to sickness, poverty, and degradation, or we can embrace health, longevity, and bounty. And all it takes is the courage to change. How will our grandchildren find themselves in 100 years? Only time will tell, but I hope that the history we are witnessing and the future that lies ahead will be to the benefit of us all.

AFTERWORD
(FOR THE SECOND EDITION)

T. Colin Campbell

As I put together the second edition of this book, the issue that stands out most for me is this: In the health care world, there is no word that is more confusing, more misunderstood, and more abused than the word "nutrition." Despite the frequency with which it is spoken, nutrition's meaning remains unfortunately elusive.

This is incredibly important because there is no medical protocol of pills and procedures that can offer more human health than does nutrition. Yet, strangely, the medical profession does not even accord nutrition the status of medical specialty (among twenty-six officially recognized medical specialties). Even more suspect, nutrition is not taught in medical schools other than a few minimalist lectures in some schools only. The world's largest biomedical research funding agency, NIH (National Institutes of Health), is composed of twenty-eight institutes, centers, and programs and not one is devoted to nutrition. In my discipline of professional research and teaching nutritional science, we struggle even now to find a definition for nutrition!

After sixty years in this field, my definition is quite simple: Nutrition is the biological expression of food that promotes health. "Malnutrition" is its opposite. But the problem is not so much the way that nutrition is defined as it is our misunderstanding of the way that nutrition functions. Traditionally, we investigate, teach, and market nutrition primarily by focusing on individual nutrients, individual mechanisms by which nutrients function, and individual outcomes. This is *reductionism*. For example, when the antioxidant beta-carotene is in food, where nutrients work together, it is associated with less lung cancer, but when it is isolated and consumed as a pill, it not only does not work, it *even increases* lung cancer and total mortality. Similar findings have been reported in recent years for several more vitamins and their effects on disease.

Detailed study of individual nutrients is helpful, but it is far from being enough to comprehend the broader health effects when nutrients are consumed as food. Nutrition works through the concept of *wholism*, which represents a powerful symphony of countless nutrients and nutrient-like chemicals working by countless mechanisms to produce a highly dynamic, almost seamless series of outcomes—good outcomes when working well, not so good when not working well.

I have come to believe that nutrition, explained wholistically, is a fact of nature. I know I have said it many times before, but I cannot say it enough because, since the first edition of this book, nothing much has changed in our understanding of nutrition, which is still seen in terms of individual nutrients, not whole foods or whole diets. We can therefore see why the nutrition provided by the whole foods, plant-based (WFPB) dietary lifestyle struggles to be heard. Not even its parent, the concept of nutrition generally, is taken seriously by health authorities!

Almost every day, I am confronted with deeply personal stories with endings far less satisfactory than what might have been were nutrition better understood. Just today, as I am writing this at our home near Ithaca, NY, my wife, Karen, and I read a front page feature story in our small town newspaper about the inspiring courage of a young boy with cancer. Diagnosed at age two with a relatively rare cancer, he has over the past seven years spent many days in the hospital getting radiation therapy, having surgery, or taking oral "chemo" medication thought to work (but only temporarily). Now he's nine years old, hanging on with that courage and with lots of love and care from family and many other people in our town and elsewhere.

An hour or so after reading this story, my wife went into town and passed an unusually large gathering of friends and neighbors and well-wishers attending an outdoor memorial service for a very popular forty-two-year-old soccer coach and school athletic director at our local high school. Just a few days ago, suddenly and without warning, he dropped dead of a massive heart attack, leaving a wife and young children. I can only imagine their breathtaking grief.

When I hear stories like these with unfortunate consequences, I can only imagine whether the results might have been more favorable had the doctors and individuals involved only have known the information that a few of my colleagues and I have come to know: the role of nutrition in the causation of disease and the restoration of health through the WFPB dietary lifestyle. It has more to offer than all pills and procedures combined.

In these two stories, timely for this occasion but like so many others seen every day, I am very much aware of the unconscionable omission of that fact in both. I see no evidence, for example, that these families knew anything about the exceptional benefits of nutrition when seen through the WFPB lens. The news item about the young boy told of a party during an interlude between radiation treatments where he and his friends "had so many cookies" to eat, which I suspect, like most cookies, were loaded with fat, sugar, and refined flour. This and a related party were reported as loving, caring events, and of course they were. They are what we all, without the knowledge of nutrition's effect on health, would choose to do. But to say that he had survived "several surgeries, chemotherapy, and radiation treatments that left [him] with facial paralysis, deafness in one ear, paralysis of one vocal cord, and an inability to swallow," then also to say that he was enjoying "so many cookies," a birthday cake, and a barbecue celebration leaves me distraught at how his short life journey so far has been all about chasing harsh pills and procedures with "courage," when it might have been able to be so much more. I cannot of course be certain that cookies, barbeque, and birthday cakes have negatively affected his prognosis, but, based on some very, very impressive evidence, I have considerable confidence that they do. Still, what distresses me even more is that almost no one even knows about the possibility of benefits that I can easily imagine.

On the young man whose coaching life was cut short so early, I can only wonder what he, too, must have been eating. Did he and his family know anything about the remarkable ability of nutrition to control and even reverse heart disease? I feel strongly that this did not need to happen, based on the evidence we now have. We know that heart disease can be not just treated, but cured. And again, the really important question is: Why does he and his family not know?

I see and hear of stories like these far too often. I am constantly reminded of them, as well, when people who have read this book tell me about their miraculous recoveries and when others ask me questions about their health problems to which I can only offer some rather impersonal scientific evidence, because I am not a licensed medical practitioner.

There's a common thread among almost all these people, whether they have benefitted from the information in this book or are just discovering it for the first time: most are puzzled as to why they have not heard this before. Almost all wonder why the information about nutrition's wholistic effects isn't better known, especially among doctors. (This is why the new program in nutrition at a major medical center, directed by my co-author son, Tom, and his wife, Erin, is so important.)

Based on my long-time position in the professional research and education community—I might as well say "science establishment"—I believe that part of the reason this knowledge remains hidden from public view is that we fail to study or even to discuss this core concept of nutrition in laboratories and lecture halls and medical clinics and policy board rooms. But worse still, efforts are constantly being made by an oligarchy composed of industry, government, academia, medical practice, and media institutions to proactively deny this knowledge to the public!

Why? It's simple. They fear that this knowledge just might offer far cheaper and more effective solutions for health problems than does their products and programs. The oligarchy wants to protect its business and, too often, they do it with abandon. It's Business 101 on a very grand scale. Knowledge is power, and these institutions have power to control that knowledge. Even more ominously, preventing that knowledge from reaching the public allows them to acquire revenue that can be used to control that knowledge further. It is self-generating power—a perpetual motion machine.

The oligarchy extracts a price from us at both ends: as taxpayers, we pay for subsidies to produce the food that is killing us, then we pay for expensive pills and procedures when we get sick.

As a professional, I know well the evidence about nutrition that makes unnecessary this foolishness. But I also know that, within this maelstrom of modern-day life, we face a difficult dilemma. The oligarchy, while doing work that makes us ill, also provides jobs for many of us. We work, sometimes unwittingly, for the oligarchy even as we suffer from consuming the products that "we" produce. Together, we work against our own best interests! In doing so, we are placing a higher priority on wealth for the few than on health for the many. We must get off this merry-go-round or we all will be paying a far greater price than just our own lives—the life of our planet and all of us living on it. The fuel that makes possible the merry-go-round of this oligarchy is knowledge, and the power that it begets is self-serving.

Our system is fundamentally illogical and immoral. It is illogical when we represent nutrition as a reductionist science (mostly for commercial purposes) instead of wholistic science. When the oligarchy actively prevents this knowledge from being provided to the public, it is immoral, especially when the public's money is used to create that knowledge. It is classical hegemony. Thanks to the oligarchy, it is almost impossible, for example, to obtain research funding to seriously and professionally study the effects of wholistic nutrition on human health and disease control, especially as provided by the WFPB dietary lifestyle. Although unusually impressive, the existing research on this dietary lifestyle is not perfect. Questions remain, especially those concerned with the applicability of this dietary lifestyle for all individuals, all circumstances, and all ailments. But before we can study these secondary questions, it requires some acceptance of the primary hypothesis.

In short, we have almost no research, no sensible discussion, and no useful information. I cringe when, telling colleagues about the merits of the

WFPB diet, they respond, "But there's not enough research"—the perfect answer for catalyzing a self-serving prophecy.

Our failure to properly study nutrition is a huge issue, for this scientific discipline is the scientific core of so many contemporary discussions of our society's problems, including environmental degradation, health care costs, personal health, and their many dependent issues.

I don't want to leave the reader believing that I am a doomsday cynic having no place to go. Since the first edition of this book, there have been some very exciting developments within a rapidly growing community of people who care about and who will do whatever it takes to advance this discussion. The 2011 documentary film *Forks Over Knives* (available on Netflix as of this writing) has been seen by a very large audience, reaching at least 20 million viewers according to one estimate of a year ago. Since then, many other documentary films have focused on particular problems related to our current dietary practices. The 2015 film *PlantPure Nation* (also available on Netflix) takes a journey into the world of government and includes firsthand footage of a debate in the Kentucky Legislature where, faced with a proposal to gain simple recognition of the benefits of a WFPB diet, members wrestle with the issue of political expediency. (The outcome is revealing.) The film *Cowspiracy* (2014), which has over 1.2 million viewers on YouTube, shows how difficult it is even to create discussion on the impact of livestock production on our imposing environmental problems. These and many newer films feel like a much-awaited awakening.

I am especially gratified by the growing interest of the medical practice community in learning the nutrition information that they did not get from their official training. Of my more than 600 lectures in the U.S. and abroad since the publication of the first edition of this book, most of the recent 200 or so have been to medical schools and medical conferences, and it is exhilarating to think of these professionals continuing to take leadership positions in health care going forward. Also, Tom's very exciting new program focused on plant-based nutrition boldly called *Program for Nutrition in Medicine* at the University of Rochester Medical Center is most welcome.

There is no question that there has been progress since the first edition of this book. But, sadly, this has not occurred within what I call "the Oligarchy," especially in academia or in government policy circles.

Still, everyday people need to know this information, not only for their personal health, but also for the health of our global community as well as our planet.

It is time that this information on nutrition be shared with the public without being sanctioned by government and academic institutions. For those scientists who question the WFPB diet as the optimal form of nutrition or who question any of the hypotheses or challenges to current dietary practices, I suggest that they organize research to disprove it—not piecemeal, but through whole food, multi-outcome intervention studies! For research-funding institutions, like NIH, I suggest they re-prioritize their budget and call for projects to explore the concept of wholism, especially as it applies to a broad range of health outcomes. For the government, cease support of the nonsensical advertising of pharmaceuticals on public TV. If not that, then at least give equal time to a discussion of nutrition's impact on health.

We can no longer accept or advance the status quo. It is well past time for government institutions and government-funded institutions to act on behalf of the public taxpayer.

The information on the benefits of the WFPB diet, in my opinion, is the most progressive news in the history of Western medicine. It may be the road less traveled, but I am confident that it will become the superhighway of the future. We have no other choice.

APPENDIX A

Q&A: Protein Effect in Experimental Rat Studies

Could the Effects Attributed to Low Dietary Protein Be Due to Other Nutrients in the Rat Diet?

Decreasing dietary protein from 20% to 5% means finding something to replace the missing 15%. We used a carbohydrate to replace the casein because it had the same energy content. As dietary protein decreased, a 1:1 mixture of starch and sucrose (sugar) increased by the same amount. The extra starch and sucrose in the low-protein diets could not have been responsible for the lower development of foci because these carbohydrates, when tested alone, actually increase focus development.[1] If anything, a little extra carbohydrate in the low-protein diet would only increase cancer incidence and offset the low-protein effect. This makes prevention of cancer by low-protein diets even more impressive.

Might the Effects Attributed to a Low-Protein Diet Actually Be Due to Lower Overall Food Consumption (i.e., Less Calorie Consumption)?

Many studies done in the 1930s, 1940s, and 1950s[2] had shown that decreasing total food intake, or total calories, decreased tumor development. A review of our many experiments, however, showed that animals fed the low-protein diets did not consume fewer calories but, on average, actually consumed more calories.[3,4] Again, this only reinforced the tumor-promoting effect observed for casein.

What Was the Overall Health of the Rats on a Low-Protein Diet?

Many researchers have long assumed that animals fed diets this low in protein would not be healthy. However, the low-protein animals were healthier by every indication. They lived longer, were more physically active, were slimmer, and had healthy hair coats at 100 weeks, while the high-protein counterpart rats were all dead. Also, animals consuming less dietary casein not only ate more calories, but they also burned off more calories. Low-protein animals consumed more oxygen, which is required to burn these calories, and had higher levels of a special tissue called brown adipose tissue,[5,6] which is especially effective in burning off calories. This occurs through a process of "thermogenesis"—the expenditure of calories as body heat. This phenomenon had already been demonstrated many years before.[7–11] *Low-protein diets enhance the burning off of calories, thus leaving fewer calories for body weight gain and perhaps also fewer for tumor growth as well.*

Was Physical Activity Related to the Consumption of the Low-Protein Diet?

To measure the physical activity of each group of rats, we compared how much they voluntarily operated an exercise wheel attached to their cages. A monitor recorded the number of times the animals turned the exercise wheel. Measured over a two-week period, the low-casein animals[12] exercised about twice as much! This observation seems to be very similar to how one feels after eating a high-protein meal: sluggish and sleepy. I have heard that a side effect of the protein-drenched Atkins Diet is fatigue. Have you ever noticed this feeling in yourself after a high-protein meal?

APPENDIX B

Experimental Design of the China Study

Sixty-five counties in twenty-four different provinces (out of twenty-seven) were selected for the survey. They represented the full range of mortality rates for seven of the more common cancers. They also provided broad geographic coverage and were within four hours' travel time of a central laboratory. The survey counties represented:

- semitropical coastal areas of southeast China;
- frigid wintry areas in northeast China, near Siberia;
- areas near the Great Gobi Desert and the northern steppes;
- and areas near or in the Himalaya Mountains ranging from the far northwest to the far southwest part of the country.

Except for suburban areas near Shanghai, most counties were located in rural China where people lived in the same place their entire lives and consumed locally produced food. Population densities varied widely, from 20,000 nomadic residents for the most remote county near the Great Gobi Desert, to 1.3 million people for the county on the outskirts of Shanghai.

This survey is referred to as an ecological or correlation study design, meaning that we are comparing diet, lifestyle, and disease characteristics of a number of sample populations, in this case the sixty-five counties. We determine how these characteristics, as county averages, correlate or associate with each other. For example, how does dietary fat relate to breast cancer rates? Or how does blood cholesterol relate to coronary heart disease? How does a certain kind of fatty acid in red blood cells relate to rice consumption? We could also compare blood testosterone levels or estrogen levels with breast cancer risk. We did thousands of different comparisons of this type.

In a study of this kind, it is important to note that only the average values for county populations are being compared. Individuals are not being compared with individuals (in reality, neither does any other epidemiological study design). As ecological studies go, this study, with its sixty-five counties, was unusually large. Most such studies only have ten to twenty such population units, at most.

Each of the sixty-five counties provided 100 adults for the survey. One-half were male and one-half female, all aged thirty-five to sixty-four years. The data were collected in the following manner:

- each person volunteered a blood sample and completed a diet and lifestyle questionnaire;
- one-half of the people provided a urine sample;
- the survey teams went to 30% of the homes to carefully measure food consumed by the family over a three-day period;
- samples of food representing the typical diets at each survey site were collected at the local marketplace and were later analyzed for dietary and nutritional factors.

One of the more important questions during the early planning stages was how to survey for diet and nutrition information. Estimating consumption of food and nutrients from memory is a common method, but this is very imprecise, especially when mixed dishes are consumed. Can you remember what foods you ate last week, or even yesterday? Can you remember how much? Another even more crude method of estimating food intake is to see how much of each food is sold in the marketplace. These findings can give reasonable estimates of diet trends over time for whole populations, but they do not account for food waste or measure individual amounts of consumption.

Although each of these relatively crude methods can be useful for certain purposes, they still are subject to considerable technical error and personal bias. And the bigger the technical error, the more difficult it is to detect significant cause–effect associations.

We wanted to do better than crudely measure which foods and how much of these foods were being consumed. Thus we decided to evaluate nutritional conditions by analyzing blood and urine samples for indicators (biomarkers) of multiple nutrient intakes. These analyses would be far more objective than having people recall what they ate.

Collecting and analyzing blood, however, was not easy to arrange, at least not in the way that we preferred. The initial problem was getting *enough* blood. For cultural reasons, rural Chinese were reluctant to provide blood samples. A finger prick seemed to be the only possibility but this was not good enough. A regular vial of blood would give 100 times as much blood and allow for analyses of many more factors.

Dr. Junshi Chen of our team, at the Institute of Nutrition and Food Hygiene in the Ministry of Health, had the unenviable task of convincing these volunteers to give a regular vial of blood. He succeeded. Sir Richard Peto at the University of Oxford of our team then made the very practical suggestion of combining the individual blood samples to make a big pool of blood for each village for each sex. This strategy gave more than 1,200–1,300 times more blood when compared with the finger prick method.

Making big pools of blood had enormous implications and made possible the China Study, as it later became known. It allowed analyses of far more indicators of diet and health. This allowed us to consider relationships in a far more comprehensive manner than would have otherwise been possible. For more detail on the theoretical and practical basis for collecting and analyzing blood in this way, the reader is referred to the original monograph of the study.[1]

After collecting the blood, we then had to decide who would do the many analyses that were possible. We wanted nothing but the best. While some analyses were conducted at our Cornell lab and at Dr. Chen's Beijing lab, the rest of the analyses, especially the more specialized types, were done in about two dozen laboratories located in six countries and on four continents. Laboratories were selected for their demonstrated expertise and interest. The participating laboratories are listed in the original monograph.[1]

HOW GOOD IS THIS STUDY?

Because this survey was a one-of-a-kind opportunity, we intended that it be the best of its kind ever undertaken. It was comprehensive, it was high quality, and its uniqueness allowed new opportunities to investigate diet and disease that were never before possible. These features of comprehensiveness, quality, and uniqueness greatly improved the credibility and reliability of the findings—by far. Indeed, the *New York Times*, in a lead Science section story, called the study "The Grand Prix" of epidemiological studies.

COMPREHENSIVENESS OF DATA

This survey was, and still is, the most comprehensive of its kind ever undertaken. After all the blood, urine, and food samples were collected, stored, and analyzed, and after the final results were tabulated and evaluated for quality (a few suspect results were not included in the final publication), we were able to study 367 variables. These represented a wide variety of dietary, lifestyle, and disease characteristics, now included in a dense 896-page monograph.[1] There were:

- disease mortality rates on more than forty-eight different kinds of disease[2];
- 109 nutritional, viral, hormonal, and other indicators in blood;
- over twenty-four urinary factors;
- almost thirty-six food constituents (nutrients, pesticides, heavy metals);
- more than thirty-six specific nutrient and food intakes measured in the household survey;
- sixty diet and lifestyle factors obtained from questionnaires; and
- seventeen geographic and climatic factors.

The study was comprehensive not only because of the sheer number of variables, but also because most of these variables varied over broad ranges, as with the cancer mortality rates. Broad ranges strengthened our ability to detect important previously undiscovered associations of variables.

QUALITY OF DATA

A number of features added quality to this study.

- The adults chosen for this survey were limited to those who were thirty-five to sixty-four years of age. This is the age range in which the diseases being investigated are more common. Information on death certificates of people older than sixty-four years was not included in the survey because this information was considered less reliable.
- In each of the sixty-five counties in the study, two villages were selected for collecting information. Having two villages in each county rather than one gives a more reliable county average. When the values of two villages are more similar to each other than to all the other counties, then this means higher-quality data.[3]
- When possible, variables were measured by more than one kind of method. For example, iron status was measured in six different ways, riboflavin (vitamin B_2) in three ways, and so forth. Also, in many cases, we could assess the quality and reliability of data by comparing variables known to have plausible biological relationships.

- The populations under study proved to be very stable. An average of 93–94% of the men in the survey were born in the county where they lived at the time of the survey; for women it was 89%. Also, according to data published by the World Bank,[4] the diets at the time of our survey were very similar to those consumed in earlier years. This was ideal because those earlier years represented the time when the diseases were initially forming.

UNIQUENESS OF DATA

One idea that makes our study unique is our use of the ecologic study design. Critics of the ecologic study design correctly assume that it is a weak design for determining cause-and-effect associations when one is interested in the effects of single causes acting on single outcomes. But this is not the way nutrition works. Rather, nutrition causes or prevents disease by multiple nutrients and other chemicals acting together, as in whole foods. An ecologic study is almost ideal if we wish to learn how an array of dietary factors act together to cause disease. It is the comprehensive effects of nutrients and other factors on disease occurrence where the most important lessons are to be learned. To investigate these comprehensive causes of disease, it was therefore necessary to record as many dietary and other lifestyle factors as possible, then formulate hypotheses and interpret data that represent comprehensiveness.

Perhaps the most unique characteristic that set this study apart concerned the nutritional characteristics of the diets consumed in rural China. Virtually every other human study on diet and health, of whatever design, has involved subjects who were consuming a rich Western diet. This is true even when vegetarians are included in the study because 90% of vegetarians still consume rather large amounts of milk, cheese, and eggs, while a significant number still consume some fish and poultry. As is shown in the accompanying chart (Chart B.1),[5] there is only a small difference in the nutritional properties of non-vegetarian and vegetarian diets as consumed in Western countries.

A strikingly different dietary situation existed in China. In America, 15–17% of our total calories is provided by protein, and upwards of 80% of this amount is animal-based. In other words, we gorge on protein and we get most of it from meat and dairy products. But in rural China, they consume less protein overall (9–10% of total calories), and only 10% of it comes from animal-based foods. This means that there are many other major nutritional differences in the Chinese and American diets, as shown in Chart B.2.[1]

Chart B.1: Vegetarian and Non-Vegetarian Diet Comparisons Among Westerners

Nutrient	Vegetarian	Non-vegetarian
Fat (% of calories)	30–36	34–38
Cholesterol (g/day)	150–300	300–500
Carbohydrates (% of calories)	50–55	<50
Total protein (% of calories)	12–14	14–18
Animal protein (% of total protein)	40–60	60–70

Chart B.2: Chinese and American Dietary Intakes

Nutrient	China	United States
Calories (kcal/kg body wt./day)	40.6	30.6
Total fat (% of calories)	14.5	34–38
Dietary fiber (g/day)	33	12
Total protein (g/day)	64	91
Animal protein (% of total calories)	0.8*	10–11
Total iron (mg/day)	34	18

*Non-fish animal protein

This was the first and only large study that investigated this range of dietary experience and its health consequences. Chinese diets ranged from rich to very rich in plant-based foods. In all other studies done on Western subjects, diets ranged from rich to very rich in animal-based foods. It was this distinction that made the China Study so different from other studies.

MAKING IT HAPPEN

Organization and conduct of a study of this size, scope, and quality was possible because of the exceptional skills of Dr. Junshi Chen. Survey sites were scattered across the far reaches of China. In American travel distances, they ranged from the Florida Keys to Seattle, Washington, and from San Diego, California, to Bangor, Maine. Travel between these places was more difficult than in the United States, and supplies and instructions for the survey had to be in place and standardized for all collection sites. And this was done before email, fax machines, and cellular phones were available.

It was important that the twenty-four provincial health teams, each composed of twelve to fifteen health workers, be trained to carry out the blood, food, and urine collections and complete the questionnaires in a systematic and standardized manner. To standardize the collection of information, Dr. Chen divided the country into regions. Each region sent trainers to Beijing for the senior training session. They, in turn, returned to their home provinces to train the provincial health teams.

Although the U.S. National Cancer Institute of the National Institutes of Health provided the initial funding for this project, the Chinese Ministry of Health paid the salaries of the approximately 350 health workers. It is my estimate that the Chinese contribution to the project was approximately $5–6 million. This compares with the U.S. contribution of about $2.9 million over a ten-year period. Were the U.S. government to have paid for this service in a similar project in the U.S., it would have cost at least ten times this amount, or $50–60 million.

APPENDIX C

The "Vitamin" D Connection

The most impressive evidence favoring plant-based diets is the way that so many food factors and biological events are integrated to maximize health and minimize disease. Although the biological processes are exceptionally complex, these factors still work together as a beautifully choreographed, self-correcting network. It is exceptionally impressive, especially the coordination and control of this network.

Perhaps a couple of analogies might help to illustrate such a process. Flocks of birds in flight or schools of fish darting about are able to shift direction in a microsecond without bumping into each other. They seem to have a collective consciousness that knows where they are going and when they will rest. Colonies of ants and swarms of bees also integrate varying labor chores with great proficiency. But as amazing as these animal activities are, have you ever thought about how their behaviors are coordinated with such finesse? I see these same characteristics, and more, in the way that the countless factors of plant-based foods work their magic to create health at all levels within our body, among our organs and between our cells, and among the enzymes and other sub-cellular particles within our cells.

For those unfamiliar with biomedical research laboratories, the walls of these labs are often covered with large posters showing thousands of biochemical reactions operating within our bodies. These are reactions that are known; far more remain to be discovered. The interdependence of these reactions is especially informative, even awesome in its implications.

An example of a very small portion of this enormous network of reactions is the effect of vitamin D and its metabolites on several of the diseases discussed in this book. This particular network illustrates a complex interconnection between the inner workings of our cells, the food we eat, and the environment in which we live (Chart C.1). Although some of the vitamin D present in our bodies may come from food, we can usually get all that we need from a few hours of sunshine each week. In fact, it is our ability to make our vitamin D that leads to the idea that it is not a vitamin; it is a hormone (i.e., made in one part of our body but functioning in another part). The sun's UV rays make vitamin D from a precursor chemical located in our skin. Provided we get adequate sunshine, this is all the vitamin D we need.[1] We can, of course, also get vitamin D from fortified milk, certain fish oils, and some vitamin supplements.

The vitamin D made in our skin then travels to our liver, where it is converted by an enzyme to a vitamin D metabolite. This metabolite's main function is to serve as the body's storage form of vitamin D (while remaining mostly in the liver but also in body fat). The next step is the crucial one. When needed, some of the storage form of vitamin D in the liver is transported to the kidneys, where another enzyme converts it into a supercharged vitamin D metabolite, which is called 1,25 D. The rate at which the storage form of vitamin D is converted to the supercharged 1,25 D is a crucial reaction in this network. The 1,25 D metabolite does most of the important work of vitamin D in our bodies.

This supercharged 1,25 D is about 1,000 times more active than the storage vitamin D. Supercharged 1,25 D only survives for six to eight hours once it is made. In contrast, our storage vitamin D survives for twenty days or more.[2,3] This demonstrates an important principle typically found in networks like this: the far greater activity, the far shorter lifetime, and the far lower amounts of the 1,25 D end product provide a very responsive system wherein the 1,25 D can quickly adjust its activity minute by minute and microsecond by microsecond as long as there is sufficient storage vitamin D to draw from. Small changes, making a big difference, can occur quickly.

The relationship between the storage form of vitamin D and the supercharged 1,25 D is like having a large tank of natural gas buried in our yard (storage vitamin D) but carefully using only a very tiny amount of gas to light the burner at our stovetop. It is critical that the amount and timing of gas (1,25 D) coming to our stovetop be carefully regulated, regardless of how much there may be in the tank, whether it is low or full. However, it is also useful that we maintain an adequate supply in our storage tank. In the same way, it is critical that the kidney enzyme in this reaction has a soft, sensitive touch, so to speak, as it produces the right amount of the 1,25 D at the right time for its very important work.

One of the more important things that vitamin D does, mostly through its conversion to supercharged 1,25 D, is to control the development of a wide variety of serious diseases. For the sake of simplicity, this is schematically represented by showing the inhibition of the conversion of healthy tissue to diseased tissue by 1,25 D.[4–12]

Chart C.1: The Vitamin D Network

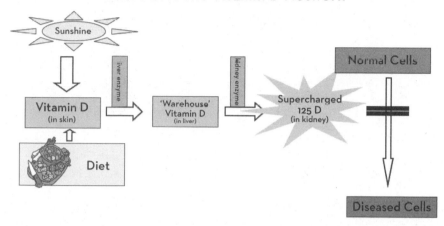

So far, we can see how adequate sunshine exposure, by ensuring enough storage form of vitamin D, helps to prevent cells from becoming diseased. This suggests that certain diseases might be more common in areas of the world where there is less sunshine, in countries nearer the North and South Poles. Indeed there is such evidence. To be more specific: *in the Northern Hemisphere, communities that are farther north tend to have more Type 1 diabetes, multiple sclerosis, rheumatoid arthritis, osteoporosis, breast cancer, prostate cancer, and colon cancer, in addition to other diseases.*

Researchers have known for eighty years that multiple sclerosis, for example, is associated with increasing latitude.[13] As you can see in Chart C.2, there is a huge difference in MS prevalence as one goes away from the equator, being over 100 times more prevalent in the far north than at the equator.[14] Similarly, in Australia, there is less sunshine and more MS as one goes farther south ($r = 91\%$).[15] MS is about sevenfold more prevalent in southern (43°S) than in northern Australia (19°S).[16]

A lack of sunshine, however, is not the only factor related to these diseases. There is a larger context. The first thing to note is the control and coordination of these vitamin D–related reactions. Control operates at several places in this network, but, as I said, it is the conversion of storage vitamin D into the supercharged 1,25 D in the kidneys that is especially critical. In considerable measure, this control is exercised by another complex network of reactions involving a "manager"-type hormone produced by the parathyroid gland located in our neck (Chart C.3).

Chart C.2: Worldwide Distribution of MS for 120 Countries

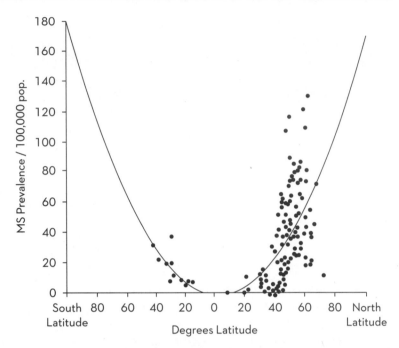

Chart C.3: Role of the Parathyroid Hormone in the Regulation of Supercharged 1,25 D

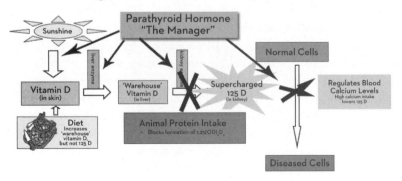

When, for example, we need more 1,25 D, parathyroid hormone induces the kidney enzyme activity to produce it. When there is enough, parathyroid hormone slows down the kidney enzyme activity. Within seconds, this hormone manages how much 1,25 D there will be at each time and place. Parathyroid hormone also acts as a conductor at several other places in this network, as shown by the several arrows in Chart C.3. By being aware of the role of each player in its "orchestra," it coordinates, controls, and finely tunes these reactions as a conductor would a symphony orchestra.

Under optimal conditions, sunshine exposure alone can supply all the vitamin D that we need to produce the all-important 1,25 D at the right time. Even the elderly, who are not able to produce as much vitamin D from sunshine, have nothing to worry about if there is enough sunshine.[17] How much is "enough"? If you know how much sunshine causes a slight redness of your skin, then one-fourth of this amount, provided two to three times per week, is more than adequate to meet our vitamin D needs and to store some in our liver and body fat.[17] If your skin becomes slightly red after about thirty minutes in the sun, then ten minutes, three times per week will be enough exposure to get plenty of vitamin D.

When and if we don't get enough sunshine, it may be helpful to consume vitamin D in our diets. Almost all of our dietary vitamin D has been artificially added to foods like milk and breakfast cereals. Along with vitamin supplements, this amount of vitamin D can be quite significant and, under certain circumstances, there is some evidence that this practice may be beneficial.[18–21]

In this scheme, sunshine and parathyroid hormone work together in a marvelously coordinated way to keep this system running smoothly, both in filling our vitamin D tank and in helping to produce from moment to moment the exact amount of 1,25 D that we need. When it comes to getting sufficient sunshine or getting vitamin D in food, taking light from the sun makes far more sense.

THROWING WRENCHES INTO THE SYSTEM

Several studies now show that if 1,25 D remains at consistently low levels, the risk of several diseases increases. So then the question is: What causes low levels of 1,25 D? Animal-protein-containing foods cause a significant decrease in 1,25 D.[22] These proteins create an acidic environment in the blood that blocks the kidney enzyme from producing this very important metabolite.[23]

A second factor that influences this process is calcium. Calcium in our blood is crucial for optimum muscle and nerve functioning, and it must be maintained within a fairly narrow range. The 1,25 D keeps the blood levels of calcium operating within this narrow range by monitoring and regulating how much calcium is absorbed from food being digested in the intestine, how much calcium is excreted in the urine and feces, and how much is exchanged with bone, the big supply tank for the body's calcium.

For example, if there is too much calcium in the blood, 1,25 D becomes less active, less calcium is absorbed, and more calcium is excreted. It is a very sensitive balancing act in our bodies. As blood calcium goes up, 1,25 D goes down, and when blood calcium goes down, 1,25 D goes up.[10,24] Here's the kicker: if calcium consumption is unnecessarily high, it lowers the activity of the kidney enzyme and, as a consequence, the level of 1,25 D.[1,25] In other words, routinely consuming high-calcium diets is not in our best interests.

The blood levels of 1,25 D therefore are depressed both by consuming too much animal protein and too much calcium. Animal-based food, with its protein, depresses 1,25 D. Cow's milk, however, is high both in protein and calcium. In fact, in one of the more extensive studies on MS that is associated with lower levels of 1,25 D, cow's milk was found to be as important a factor as latitude mentioned earlier.[26] For example, the association of MS with latitude and sunshine shown in Chart C.2 is also seen with animal-based foods, as shown in Chart C.4.[14]

One could hypothesize that diseases like MS are due, at least in part, to a lack of sunshine and lower vitamin D status. This is supported by the observation that northern people living along coastlines (e.g., Norway and Japan)[26] who consume lots of vitamin D–rich fish have less MS than people living inland. However, in these fish-eating communities with lower rates of disease, much less cow's milk is consumed. Consuming cow's milk has been shown to associate with MS[26] and Type 1 diabetes[27] independent of fish intake.

In another reaction associated with this network, increased intake of animal protein also enhances the production of insulin-like growth factor (IGF-1, first introduced in chapter eight), and this enhances cancer cell growth.[5] In effect, there are many reactions acting in a coordinated and mutually consistent way to cause disease when a diet high in animal protein is consumed. When blood levels of 1,25 D are depressed, IGF-1 simultaneously becomes more active. Together, these factors increase the birth of new cells while simultaneously inhibiting the removal of old cells, both of which favor the development of cancer, as seven studies have described.[28] For example, people with higher-than-normal blood levels of IGF-1 have been shown to have 5.1 times the risk of advanced-stage prostate cancer.[28] If combined with low blood levels of a protein that inactivates IGF-I[29] (i.e., more IGF-1 activity), there is *9.5 times the risk of advanced-stage prostate cancer.*[28] This level of disease risk is alarming. Fundamental to it all is the fact that animal-based foods like meat and dairy[30–32] lead to more IGF-I and less 1,25 D, both of which increase cancer risk.

These are only a few of the factors and events associated with this vitamin D network. With the right food and environment, these events and reactions cooperate in an integrated manner to produce health benefits. In

Chart C.4 Worldwide Distribution of Calorie Consumption from Animal-Based Foods for 120 Countries[14]

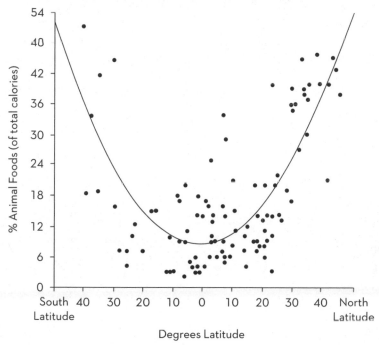

contrast, when the wrong food is consumed, its adverse effects are mediated by not one, but many, of the reactions within this network. Also, many factors in such foods, even beyond the protein and calcium, participate in causing the problem. And, finally, it often is not one disease but many that are likely to occur.

What impresses me about this and other networks is the convergence of so many disease-causing factors operating through so many different reactions to produce a common result. When that common result is more than one disease, it is even more impressive. When these various factors are found in one type of food and this food is epidemiologically related to one or more of these diseases, the associations become still more impressive. This example begins to explain why dairy foods would be expected to increase the risk of these diseases. There is no way that so many intricate mechanisms, operating in such synchrony to produce the same result, are only a random unimportant happenstance. Nature would not have been so devious as to refine such a useless, internally conflicting maze. Networks like this exist throughout the body and within the cells. But of even more importance, they are highly integrated into a far larger dynamic called "life."

REFERENCES

PART I

Chapter 1

1. American Cancer Society. "Cancer Facts and Figures—1998." Atlanta, GA: American Cancer Society, 1998.

2. American Cancer Society. "Cancer Facts & Figures 2015." Atlanta, GA: American Cancer Society, 2015.

3. Flegal KM, Carroll MD, Ogden CL, et al. "Prevalence and trends in obesity among U.S. adults, 1999–2000." *JAMA* 288 (2002): 1723–1727.

4. National Center for Health Statistics. "Obesity and Overweight." Accessed September 2, 2016 at http://www.cdc.gov/nchs/fastats/obesity-overweight.htm.

5. Lin B-H, Guthrie J, and Frazao E. "Nutrient Contribution of Food Away from Home." In: E. Frazao (ed.), *America's Eating Habits: Changes and Consequences*. Washington, DC: Economic Research Service, USDA, 1999. Cited on p. 138 in: *Information Plus. Nutrition: a key to good health*. Wylie, TX: Information Plus, 1999.

6. Mokdad AH, Ford ES, Bowman BA, et al. "Diabetes trends in the U.S.: 1990 1998." *Diabetes Care* 23 (2000): 1278–1283.

7. Centers for Disease Control and Prevention. "National Diabetes Fact Sheet: National Estimates and General Information on Diabetes in the United States, Revised Edition." Atlanta, GA: Centers for Disease Control and Prevention, 1998.

8. American Diabetes Association. "Economic consequences of diabetes mellitus in the U.S. in 1997." *Diabetes Care* 21 (1998): 296–309. Cited in: Mokdad AH, Ford ES, Bowman BA, et al. "Diabetes trends in the U.S.: 1990–1998." *Diabetes Care* 23 (2000): 1278–1283.

9. American Diabetes Association. "Statistics about Diabetes. Data from the National Diabetes Statistics Report." Alexandria, VA: American Diabetes Association, 2014.

10. American Heart Association. "Heart Disease and Stroke Statistics—2003 Update." Dallas: American Heart Association, 2002.

11. Ornish D, Brown SE, Scherwitz LW, et al. "Can lifestyle changes reverse coronary heart disease?" *Lancet* 336 (1990): 129–133.

12. Esselstyn CB, Ellis SG, Medendorp SV, et al. "A strategy to arrest and reverse coronary artery disease: a 5-year longitudinal study of a single physician's practice." *J. Family Practice* 41 (1995): 560–568.

13. Starfield B. "Is U.S. health really the best in the world?" *JAMA* 284 (2000): 483–485.

14. Anderson RN. "Deaths: leading causes for 2000." *National Vital Statistics Reports* 50 (16) (2002).

15. Phillips D, Christenfeld N, and Glynn L. "Increase in U.S. medication-error death between 1983 and 1993." *Lancet* 351 (1998): 643–644.

16. U.S. Congressional House Subcommittee Oversight Investigation. "Cost and quality of health care: unnecessary surgery." Washington, DC: 1976. Cited by: Leape, L. "Unnecessary surgery." *Ann. Rev. Publ. Health* 13 (1992): 363–383.

17. Lazarou J, Pomeranz B, and Corey PN. "Incidence of adverse drug reactions in hospitalized patients." *JAMA* 279 (1998): 1200–1205.

18. World Health Organization. Technical Report Series No. 425. "International Drug Monitoring: the Role of the Hospital." Geneva, Switzerland: World Health Organization, 1966.

19. James JT. "A new, evidence-based estimate of patient harms associated with hospital care." *J Patient Safety* 9 (2013): 122–128.

20. Health Insurance Association of America. *Source Book of Health Insurance Data*: 1999–2000. Washington, DC, 1999.

21. National Center for Health Statistics. *Health, United States, 2000 with Adolescent Health Chart-book*. Hyattsville, MD: National Center for Health Statistics, 2000.

22. Starfield B. *Primary Care: Balancing Health Needs, Services, and Technology*. New York: Oxford University Press, 1998.

23. World Health Organization. World Health Report 2000: Press release. "World Health Organization assesses the world's health systems." June 21, 2000. Geneva. Accessed at http://www.who.int.

24. PricewaterhouseCoopers. "Behind the Numbers: Slight Uptick in Expected Growth Rate Ends Five-Year Contraction." London: PricewaterhouseCoopers, 2014.

25. de Rugy V. "US health care spending more than twice the average for developed countries." Arlington, VA: Mercatus Center, George Mason University, 2013. Accessed at http://mercatus.org/publication/us-health-care-spending-more-twice-average-developed-countries.

26. Centers for Medicare and Medicaid Services. "National Health Expenditure Projections 2012–2022." Baltimore, MD: Centers for Medicare and Medicaid Services, 2014. Accessed at https://www.cms.gov/research-statistics-data-and-systems/statistics-trends-and-reports/nationalhealthexpenddata/downloads/proj2012.pdf.

27. Shiller R. "US inflation rate by year." 2015. Accessed at http://www.multpl.com/inflation/table.

28. Campbell, TC. Re: "Seize the ACA: The innovator's guide to the Affordable Care Act (executive summary)." [Blog comment]. Clayton Christensen Institute for Disruptive Innovation, November 23, 2014. Accessed at http://www.christenseninstitute.org/publications/aca/#comment-159005; PricewaterhouseCoopers. "Behind the Numbers: Slight Uptick in Expected Growth Rate Ends Five-Year Contraction." London: PricewaterhouseCoopers, 2014.

29. Coble YD. American Medical Association press release. "AMA decries rise in number of uninsured Americans." September 30, 2003. Chicago, IL. Accessed at http://www.ama-assn.org/ama/pub/article/1617–8064.html.

30. Cohen RA, and Martinez ME. "Health insurance coverage: early release of estimates from the National Health Interview Survey, January–March 2015." Rockville, MD: National Health Interview Survey Early Release Program, U.S. Centers for Disease

Control and Prevention, August 2015. Accessed at http://www.cdc.gov/nchs/data/nhis/earlyrelease/insur201508.pdf.

31. Campbell TC. "Present day knowledge on aflatoxin." *Phil. J. Nutr.* 20 (1967): 193–201.

32. Campbell TC, Caedo JP, Jr., Bulatao-Jayme J, et al. "Aflatoxin M$_1$ in human urine." *Nature* 227 (1970): 403–404.

33. This program was conducted in collaboration with the Philippine Department of Health and was funded by the United States Agency for International Development (USAID). USAID paid my full salary for six years and resulted in 110 "mothercraft centers" distributed around much of the Philippines. Progress on this contract was prepared as monthly reports to USAID by Associate Dean C. W. Engel at Virginia Tech.

34. Hu J, Zhao X, Jia J, et al. "Dietary calcium and bone density among middle-aged and elderly women in China." *Am. J. Clin. Nutr.* 58 (1993): 219–227.

35. Hu J, Zhao X, Parpia B, et al. "Dietary intakes and urinary excretion of calcium and acids: a cross-sectional study of women in China." *Am. J. Clin. Nutr.* 58 (1993): 398–406.

36. Hu J, Zhao X, Parpia B, et al. "Assessment of a modified household food weighing method in a study of bone health in China." *European J. Clin. Nutr.* 48 (1994): 442–452.

37. Potischman N, McCulloch CE, Byers T, et al. "Breast cancer and dietary and plasma concentrations of carotenoids and vitamin A." *Am. J. Clin. Nutr.* 52 (1990): 909–915.

38. Potischman N, McCulloch CE, Byers T, et al. "Associations between breast cancer, triglycerides and cholesterol." *Nutr. Cancer* 15 (1991): 205–215.

39. Chen J, Campbell TC, Li J, et al. *Diet, life-style and mortality in China. A study of the characteristics of 65 Chinese counties.* Oxford, UK; Ithaca, NY; Beijing, PRC: Oxford University Press; Cornell University Press; People's Medical Publishing House, 1990.

40. Campbell TC, and Chen J. "Diet and chronic degenerative diseases: perspectives from China." *Am. J. Clin. Nutr.* 59 (Suppl.) (1994): 1153S–1161S.

41. Campbell TC. "The dietary causes of degenerative diseases: nutrients vs foods." In: N. J. Temple and D. P. Burkitt (eds.), *Western diseases: their dietary prevention and reversibility*, pp. 119–152. Totowa, NJ: Humana Press, 1994.

42. Campbell TC, and Chen J. "Diet and chronic degenerative diseases: a summary of results from an ecologic study in rural China." In: N. J. Temple and D. P. Burkitt (eds.), *Western diseases: their dietary prevention and reversibility*, pp. 67–118. Totowa, NJ: Humana Press, 1994.

43. Chittenden RH. *Physiological economy in nutrition.* New York: F.A. Stokes, 1904.

44. Chittenden RH. *The nutrition of man.* New York: F. A. Stokes, 1907.

Chapter 2

1. Mulder GJ. *The Chemistry of Vegetable & Animal Physiology* (translated by PFH Fromberg). Edinburgh, Scotland: W. Blackwood & Sons, 1849.

2. Stillings BR. "World supplies of animal protein." In: JWG Porter and BA Rolls (eds.), *Proteins in Human Nutrition*, pp. 11–33. London: Academic Press, 1973.

3. Campbell TC, Warner RG, and Loosli JK. "Urea and biuret for ruminants." In: Cornell Nutrition Conference, Buffalo, NY, 1960, pp. 96–103.

4. Campbell TC, Loosli JK, Warner RG, et al. "Utilization of biuret by ruminants." *J. Animal Science* 22 (1963): 139–145.

5. Autret M. "World protein supplies and needs. Proceedings of the Sixteenth Easter School in Agricultural Science, University of Nottingham, 1969." In: R. A. Laurie (ed.), *Proteins in Human Food*, pp. 3–19. Westport, CT: Avi Publishing Company, 1970.

6. Scrimshaw NS, and Young VR. "Nutritional evaluation and the utilization of protein resources." In: C. E. Bodwell (ed.), *Evaluation of Proteins for Humans*, pp. 1–10. Westport, CT: The Avi Publishing Co., 1976.

7. Jalil ME, and Tahir WM. "World supplies of plant proteins." In: J. W. G. Porter and B. A. Rolls (eds.), *Proteins in Human Nutrition*, pp. 35–46. London: Academic Press, 1973.

8. Blount WP. "Turkey 'X' Disease." *Turkeys* 9 (1961): 52, 55–58, 61, 77.

9. Sargeant K, Sheridan A, O'Kelly J, et al. "Toxicity associated with certain samples of groundnuts." *Nature* 192 (1961): 1096–1097.

10. Lancaster MC, Jenkins FP, and Philp JM. "Toxicity associated with certain samples of groundnuts." *Nature* 192 (1961): 1095–1096.

11. Wogan GN, and Newberne PM. "Dose-response characteristics of aflatoxin B_1 carcinogenesis in the rat." *Cancer Res.* 27 (1967): 2370–2376.

12. Wogan GN, Paglialunga S, and Newberne PM. "Carcinogenic effects of low dietary levels of aflatoxin B_1 in rats." *Food Cosmet. Toxicol.* 12 (1974): 681–685.

13. Campbell TC, Caedo JP, Jr., Bulatao-Jayme J, et al. "Aflatoxin M_1 in human urine." *Nature* 227 (1970): 403–404.

14. Madhavan TV, and Gopalan C. "The effect of dietary protein on carcinogenesis of aflatoxin." *Arch. Path.* 85 (1968): 133–137.

Chapter 3

1. Natural Resources Defense Council. "Intolerable risk: pesticides in our children's food." New York: Natural Resources Defense Council, February 27, 1989.

2. Winter C, Craigmill A, and Stimmann M. "Food Safety Issues II. NRDC report and Alar." *UC Davis Environmental Toxicology Newsletter* 9(2) (1989): 1.

3. Lieberman AJ, and Kwon SC. "Fact versus fears: a review of the greatest unfounded health scares of recent times." New York: American Council on Science and Health, June, 1998.

4. Whelan EM, and Stare FJ. *Panic in the pantry: facts and fallacies about the food you buy*. Buffalo, NY: Prometheus Books, 1992.

5. U.S. Apple Association. "News release: synopsis of U.S. Apple Press Conference." McLean, VA: U.S. Apple Association, February 25, 1999.

6. Cassens RG. *Nitrite-cured meat: a food safety issue in perspective*. Trumbull, CT: Food and Nutrition Press, Inc., 1990.

7. Lijinsky W, and Epstein SS. "Nitrosamines as environmental carcinogens." *Nature* 225 (1970): 21–23.

8. National Toxicology Program. "Ninth report on carcinogens, revised January 2001." Washington, DC: U.S. Department of Health and Human Services, Public Health Service, January, 2001.

9. International Agency for Cancer Research. *IARC Monographs on the Evaluation of the Carcinogenic Risk of Chemicals to Humans: Some N-Nitroso Compounds*. Vol. 17. Lyon, France: International Agency for Research on Cancer, 1978.

10. Druckrey H, Janzowski R, and Preussmann R. "Organotrope carcinogene wirkungen bei 65 verschiedenen N-nitroso-verbindungen an BD-ratten." *Z. Krebsforsch.* 69 (1967): 103–201.

11. Thomas C, and So BT. "Zur morphologie der durch N-nitroso-verbindungen erzeugten tumoren im oberen verdauungstrakt der ratte." *Arzneimittelforsch.* 19 (1969): 1077–1091.

12. Eisenbrand G, Spiegelhalder B, Janzowski C, et al. "Volatile and non-volatile N-nitroso compounds in foods and other environmental media." *IARC Sci. Publi.* 19 (1978): 311–324.

13. National Archives and Records Administration. "Code of Federal Regulations: Title 9, Animals and Animal Products, Section 319.180 (9CFR319.180)." Washington, DC: Government Printing Office, 2001.

14. Kanfer S. October 2, 1972. "The decline and fall of the American hot dog." *Time*: 86.

15. Newberne P. "Nitrite promotes lymphoma incidence in rats." *Science* 204 (1979): 1079–1081.

16. Madhavan TV, and Gopalan C. "The effect of dietary protein on carcinogenesis of aflatoxin." *Arch. Path.* 85 (1968): 133–137.

17. If this defect becomes part of the first round of daughter cells, then this will be passed on to all subsequent generations of cells, with the potential to eventually become clinically detectable cancer. However, this is an oversimplification of a very complex process. Perhaps two of the more significant omissions are the hypotheses that (1) more than one mutation may be required to initiate and promote cancer, and (2) not all genetic defects result in cancer.

18. Mgbodile MUK, and Campbell TC. "Effect of protein deprivation of male weanling rats on the kinetics of hepatic microsomal enzyme activity." *J. Nutr.* 102 (1972): 53–60.

19. Hayes JR, Mgbodile MUK, and Campbell TC. "Effect of protein deficiency on the inducibility of the hepatic microsomal drug-metabolizing enzyme system. I. Effect on substrate interaction with cytochrome P-450." *Biochem. Pharmacol.* 22 (1973): 1005–1014.

20. Mgbodile MUK, Hayes JR, and Campbell TC. "Effect of protein deficiency on the inducibility of the hepatic microsomal drug-metabolizing enzyme system. II. Effect on enzyme kinetics and electron transport system." *Biochem. Pharmacol.* 22 (1973): 1125–1132.

21. Hayes JR, and Campbell TC. "Effect of protein deficiency on the inducibility of the hepatic microsomal drug-metabolizing enzyme system. III. Effect of 3-methylcholanthrene induction on activity and binding kinetics." *Biochem. Pharmacol.* 23 (1974): 1721–1732.

22. Campbell TC. "Influence of nutrition on metabolism of carcinogens (Martha Maso Honors Thesis)." *Adv. Nutr. Res.* 2 (1979): 29–55.

23. Preston RS, Hayes JR, and Campbell TC. "The effect of protein deficiency on the in vivo binding of aflatoxin B_1 to rat liver macromolecules." *Life Sci.* 19 (1976): 1191–1198.

24. Portman RS, Plowman KM, and Campbell TC. "On mechanisms affecting species susceptibility to aflatoxin." *Biochim. Biophys. Acta* 208 (1970): 487–495.

25. Prince LO, and Campbell TC. "Effects of sex difference and dietary protein level on the binding of aflatoxin B_1 to rat liver chromatin proteins in vivo." *Cancer Res.* 42 (1982): 5053–5059.

26. Mainigi KD, and Campbell TC. "Subcellular distribution and covalent binding of aflatoxins as functions of dietary manipulation." *J Toxicol. Eviron. Health* 6 (1980): 659–671.

27. Nerurkar LS, Hayes JR, and Campbell TC. "The reconstitution of hepatic microsomal mixed function oxidase activity with fractions derived from weanling rats fed different levels of protein." *J. Nutr.* 108 (1978): 678–686.

28. Gurtoo HL, and Campbell TC. "A kinetic approach to a study of the induction of rat liver microsomal hydroxylase after pretreatment with 3,4-benzpyrene and aflatoxin B_1." *Biochem. Pharmacol.* 19 (1970): 1729–1735.

29. Adekunle AA, Hayes JR, and Campbell TC. "Interrelationships of dietary protein level, aflatoxin B_1 metabolism, and hepatic microsomal epoxide hydrase activity." *Life Sci.* 21 (1977): 1785–1792.

30. Mainigi KD, and Campbell TC. "Effects of low dietary protein and dietary aflatoxin on hepatic glutathione levels in F-344 rats." *Toxicol. Appl. Pharmacol.* 59 (1981): 196–203.

31. Farber E, and Cameron R. "The sequential analysis of cancer development." *Adv. Cancer Res.* 31 (1980): 125–226.

32. Foci response for the various charts in this chapter mostly reflect "% of liver volume," which integrates "number of foci" and "size of foci," both of which indicate tumor-forming tendency. So that the responses from individual experiments can be compared among each other, the data are adjusted to a common scale that reflects the response produced by a standard dose of aflatoxin and by feeding a 20% protein diet.

33. Appleton BS, and Campbell TC. "Inhibition of aflatoxin-initiated preneoplastic liver lesions by low dietary protein." *Nutr. Cancer* 3 (1982): 200–206.

34. Dunaif GE, and Campbell TC. "Relative contribution of dietary protein level and Aflatoxin B_1 dose in generation of presumptive preneoplastic foci in rat liver." *J. Natl. Cancer Inst.* 78 (1987): 365–369.

35. Youngman LD, and Campbell TC. "High protein intake promotes the growth of preneoplastic foci in Fischer #344 rats: evidence that early remodeled foci retain the potential for future growth." *J. Nutr.* 121 (1991): 1454–1461.

36. Youngman LD, and Campbell TC. "Inhibition of aflatoxin B_1-induced gamma-glutamyl transpeptidase positive (GGT+) hepatic preneoplastic foci and tumors by low protein diets: evidence that altered GGT+ foci indicate neoplastic potential." *Carcinogenesis* 13 (1992): 1607–1613.

37. Dunaif GE, and Campbell TC. "Dietary protein level and aflatoxin B_1-induced preneoplastic hepatic lesions in the rat." *J. Nutr.* 117 (1987): 1298–1302.

38. Horio F, Youngman LD, Bell RC, et al. "Thermogenesis, low-protein diets, and decreased development of AFB1-induced preneoplastic foci in rat liver." *Nutr. Cancer* 16 (1991): 31–41.

39. About 12% dietary protein is required to maximize growth rate, according to the National Research Council of the National Academy of Sciences.

40. Subcommittee on Laboratory Animal Nutrition. *Nutrient requirements of laboratory animals.* 2nd revised edition, number 10. Washington, DC: National Academy Press, 1972.

41. National Research Council. *Recommended dietary allowances.* 10th ed. Washington, DC: National Academy Press, 1989.

42. Schulsinger DA, Root MM, and Campbell TC. "Effect of dietary protein quality on development of aflatoxin B_1-induced hepatic preneoplastic lesions." *J. Natl. Cancer Inst.* 81 (1989): 1241–1245.

43. Youngman LD. *The growth and development of aflatoxin B₁-induced preneoplastic lesions, tumors, metastasis, and spontaneous tumors as they are influenced by dietary protein level, type, and intervention.* Ithaca, NY: Cornell University, PhD Thesis, 1990.

44. Beasley RP. "Hepatitis B virus as the etiologic agent in hepatocellular carcinoma-epidemiologic considerations." *Hepatol.* 2 (1982): 21S–26S.

45. Blumberg BS, Larouze B, London WT, et al. "The relation of infection with the hepatitis B agent to primary hepatic carcinoma." *Am. J. Pathol.* 81 (1975): 669–682.

46. Chisari FV, Ferrari C, and Mondelli MU. "Hepatitis B virus structure and biology." *Microbiol. Pathol.* 6 (1989): 311–325.

47. Hu J, Cheng Z, Chisari FV, et al. "Repression of hepatitis B virus (HBV) transgene and HBV-induced liver injury by low protein diet." *Oncogene* 15 (1997): 2795–2801.

48. Cheng Z, Hu J, King J, et al. "Inhibition of hepatocellular carcinoma development in hepatitis B virus transfected mice by low dietary casein." *Hepatology* 26 (1997): 1351–1354.

49. Hawrylewicz EJ, Huang HH, Kissane JQ, et al. "Enhancement of the 7,12-dimethylbenz(a)anthracene (DMBA) mammary tumorigenesis by high dietary protein in rats." *Nutr. Reps. Int.* 26 (1982): 793–806.

50. Hawrylewicz EJ. "Fat-protein interaction, defined 2-generation studies." In: C. Ip, D. F. Birt, A. E. Rogers, and C. Mettlin (eds.), *Dietary fat and cancer*, pp. 403–434. New York: Alan R. Liss, 1986.

51. Huang HH, Hawrylewicz EJ, Kissane JQ, et al. "Effect of protein diet on release of prolactin and ovarian steroids in female rats." *Nutr. Rpts. Int.* 26 (1982): 807–820.

52. O'Connor TP, Roebuck BD, and Campbell TC. "Dietary intervention during the post-dosing phase of L-azaserine-induced preneoplastic lesions." *J Natl Cancer Inst* 75 (1985): 955–957.

53. O'Connor TP, Roebuck BD, Peterson F, et al. "Effect of dietary intake of fish oil and fish protein on the development of L-azaserine-induced preneoplastic lesions in rat pancreas." *J Natl Cancer Inst* 75 (1985): 959–962.

54. He Y. *Effects of carotenoids and dietary carotenoid extracts on aflatoxin B₁-induced mutagenesis and hepatocarcinogenesis.* Ithaca, NY: Cornell University, PhD Thesis, 1990.

55. He Y, and Campbell TC. "Effects of carotenoids on aflatoxin B₁-induced mutagenesis in S. typhimurium TA 100 and TA 98." *Nutr. Cancer* 13 (1990): 243–253.

Chapter 4

1. Li J-Y, Liu B-Q, Li G-Y, et al. "Atlas of cancer mortality in the People's Republic of China. An aid for cancer control and research." *Int. J. Epid.* 10 (1981): 127–133.

2. Higginson J. "Present trends in cancer epidemiology." *Proc. Can. Cancer Conf.* 8 (1969): 40–75.

3. Wynder EL, and Gori GB. "Contribution of the environment to cancer incidence: an epidemiologic exercise." *J. Natl. Cancer Inst.* 58 (1977): 825–832.

4. Doll R, and Peto R. "The causes of cancer: Quantitative estimates of avoidable risks of cancer in the United States today." *J Natl Cancer Inst* 66 (1981): 1192–1265.

5. Fagin D. News release. "Breast cancer cause still elusive study: no clear link between pollution, breast cancer on LI." August 6, 2002. Newsday.com. Accessed

at http://www.newsday.com/news/local/longisland/nylicanc062811887aug06. story?coll=ny%2Dtop%2Dheadlines.

6. There were 82 mortality rates, but about a third of these rates were duplicates of the same disease for different-aged people.

7. Hu FB, Stampfer MJ, Manson JE, et al. "Dietary protein and risk of ischemic heart disease in women." *Am. J. Clin. Nutr.* 70 (1999): 221–227.

8. Chen J, Campbell TC, Li J, et al. *Diet, life-style and mortality in China. A study of the characteristics of 65 Chinese counties.* Oxford, UK; Ithaca, NY; Beijing, PRC: Oxford University Press; Cornell University Press; People's Medical Publishing House, 1990.

9. Calorie intake in China is for a 65 kg adult male doing "light physical work." Comparable data for the American male is adjusted for a body weight of 65 kg.

10. SerVaas C. "Diets that protected against cancers in China." *The Saturday Evening Post* October 1990: 26–28.

11. All the available disease mortality rates were arranged in a matrix so that it was possible to readily determine the relationship of each rate with every other rate. Each comparison was then assigned a plus or minus, depending on whether they were directly or inversely correlated. All plus correlations were assembled in one list and all minus correlations were assembled in a second list. Each individual entry in either list was therefore positively related to entries in its own list but inversely related to diseases in the opposite list. Most, but not all, of these correlations were statistically significant.

12. Campbell TC, Chen J, Brun T, et al. "China: from diseases of poverty to diseases of affluence. Policy implications of the epidemiological transition." *Ecol. Food Nutr.* 27 (1992): 133–144.

13. Chen J, Campbell TC, Li J, et al. *Diet, life-style and mortality in China. A study of the characteristics of 65 Chinese counties.* Oxford, UK; Ithaca, NY; Beijing, PRC: Oxford University Press; Cornell University Press; People's Medical Publishing House, 1990.

14. Campbell TC, Chen J, Brun T, et al. "China: from diseases of poverty to diseases of affluence. Policy implications of the epidemiological transition." *Ecol Food Nutr* 27 (1992): 133–144.

15. Lipid Research Clinics Program Epidemiology Committee. "Plasma lipid distributions in selected North American Population. The Lipid Research Clinics Program Prevalence Study." *Circulation* 60 (1979): 427–439.

16. Campbell TC, Parpia B, and Chen J. "Diet, lifestyle, and the etiology of coronary artery disease: The Cornell China Study." *Am. J. Cardiol.* 82 (1998): 18T-21T.

17. These data are for villages SA, LC, and RA for women and SA, QC, and NB for men, as seen in the monograph (Chen, et al. 1990).

18. Sirtori CR, Noseda G, and Descovich GC. "Studies on the use of a soybean protein diet for the management of human hyperlipoproteinemias." In: MJ Gibney and D Kritchevsky (eds.), *Current Topics in Nutrition and Disease, Volume 8: Animal and Vegetable Proteins in Lipid Metabolism and Atherosclerosis*, pp. 135–148. New York: Alan R. Liss, 1983.

19. Carroll KK. "Dietary proteins and amino acids—their effects on cholesterol metabolism." In: M. J. Gibney and D. Kritchevsky (eds.), *Animal and Vegetable Proteins in Lipid Metabolism and Atherosclerosis, Volume 8: Animal and Vegetable Proteins in Lipid Metabolism and Atherosclerosis*, pp. 9–17. New York: Alan R. Liss, 1983.

20. Terpstra AHM, Hermus RJJ, and West CE. "Dietary protein and cholesterol metabolism in rabbits and rats." In: MJ Gibney and D Kritchevsky (eds.), *Animal and Vegetable Proteins in Lipid Metabolism and Atherosclerosis, Volume 8: Animal and Vegetable*

Proteins in Lipid Metabolism and Atherosclerosis, pp. 19–49. New York: Alan R. Liss, 1983.

21. Kritchevsky D, Tepper SA, Czarnecki SK, et al. "Atherogenicity of animal and vegetable protein. Influence of the lysine to arginine ratio." *Atherosclerosis* 41 (1982): 429–431.

22. Dietary fat can be expressed as percent of total weight of the diet or as percent of total calories. Most commentators and researchers express fat as percent of total calories because we primarily consume food to satisfy our need for calories, not our need for weight. I will do the same throughout this book.

23. National Research Council. *Diet, Nutrition and Cancer*. Washington, DC: National Academy Press, 1982.

24. United States Department of Health and Human Services. *The Surgeon General's Report on Nutrition and Health*. Washington, DC: Superintendent of Documents, U.S. Government Printing Office, 1988.

25. National Research Council, and Committee on Diet and Health. *Diet and health: implications for reducing chronic disease risk*. Washington, DC: National Academy Press, 1989.

26. Expert Panel. *Food, nutrition and the prevention of cancer, a global perspective*. Washington, DC: American Institute for Cancer Research/World Cancer Research Fund, 1997.

27. Exceptions include those foods artificially stripped of their fat, such as nonfat milk.

28. Armstrong D, and Doll R. "Environmental factors and cancer incidence and mortality in different countries, with special reference to dietary practices." *Int. J. Cancer* 15 (1975): 617–631.

29. U.S. Senate. "Dietary goals for the United States, 2nd Edition." Washington, DC: U.S. Government Printing Office, 1977.

30. Committee on Diet Nutrition and Cancer. *Diet, nutrition and cancer: directions for research*. Washington, DC: National Academy Press, 1983.

31. There also were a number of other policy statements and large human studies that were begun at about this time that were to receive much public discussion and that were founded and/or interpreted in relation to dietary fat and these diseases. These included the initiation of the U.S. Dietary Guidelines report series begun in 1980, the Harvard Nurses' Health Study in 1984, the initial reports of the Framingham Heart Study in the 1960s, the Seven Countries Study of Ancel Keys, the Multiple Risk Factor Intervention Trial (MRFIT), and others.

32. Carroll KK, Braden LM, Bell JA, et al. "Fat and cancer." *Cancer* 58 (1986): 1818–1825.

33. Drasar BS, and Irving D. "Environmental factors and cancer of the colon and breast." *Br. J. Cancer* 27 (1973): 167–172.

34. Haenszel W, and Kurihara M. "Studies of Japanese migrants: mortality from cancer and other disease among Japanese and the United States." *J. Natl. Cancer. Inst.* 40 (1968): 43–68.

35. Higginson J, and Muir CS. "Epidemiology in Cancer." In: J. F. Holland and E. Frei (eds.), *Cancer Medicine*, pp. 241–306. Philadelphia: Lea and Febiger, 1973.

36. The correlation of fat intake with animal protein intake is 84% for grams of fat consumed and 70% for fat as a percent of calories.

37. Kelsey JL, Gammon MD, and Esther MJ. "Reproductive factors and breast cancer." *Epidemiol. Revs.* 15 (1993): 36–47.

38. de Stavola BL, Wang DY, Allen DS, et al. "The association of height, weight, menstrual and reproductive events with breast cancer: results from two prospective studies on the island of Guernsey (United Kingdom)." *Cancer Causes and Control* 4 (1993): 331–340.

39. Rautalahti M, Albanes D, Virtamo J, et al. "Lifetime menstrual activity—indicator of breast cancer risk." (1993): 17–25

40. It was not possible to statistically detect an association of blood hormone levels with breast cancer risk within this group of women because their blood samples were taken at random times of their menstrual cycles and breast cancer rates were so low, thus minimizing the ability to detect such an association, even when real.

41. Key TJA, Chen J, Wang DY, et al. "Sex hormones in women in rural China and in Britain." *Brit. J. Cancer* 62 (1990): 631–636.

42. These biomarkers include plasma copper, urea nitrogen, estradiol, prolactin, testosterone and, inversely, sex hormone binding globulin, each of which has been known to be associated with animal protein intake from previous studies.

43. For the total dietary fiber (TDF), the averages for China and the U.S. were 33.3 and 11.1 grams per day, respectively. The range of the county averages are 7.7–77.6 grams per day in China, compared with a range of 2.4–26.6 grams per day for the middle 90% of American males.

44. The correlation for plant protein was +0.53[III] and for animal protein was +0.12.

45. In principle, using "cancer prevalence within families" as the outcome measurement more effectively controls for the various causes of cancer that associate with different kinds of cancer, thus permitting study of an isolated effect of the dietary factor.

46. Guo W, Li J, Blot WJ, et al. "Correlations of dietary intake and blood nutrient levels with esophageal cancer mortality in China." *Nutr. Cancer* 13 (1990): 121–127.

47. The full effects of these fat-soluble antioxidants can be demonstrated only when antioxidant concentrations are adjusted for the levels of LDL for individual subjects. This was not known at the time of the survey; thus provisions were not made for this adjustment.

48. Kneller RW, Guo W, Hsing AW, et al. "Risk factors for stomach cancer in sixty-five Chinese counties." *Cancer Epi. Biomarkers Prev.* 1 (1992): 113–118.

49. Campbell TC (with Jacobson H). *The low-carb fraud.* Dallas: BenBella Books, 2013.

50. Campbell TC (with Jacobson H). *Whole: rethinking the science of nutrition.* Dallas: BenBella Books, 2013.

51. Perlmutter D. *Grain brain.* New York: Little, Brown, 2013, p. 323.

52. Information Plus. *Nutrition: a key to good health.* Wylie, TX: Information Plus, 1999.

53. Westman EC, Yancy WS, Edman JS, et al. "Carbohydrate Diet Program." *Am. J. Med.* 113 (2002): 30–36.

54. Atkins RC. *Dr. Atkins' New Diet Revolution.* New York: Avon Books, 1999.

55. Wright JD, Kennedy-Stephenson J, Wang CY, et al. "Trends in Intake of Energy and Macronutrients—United States, 1971–2000." *Morbidity and Mortality Weekly Report* 53 (February 6, 2004): 80–82.

56. Noakes M, and Clifton PM. "Weight loss and plasma lipids." *Curr. Opin. Lipidol.* 11 (2000): 65–70.

57. Bilsborough SA, and Crowe TC. "Low-carbohydrate diets: what are the potential short- and long-term health implications?" *Asia Pac. J. Clin. Nutr.* 12 (2003): 396–404.

58. Stevens A, Robinson DP, Turpin J, et al. "Sudden cardiac death of an adolescent during dieting." *South. Med. J.* 95 (2002): 1047–1049.

59. Patty A. "Low-carb fad claims teen's life - Star diet blamed in death." *The Daily Telegraph* (Sidney, Australia) November 2, 2002: 10.

60. Smith MJ, Trexler E, Sommer A, Starkoff B, and Devor S. "Unrestricted Paleolithic diet is associated with unfavorable changes to blood lipids in healthy subjects." *Int. J. Exerc. Sci.* 7 (2014): 128–139.

61. Noto H, Goto A, Tsujimoto T, and Noda M. "Low-carbohydrate diets and all-cause mortality: a systematic review and meta-analysis of observational studies." *PLoS ONE* 8 (2013): 1–10.

62. Carroll KK, Gammal EB, & Plunkett ER. "Dietary fat and mammary cancer." *Can. Med. Assoc. J.* 98 (1968): 590–594.

63. Drasar BS, and Irving D. "Environmental factors and cancer of the colon and breast." *Br. J. Cancer* 27 (1973): 167–172; Armstrong D, and Doll R. "Environmental factors and cancer incidence and mortality in different countries, with special reference to dietary practices." *Int. J. Cancer* 15 (1975): 617–631.

64. Keys A. "Coronary heart disease in seven countries." *Circulation* 41, suppl. (1970): I1–I211.

65. Atkins, 1999. Page 275.

66. Atkins claims that an antioxidant cocktail can protect against heart disease, cancer, and aging, a claim refuted by several large trials recently completed (see chapter 11).

67. Atkins, 1999. Page 103.

68. Bone J. "Diet doctor Atkins 'obese,' had heart problems: coroner: widow angrily denies that opponents' claims that heart condition caused by controversial diet." *Ottawa Citizen* February 11, 2004: A11.

69. Welsh JA, Sharma AJ, Grellinger L, & Vos MB. "Consumption of added sugars is decreasing in the United States." *Am J Clin Nutr* 94 (2011): 726–734.

70. Campbell TC. "Energy balance: interpretation of data from rural China." *Toxicological Sciences* 52 (1999): 87–94.

71. Horio F, Youngman LD, Bell RC, et al. "Thermogenesis, low-protein diets, and decreased development of AFB1-induced preneoplastic foci in rat liver." *Nutr. Cancer* 16 (1991): 31–41.

72. Krieger E, Youngman LD, and Campbell TC. "The modulation of aflatoxin (AFB1) induced preneoplastic lesions by dietary protein and voluntary exercise in Fischer 344 rats." *FASEB J.* 2 (1988): 3304 Abs.

73. The cited associations of total animal and plant protein intakes are taken from manuscript under review.

74. Campbell TC, Chen J, Liu C, et al. "Non-association of aflatoxin with primary liver cancer in a cross-sectional ecologic survey in the People's Republic of China." *Cancer Res.* 50 (1990): 6882–6893.

75. Campbell TC (with Jacobson H). *Whole: Rethinking the Science of Nutrition.* Dallas: BenBella Books, 2013.

PART II

Chapter 5

1. Adams CF. "How many times does your heart beat per year?" Accessed October 20, 2003. Accessed at http://www.straightdope.com/classics/a1_088a.html.

2. National Heart, Lung, and Blood Institute. "Morbidity and Mortality: 2002 Chart Book on Cardiovascular, Lung, and Blood Diseases." Bethesda, MD: National Institutes of Health, 2002.

3. American Heart Association. "Heart Disease and Stroke Statistics—2003 Update." Dallas: American Heart Association, 2002.

4. Braunwald E. "Shattuck lecture—cardiovascular medicine at the turn of the millennium: triumphs, concerns and opportunities." *New Engl. J. Med.* 337 (1997): 1360–1369.

5. American Cancer Society. "Cancer Facts and Figures—1998." Atlanta: American Cancer Society, 1998.

6. Anderson RN. "Deaths: leading causes for 2000." *National Vital Statistics Reports* 50 (16) (2002).

7. Enos WE, Holmes RH, and Beyer J. "Coronary disease among United States soldiers killed in action in Korea." *JAMA* 152 (1953): 1090–1093.

8. Esselstyn CJ. "Resolving the coronary artery disease epidemic through plant-based nutrition." *Prev. Cardiol.* 4 (2001): 171–177.

9. Antman EM, and Braunwald E. "Acute myocardial infarction." In: E Braunwald (ed.), *Heart Disease, a Textbook of Cardiovascular Disease, Vol. II (5th ed.)*, pp. 1184–1288. Philadelphia: W. B. Saunders Company, 1997.

10. Esselstyn CJ. "Lecture: reversing heart disease." December 5, 2002. Ithaca, NY: Cornell University, 2002.

11. Ambrose JA, and Fuster V. "Can we predict future acute coronary events in patients with stable coronary artery disease?" *JAMA* 277 (1997): 343–344.

12. Ellulu MS, Patimah I, Khaza'ai H, Rahmat A, Abed Y, and Ali F. "Atherosclerotic cardiovascular disease: a review of initiators and protective factors." *Inflammopharmacology* 24 (2016): 1–10, doi:10.1007/s10787-015-0255-y.

13. Forrester JS, and Shah PK. "Lipid lowering versus revascularization: an idea whose time (for testing) has come." *Circulation* 96 (1997): 1360–1362.

14. Now named the National Heart, Lung, and Blood Institute of the National Institutes of Health in Bethesda, Maryland.

15. Gofman JW, Lindgren F, Elliot H, et al. "The role of lipids and lipoproteins in atherosclerosis." *Science* 111 (1950): 166.

16. Kannel WB, Dawber TR, Kagan A, et al. "Factors of risk in the development of coronary heart disease—six-year follow-up experience." *Ann. Internal Med.* 55 (1961): 33–50.

17. Jolliffe N, and Archer M. "Statistical associations between international coronary heart disease death rates and certain environmental factors." *J. Chronic Dis.* 9 (1959): 636–652.

18. Scrimgeour EM, McCall MG, Smith DE, et al. "Levels of serum cholesterol, triglyceride, HDL cholesterol, apolipoproteins A-1 and B, and plasma glucose, and prevalence of diastolic hypertension and cigarette smoking in Papua New Guinea Highlanders." *Pathology* 21 (1989): 46–50.

19. Campbell TC, Parpia B, and Chen J. "Dict, lifestyle, and the etiology of coronary artery disease: The Cornell China Study." *Am. J. Cardiol.* 82 (1998): 18T–21T.

20. Kagan A, Harris BR, Winkelstein W, et al. "Epidemiologic studies of coronary heart disease and stroke in Japanese men living in Japan, Hawaii and California." *J. Chronic Dis.* 27 (1974): 345–364.

21. Kato H, Tillotson J, Nichaman MZ, et al. "Epidemiologic studies of coronary heart disease and stroke in Japanese men living in Japan, Hawaii and California: serum lipids and diet." *Am. J. Epidemiol.* 97 (1973): 372–385.

22. Morrison LM. "Arteriosclerosis." *JAMA* 145 (1951): 1232–1236.

23. Morrison LM. "Diet in coronary atherosclerosis." *JAMA* 173 (1960): 884–888.

24. Lyon TP, Yankley A, Gofman JW, et al. "Lipoproteins and diet in coronary heart disease." *California Med.* 84 (1956): 325–328.

25. Gibney MJ, and Kritchevsky D, eds. *Current Topics in Nutrition and Disease, Volume 8: Animal and Vegetable Proteins in Lipid Metabolism and Atherosclerosis.* New York: Alan R. Liss, 1983.

26. Sirtori CR, Noseda G, and Descovich GC. "Studies on the use of a soybean protein diet for the management of human hyperlipoproteinemias." In: MJ Gibney and D Kritchevsky (eds.), *Current Topics in Nutrition and Disease, Volume 8: Animal and Vegetable Proteins in Lipid Metabolism and Atherosclerosis,* pp. 135–148. New York: Alan R. Liss, 1983.

27. Meeker DR, and Kesten HD. "Experimental atherosclerosis and high protein diets. *Proc. Soc. Exp. Biol. Med.* 45 (1940): 543–545; Meeker DR, and Kesten HD. "Effect of high protein dicts on experimental atherosclerosis of rabbits." *Arch. Pathol.* 31 (1941): 147–162.

28. Kritchevsky D, and Czarnecki SK. "Animal and vegetable proteins in lipid metabolism and atherosclerosis." In: MJ Gibney and D Kritchevsky (eds.), *Current Topics in Nutrition and Disease, Volume 8: Animal and Vegetable Proteins in Lipid Metabolism and Atherosclerosis,* pp. 1–7. New York: Alan R. Liss, 1983; Newburgh LH. "The production of Bright's disease by feeding high protein diets." *Arch. Intern. Med.* 24 (1919): 359–377; Newburgh LH, and Clarkson S. "Production of atherosclerosis in rabbits by diet rich in animal protein." *JAMA* 79 (1922): 1106–1108; Newburgh LH, and Clarkson S. "The production of arteriosclerosis in rabbits by feeding diets rich in meat." *Arch. Intern. Med.* 31 (1923): 653–676.

29. Ignatowski A. "Uber die Wirbung des tierischen eiweiss auf die aorta und die parenchymatosen organe der kaninchen." *Vrichows. Arch. Pathol. Anat. Physiol. Klin. Med.* 198 (1909): 248–270.

30. Newburgh LH, and Clarkson S. "Production of atherosclerosis in rabbits by diet rich in animal protein." *JAMA* 79 (1922): 1106–1108; Newburgh LH, and Clarkson S. "The production of arteriosclerosis in rabbits by feeding diets rich in meat." *Arch. Intern. Med.* 31 (1923): 653–676.

31. GS Myers, personal communication, cited by Groom D. "Population studies of atherosclerosis." *Ann. Intern. Med.* 55 (1961): 51–62.

32. Centers for Disease Control. "Smoking and health: a national status report." *Morbidity and Mortality Weekly Report* 35 (1986): 709–711.

33. Centers for Disease Control. "Cigarette smoking among adults—United States, 2000." *Morbidity and Mortality Weekly Report* 51 (2002): 642–645.

34. Age-adjusted, ages 25–74.

35. Mentias A, Barakat A, Raza M, et al. "An alarming trend: change in risk profile of patients with ST elevation myocardial infarction over the last two decades." *J. Am. Coll. Cardiol.* 67 (2016): 659.

36. Marwick C. "Coronary bypass grafting economics, including rehabilitation. Commentary." *Curr. Opin. Cardiol.* 9 (1994): 635–640.

37. Page 1319 in Gersh BJ, Braunwald E, and Rutherford JD. "Chronic coronary artery disease." In: E Braunwald (ed.), *Heart Disease: A Textbook of Cardiovascular Medicine, Vol. 2 (5th ed.)*, pp. 1289–1365. Philadelphia: W. B. Saunders, 1997.

38. Ornish D. "Avoiding revascularization with lifestyle changes: the Multicenter Lifestyle Demonstration Project." *Am. J. Cardiol.* 82 (1998): 72T–76T.

39. Roger VL, et al. "Heart disease and stroke statistics—2011 update: a report from the American Heart Association." *Circulation* 123 (2011): e18–e20.

40. Shaw PJ, Bates D, Cartlidge NEF, et al. "Early intellectual dysfunction following coronary bypass surgery." *Quarterly J. Med.* 58 (1986): 59–68.

41. Cameron AAC, Davis KB, and Rogers WJ. "Recurrence of angina after coronary artery bypass surgery. Predictors and prognosis (CASS registry)." *J. Am. Coll. Cardiol.* 26 (1995): 895–899.

42. Page 1320 in Gersh BJ, Braunwald E, and Rutherford JD. "Chronic coronary artery disease." In: E Braunwald (ed.), *Heart Disease: A Textbook of Cardiovascular Medicine, Vol. 2 (5th ed.)*, pp. 1289–1365. Philadelphia: W. B. Saunders, 1997.

43. Kirklin JW, Naftel DC, Blackstone EH, et al. "Summary of a consensus concerning death and ischemic events after coronary artery bypass grafting." *Circulation* 79 (Suppl 1) (1989): I81–I91.

44. Waldman P, Armstrong D, and Freedberg SP. "Deaths linked to cardiac stents rise as overuse seen." *Bloomberg* (2013, September 26). Accessed at http://www.bloomberg.com/news/articles/2013-09-26/deaths-linked-to-cardiac-stents-rise-as-overuse-seen.

45. Garg S, Serruys PW. "Coronary stents: current status." *J. Am. Coll. Cardiol.* 56 (2010): S1–S42

46. Stergiopoulos K, Brown DL. "Initial coronary stent implantation with medical therapy vs medical therapy alone for stable coronary artery disease: meta-analysis of randomized controlled trials." *Arch. Intern. Med.* 172 (2012): 312–319.

47. Waldman P, Armstrong D, and Freedberg SP. "Deaths linked to cardiac stents rise as overuse seen." *Bloomberg* (2013, September 26). Accessed at http://www.bloomberg.com/news/articles/2013-09-26/deaths-linked-to-cardiac-stents-rise-as-overuse-seen.

48. Information Plus. *Nutrition: A Key to Good Health.* Wylie, TX: Information Plus, 1999.

49. Naifeh SW. *The Best Doctors in America*, 1994–1995. Aiken, SC: Woodward & White, 1994.

50. Esselstyn CB, Jr. "Foreword: changing the treatment paradigm for coronary artery disease." *Am. J. Cardiol.* 82 (1998): 2T–4T.

51. Esselstyn CB, Ellis SG, Medendorp SV, et al. "A strategy to arrest and reverse coronary artery disease: a 5-year longitudinal study of a single physician's practice." *J. Family Practice* 41 (1995): 560–568.

52. Esselstyn CJ. "Introduction: more than coronary artery disease." *Am. J. Cardiol.* 82 (1998): 5T–9T.

53. The flow of blood is related to the fourth power of the radius. Thus, a reduction of seven percent is approximately related to a 30% greater blood flow, although it is not possible to obtain by calculation a more precise determination of this number.

54. Personal communication with Dr. Esselstyn, September 15, 2003.

55. Esselstyn CBJ, Gendy G, Doyle J, et al. "A way to reverse CAD?" *J. Fam. Pract.* 63 (2014): 356–364b; Esselstyn C, and Golubic M. "The nutritional reversal of cardiovascular disease, fact or fiction? Three case reports." *Exp. Clin. Cardiol.* 20 (2014): 1901–1908.

56. Fulkerson, Lee, director. *Forks Over Knives.* Monica Beach Media, 2011.

57. Ornish D, Brown SE, Scherwitz LW, et al. "Can lifestyle changes reverse coronary heart disease?" *Lancet* 336 (1990): 129–133.

58. DeFrances CJ, Licas CA, Vuie VC, and Golosinskiy A. "2006 National Hospital discharge survey." Hyattsville, MD: National Center for Health Statistics, 2008.

59. Epstein, AJ, Polsky D, Yang F, Yang L, and Groeneveld PW. "Coronary revascularization trends in the United States, 2001–2008." *JAMA* 305 (2011): 1769–1776.

60. Boyles S. "Heart bypass surgery rate is declining." WebMD Health News (2011).

61. Wani M. "How much does a heart stent cost?" Buzzle (2013). Accessed at http://www.buzzle.com/articles/how-much-does-a-heart-stent-cost.html "Heart stent cost." CostHelperHealth. Accessed at http://health.costhelper.com/stents.html.

62. "Heart bypass surgery cost." CostHelperHealth. Accessed at http://health.costhelper.com/bypass.html.

63. Esselstyn, C. Personal communication, 2014.

64. Cooper, R. "Statins: the drug firms' goldmine." *Telegraph* (2011, January 19). Accessed at http://www.telegraph.co.uk/news/health/news/8267876/Statins-the-drug-firms-goldmine.html.

65. Heidenreich PA, et al. "Forecasting the future of cardiovascular disease in the United States: a policy statement from the American Heart Association." *Circulation* 123 (2011): 933–944.

66. Wikipedia. "List of countries by GDP (nominal)." (2016, July 7). Accessed at https://en.wikipedia.org/wiki/List_of_countries_by_GDP_(nominal).

67. Dmyterko, K. "Circ: costs to treat heart disease will triple to $818B by 2030." *Cardiovasc Business* (2011). Accessed at http://www.cardiovascularbusiness.com/topics/heart-failure/circ-costs-treat-heart-disease-will-triple-818b-2030.

68. Ratliff NB. "Of rice, grain, and zeal: lessons from Drs. Kempner and Esselstyn." *Cleveland Clin. J. Med.* 67 (2000): 565–566.

69. American Heart Association. "AHA Dietary Guidelines. Revision 2000: A Statement for Healthcare Professionals from the Nutrition Committee of the American Heart Association." *Circulation* 102 (2000): 2296–2311.

70. National Cholesterol Education Program. "Third report of the National Cholesterol Education Program (NCEP) expert panel on detection, evaluation and treatment of high blood cholesterol in adult (adult treatment panel III): executive summary." Bethesda, MD: National Institutes of Health, 2001.

71. Castelli W. "Take this letter to your doctor." *Prevention* 48 (1996): 61–64.

72. Schuler G, Hambrecht R, Schlierf G, et al. "Regular physical exercise and low-fat diet." *Circulation* 86 (1992): 1–11.

Chapter 6

1. Flegal KM, Carroll MD, Ogden CL, et al. "Prevalence and trends in obesity among U.S. adults, 1999–2000." *JAMA* 288 (2002): 1723–1727.

2. Centers for Disease Control and Prevention. "Childhood obesity facts." (2015, August 27). Accessed at https://www.cdc.gov/healthyschools/obesity/facts.htm.

3. Ogden CL, Flegal KM, Carroll MD, et al. "Prevalence and trends in overweight among U.S. children and adolescents." *JAMA* 288 (2002): 1728–1732.

4. Dietz WH. "Health consequences of obesity in youth: childhood predictors of adult disease." *Pediatrics* 101 (1998): 518–525.

5. Fontaine KR, and Barofsky I. "Obesity and health-related quality of life." *Obesity Rev.* 2 (2001): 173–182.

6. Colditz GA. "Economic costs of obesity and inactivity." *Med. Sci. Sports Exerc.* 31 (1999): S663–S667.

7. Adcox S. "New state law seeks to cut down obesity." *Ithaca J.* Sept. 21, 2002: 5A.

8. Centers for Disease Control and Prevention. "Childhood obesity facts." (2015, August 27). Accessed at https://www.cdc.gov/healthyschools/obesity/facts.htm.

9. Williams G. "The heavy price of losing weight." *U.S. News and World Report* (2013, January 2). Accessed at http://money.usnews.com/money/personal-finance/articles/2013/01/02/the-heavy-price-of-losing-weight.

10. Ellis FR, and Montegriffo VME. "Veganism, clinical findings and investigations." *Am. J. Clin. Nutr.* 23 (1970): 249–255.

11. Berenson G, Srinivasan S, Bao W, Newman WPR, Tracy, RE, and Wattigney WA. "Association between multiple cardiovascular risk factors and atherosclerosis to children and young adults. The Bogalusa Heart Study." *New Engl. J. Med.* 338 (1998): 1650–1656.

12. Key TJ, Fraser GE, Thorogood M, et al. "Mortality in vegetarians and nonvegetarians: detailed findings from a collaborative analysis of 5 prospective studies." *Am. J. Clin. Nutr.* 70 (Suppl.) (1999): 516S–524S.

13. Bergan JG, and Brown PT. "Nutritional status of 'new' vegetarians." *J. Am. Diet. Assoc.* 76 (1980): 151–155.

14. Appleby PN, Thorogood M, Mann J, et al. "Low body mass index in non-meat eaters: the possible roles of animal fat, dietary fibre, and alcohol." *Int J. Obes.* 22 (1998): 454–460.

15. Dwyer JT. "Health aspects of vegetarian diets." *Am. J. Clin. Nutr.* 48 (1988): 712–738.

16. Key TJ, and Davey G. "Prevalence of obesity is low in people who do not eat meat." *Brit. Med. J.* 313 (1996): 816–817.

17. Shintani TT, Hughes CK, Beckham S, et al. "Obesity and cardiovascular risk intervention through the ad libitum feeding of traditional Hawaiian diet." *Am. J. Clin. Nutr.* 53 (1991): 1647S–1651S.

18. Barnard RJ. "Effects of life-style modification on serum lipids." *Arch. Intern. Med.* 151 (1991): 1389–1394.

19. McDougall J, Litzau K, Haver E, et al. "Rapid reduction of serum cholesterol and blood pressure by a twelve-day, very low fat, strictly vegetarian diet." *J. Am. Coll. Nutr.* 14 (1995): 491–496.

20. Ornish D, Scherwitz LW, Doody RS, et al. "Effects of stress management training and dietary changes in treating ischemic heart disease." *JAMA* 249 (1983): 54–59.

21. Shintani TT, Beckham S, Brown AC, et al. "The Hawaii diet: ad libitum high carbohydrate, low fat multi-cultural diet for the reduction of chronic disease risk factors: obesity, hypertension, hypercholesterolemia, and hyperglycemia." *Hawaii Med. J.* 60 (2001): 69–73.

22. Nicholson AS, Sklar M, Barnard ND, et al. "Toward improved management of NIDDM: a randomized, controlled, pilot intervention using a lowfat, vegetarian diet." *Prev. Med.* 29 (1999): 87–91.

23. Ornish D, Scherwitz LW, Billings JH, et al. "Intensive lifestyle changes for reversal of coronary heart disease." *JAMA* 280 (1998): 2001–2007.

24. Astrup A, Toubro S, Raben A, et al. "The role of low-fat diets and fat substitutes in body weight management: what have we learned from clinical studies?" *J. Am. Diet. Assoc.* 97(suppl) (1997): S82–S87.

25. Burkitt L. "As obesity rises, Chinese kids are almost as fat as Americans." *Wall Street Journal China Real Time Report* (2014, May 29). Accessed at http://blogs.wsj.com/chinarealtime/2014/05/29/as-obesity-rises-chinese-kids-are-almost-as-fat-as-americans/.

26. Duncan KH, Bacon JA, and Weinsier RL. "The effects of high and low energy density diets on satiety, energy intake, and eating time of obese and nonobese subjects." *Am. J. Clin. Nutr.* 37 (1983): 763–767.

27. Heaton KW. "Food fibre as an obstacle to energy intake." *Lancet* (1973): 1418–1421.

28. Levin N, Rattan J, and Gilat T. "Energy intake and body weight in ovo-lacto vegetarians." *J. Clin. Gastroenterol.* 8 (1986): 451–453.

29. Campbell TC. "Energy balance: interpretation of data from rural China." *Toxicological Sciences* 52 (1999): 87–94.

30. Poehlman ET, Arciero PJ, Melby CL, et al. "Resting metabolic rate and postprandial thermogenesis in vegetarians and nonvegetarians." *Am. J. Clin. Nutr.* 48 (1988): 209–213.

31. The study by Poehlman et al. showed high oxygen consumption and higher resting metabolic rate but was badly misinterpreted by the authors. We had very similar results with experimental rats.

32. Campbell TC. "Energy balance: interpretation of data from rural China." *Toxicological Sciences* 52 (1999): 87–94.

33. Fogelholm M, and Kukkonen-Harjula K. "Does physical activity prevent weight gain—a systematic review." *Obesity Rev.* 1 (2000): 95–111.

34. Ravussin E, Lillioja S, Anderson TE, et al. "Determinants of 24-hour energy expenditure in man. Methods and results using a respiratory chamber." *J. Clin. Invest.* 78 (1986): 1568–1578.

35. Thorburn AW, and Proietto J. "Biological determinants of spontaneous physical activity." *Obesity Rev.* 1 (2000): 87–94.

36. Krieger E, Youngman LD, and Campbell TC. "The modulation of aflatoxin (AFB1) induced preneoplastic lesions by dietary protein and voluntary exercise in Fischer 344 rats." *FASEB J.* 2 (1988): 3304 Abs.

37. Heshka S, and Allison DB. "Is obesity a disease?" *Int. J. Obesity Rel. Dis.* 25 (2001): 1401–1404.

38. Kopelman PG, and Finer N. "Reply: is obesity a disease?" *Int J. Obes.* 25 (2001): 1405–1406.

39. Campbell TC. "Are your genes hazardous to your health?" Nutrition Advocate 1 (1995): 1–2, 8.

40. Campbell TC. "Genetic seeds of disease. How to beat the odds." *Nutrition Advocate* 1 (1995): 1–2, 8.

41. Campbell TC. "The 'Fat Gene' dream machine." *Nutrition Advocate* 2 (1996): 1–2.

Chapter 7

1. Mokdad AH, Ford ES, Bowman BA, et al. "Diabetes trends in the U.S.: 1990–1998." *Diabetes Care* 23 (2000): 1278–1283.

2. American Diabetes Association. "Statistics about diabetes. Overall numbers, diabetes and prediabetes." (2016, April 1). Accessed at http://www.diabetes.org/diabetes-basics/statistics/.

3. Centers for Disease Control and Prevention. "National Diabetes Fact Sheet: General Information and National Estimates on Diabetes in the United States, 2000." Atlanta, GA: Centers for Disease Control and Prevention.

4. Griffin KL. "New lifestyles: new lifestyles, hope for kids with diabetes." *Milwaukee Journal Sentinel* July 22, 2002: 1G.

5. American Diabetes Association. "Type 2 diabetes in children and adolescents." *Diabetes Care* 23 (2000): 381–389.

6. American Diabetes Association. "The cost of diabetes." (2015, June 22). Accessed at http://www.diabetes.org/advocacy/news-events/cost-of-diabetes.html.

7. Himsworth HP. "Diet and the incidence of diabetes mellitus." *Clin. Sci.* 2 (1935): 117–148.

8. West KM, and Kalbfleisch JM. "Glucose tolerance, nutrition, and diabetes in Uruguay, Venezuela, Malaya, and East Pakistan." *Diabetes* 15 (1966): 9–18.

9. West KM, and Kalbfleisch JM. "Influence of nutritional factors on prevalence of diabetes." *Diabetes* 20 (1971): 99–108.

10. Fraser GE. "Associations between diet and cancer, ischemic heart disease, and all-cause mortality in non-Hispanic white California Seventh-day Adventists." *Am. J. Clin. Nutr.* 70 (Suppl.) (1999): 532S–538S.

11. Snowdon DA, and Phillips RL. "Does a vegetarian diet reduce the occurrence of diabetes?" *Am. J. Publ. Health* 75 (1985): 507–512.

12. Tsunehara CH, Leonetti DL, and Fujimoto WY. "Diet of second generation Japanese-American men with and without non-insulin-dependent diabetes." *Am. J. Clin. Nutri.* 52 (1990): 731–738.

13. Marshall J, Hamman RF, and Baxter J. "High-fat, low-carbohydrate diet and the etiology of non-insulin-dependent diabetes mellitus: the San Luis Valley Study." *Am. J. Epidemiol.* 134 (1991): 590–603.

14. Kittagawa T, Owada M, Urakami T, et al. "Increased incidence of non-insulin-dependent diabetes mellitus among Japanese schoolchildren correlates with an increased intake of animal protein and fat." *Clin. Pediatr.* 37 (1998): 111–116.

15. Trowell H. "Diabetes mellitus death-rates in England and Wales 1920–1970 and food supplies." *Lancet* 2 (1974): 998–1002.

16. Meyer KA, Kushi LH, Jacobs DR, Jr., et al. "Carbohydrates, dietary fiber, and incident Type 2 diabetes in older women." *Am. J. Clin. Nutri.* 71 (2000): 921–930.

17. Anderson JW. "Dietary fiber in nutrition management of diabetes." In: GV Vahouny, and D. Kritchevsky (eds.), *Dietary Fiber: Basic and Clinical Aspects*, pp. 343–360. New York: Plenum Press, 1986.

18. Anderson JW, Chen WL, and Sieling B. "Hypolipidemic effects of high-carbohydrate, high fiber diets." *Metabolism* 29 (1980): 551–558.

19. Story L, Anderson JW, Chen WL, et al. "Adherence to high-carbohydrate, high-fiber diets: long-term studies of non-obese diabetic men." *J. Am. Diet. Assoc.* 85 (1985): 1105–1110.

20. Barnard RJ, Lattimore L, Holly RG, et al. "Response of non-insulin-dependent diabetic patients to an intensive program of dict and cxcrcisc." *Diabetes Care* 5 (1982): 370–374.

21. Barnard RJ, Massey MR, Cherny S, et al. "Long-term use of a high-complex-carbohydrate, high-fiber, low-fat diet and exercise in the treatment of NIDDM patients." *Diabetes Care* 6 (1983): 268–273.

22. Anderson JW, Gustafson NJ, Bryant CA, et al. "Dietary fiber and diabetes: a comprehensive review and practical application." *J. Am. Diet. Assoc.* 87 (1987): 1189–1197.

23. Jenkins DJA, Wolever TMS, Bacon S, et al. "Diabetic diets: high carbohydrate combined with high fiber." *Am. J. Clin. Nutri.* 33 (1980): 1729–1733.

24. Barnard N, Cohen J, and Ferdowsian H. "A low-fat vegan diet and a conventional diabetes diet in the treatment of type 2 diabetes: a randomized, controlled, 74-wk clinical trial." *Am. J. Clin. Nutr.* 89 (2009): 1588S–1596S.

25. Kiehm, T. G., Anderson, J. W., and Ward, K. "Beneficial effects of a high carbohydrate, high fiber diet on hyperglycemic diabetic men." *Am. J. Clin. Nutr.* 29, 895–899 (1976).

26. Diabetes Prevention Program Research Group. "Reduction in the incidence of Type 2 diabetes with lifestyle intervention or Metformin." *New Engl. J. Med.* 346 (2002): 393–403.

27. Tuomilehto J, Lindström J, Eriksson JG, et al. "Prevention of Type 2 diabetes mellitus by changes in lifestyle among subjects with impaired glucose tolerance." *New Engl. J. Med.* 344 (2001): 1343–1350.

Chapter 8

1. Estrogen present in its free, unbound form.

2. Estrogen activity is due to more than one analogue, but usually refers to estradiol. I will use the general term "estrogen" to include all steroid and related female hormones whose effects parallel estradiol activity. A small amount of testosterone in women also shows the same effect.

3. Wu AH, Pike MC, and Stram DO. "Meta-analysis: dietary fat intake, serum estrogen levels, and the risk of breast cancer." *J. Nat. Cancer Inst.* 91 (1999): 529–534.

4. Bernstein L, and Ross RK. "Endogenous hormones and breast cancer risk." *Epidemiol. Revs.* 15 (1993): 48–65.

5. Pike MC, Spicer DV, Dahmoush L, et al. "Estrogens, progestogens, normal breast cell proliferation, and breast cancer risk." *Epidemiol. Revs.* 15 (1993): 17–35.

6. Bocchinfuso WP, Lindzey JK, Hewitt SC, et al. "Induction of mammary gland development in estrogen receptor-alpha knockout mice." *Endocrinology* 141 (2000): 2982–2994.

7. Atwood CS, Hovey RC, Glover JP, et al. "Progesterone induces side-branching of the ductal epithelium in the mammary glands of peripubertal mice." *J. Endocrinol.* 167 (2000): 39–52.

8. Rose DP, and Pruitt BT. "Plasma prolactin levels in patients with breast cancer." *Cancer* 48 (1981): 2687–2691.

9. Dorgan JF, Longcope C, Stephenson HE, Jr., et al. "Relation of prediagnostic serum estrogen and androgen levels to breast cancer risk." *Cancer Epidemiol Biomarkers Prev* 5 (1996): 533–539.

10. Dorgan JF, Stanczyk FZ, Longcope C, et al. "Relationship of serum dehydroepiandrosterone (DHEA), DHEA sulfate, and 5-androstene-3 beta, 17 beta-diol to risk of breast cancer in postmenopausal women." *Cancer Epidemiol Biomarkers Prev* 6 (1997): 177–181.

11. Thomas HV, Key TJ, Allen DS, et al. "A prospective study of endogenous serum hormone concentrations and breast cancer risk in post-menopausal women on the island of Guernsey." *Brit. J. Cancer* 76 (1997): 410–415.

12. Hankinson SE, Willett W, Manson JE, et al. "Plasma sex steroid hormone levels and risk of breast cancer in postmenopausal women." *J. Nat. Cancer Inst.* 90 (1998): 1292–1299.

13. Rosenthal MB, Barnard RJ, Rose DP, et al. "Effects of a high-complex-carbohydrate, low-fat, low-cholesterol diet on levels of serum lipids and estradiol." *Am. J. Med.* 78 (1985): 23–27.

14. Adlercreutz H. "Western diet and Western diseases: some hormonal and biochemical mechanisms and associations." *Scand. J. Clin. Lab. Invest.* 50 (Suppl. 201) (1990): 3–23.

15. Heber D, Ashley JM, Leaf DA, et al. "Reduction of serum estradiol in postmenopausal women given free access to low-fat high-carbohydrate diet." *Nutrition* 7 (1991): 137–139.

16. Rose DP, Goldman M, Connolly JM, et al. "High-fiber diet reduces serum estrogen concentrations in premenopausal women." *Am. J. Clin. Nutr.* 54 (1991): 520–525.

17. Rose DP, Lubin M, and Connolly JM. "Effects of diet supplementation with wheat bran on serum estrogen levels in the follicular and luteal phases of the menstrual cycle." *Nutrition* 13 (1997): 535–539.

18. Tymchuk CN, Tessler SB, and Barnard RJ. "Changes in sex hormone-binding globulin, insulin, and serum lipids in postmenopausal women on a low-fat, high-fiber diet combined with exercise." *Nutr. Cancer* 38 (2000): 158–162.

19. Key TJA, Chen J, Wang DY, et al. "Sex hormones in women in rural China and in Britain." *Brit. J. Cancer* 62 (1990): 631–636.

20. Prentice R, Thompson D, Clifford C, et al. "Dietary fat reduction and plasma estradiol concentration in healthy postmenopausal women." *J. Natl. Cancer Inst.* 82 (1990): 129–134.

21. Boyar AP, Rose DP, and Wynder EL. "Recommendations for the prevention of chronic disease: the application for breast disease." *Am. J. Clin. Nutr.* 48 (3 Suppl) (1988): 896–900.

22. Nandi S, Guzman RC, and Yang J. "Hormones and mammary carcinogenesis in mice, rats and humans: a unifying hypothesis." *Proc. National Acad. Sci.* 92 (1995): 3650–3657.

23. Peto J, Easton DF, Matthews FE, et al. "Cancer mortality in relatives of women with breast cancer, the OPCS study." *Int. J. Cancer* 65 (1996): 275–283.

24. Colditz GA, Willett W, Hunter DJ, et al. "Family history, age, and risk of breast cancer. Prospective data from the Nurses' Health Study." *JAMA* 270 (1993): 338–343.

25. National Human Genome Research Institute. "Learning About Breast Cancer." Accessed at http://www.genome.gov/10000507#ql.

26. Futreal PA, Liu Q, Shattuck-Eidens D, et al. "BRCA1 mutations in primary breast and ovarian carcinomas." *Science* 266 (1994): 120–122.

27. Miki Y, Swensen J, Shatttuck-Eidens D, et al. "A strong candidate for the breast and ovarian cancer susceptibility gene BRCA1." *Science* 266 (1994): 66–71.

28. Wooster R, Bignell G, Lancaster J, et al. "Identification of the breast cancer susceptibility gene BRCA2." *Nature* 378 (1995): 789–792.

29. Tavtigian SV, Simard J, Rommens J, et al. "The complete BRCA2 gene and mutations in chromosome 13q-linked kindreds." *Nat. Genet.* 12 (1996): 333–337.

30. Ford D, Easton D, Bishop DT, et al. "Risks of cancer in BRCA1 mutation carriers." *Lancet* 343 (1994): 692–695.

31. Antoniou A, Pharoah PDP, Narod S, et al. "Average risks of breast and ovarian cancer associated with BRCA1 or BRCA2 mutations detected in case series unselected for family history: a combined analysis of 22 studies." *Am. J. Hum. Genet.* 72 (2003): 1117–1130.

32. Newman B, Mu H, Butler LM, et al. "Frequency of breast cancer attributable to BRCA1 in a population-based series of American women." *JAMA* 279 (1998): 915–921.

33. Peto J, Collins N, Barfoot R, et al. "Prevalence of BRCA1 and BRCA2 gene mutations in patients with early-onset breast cancer." *J. Nat. Cancer Inst.* 91 (1999): 943–949.

34. Tabar L, Fagerberg G, Chen HH, et al. "Efficacy of breast cancer screening by age. New results from the Swedish Two-County Trial." *Cancer* 75 (1995): 2507–2517.

35. Bjurstram N, Bjorneld L, Duffy SW, et al. "The Gothenburg Breast Cancer Screening Trial: first results on mortality, incidence, and mode of detection for women ages 39–49 years at randomization." *Cancer* 80 (1997): 2091–2099.

36. Frisell J, Lidbrink E, Hellström L, and Rutqvist LE. "Follow-up after 11 years: update of mortality results in the Stockholm mammographic screening trial." *Breast Cancer Res. Treat* 45 (1997): 263–270.

37. Greenlee RT, Hill-Harmon MB, Murray T, et al. "Cancer statistics, 2001." *CA Cancer J. Clin.* 51 (2001): 15–36.

38. Cairns J. "The treatment of diseases and the war against cancer." *Sci. Am.* 253 (1985): 31–39.

39. Cuzick J, and Baum M. "Tamoxifen and contralateral breast cancer." *Lancet* 2 (1985): 282.

40. Cuzick J, Wang DY, and Bulbrook RD. "The prevention of breast cancer." *Lancet* 1 (1986): 83–86.

41. Fisher B, Costantino JP, Wickerham DL, et al. "Tamoxifen for prevention of breast cancer: report of the National Surgical Adjuvant Breast and Bowel Project P-1 Study." *J. Nat. Cancer Inst.* 90 (1998): 1371–1388.

42. Freedman AN, Graubard BI, Rao SR, et al. "Estimates of the number of U.S. women who could benefit from tamoxifen for breast cancer chemoprevention." *J. Nat. Cancer Inst.* 95 (2003): 526–532.

43. Powles T, Eeles R, Ashley S, et al. "Interim analysis of the incidence of breast cancer in the Royal Marsden Hospital tamoxifen randomised chemoprevention trial." *Lancet* 352 (1998): 98–101.

44. Veronesi U, Maisonneuve P, Costa A, et al. "Prevention of breast cancer with tamoxifen: preliminary findings from the Italian randomised trial among hysterectomised women." *Lancet* 352 (1998): 93–97.

45. Cuzick J. "A brief review of the current breast cancer prevention trials and proposals for future trials." *Eur. J. Cancer* 36 (2000): 1298–1302.

46. Cummings SR, Eckert S, Krueger KA, et al. "The effect of raloxifene on risk of breast cancer in postmenopausal women: results from the MORE randomized trial." *JAMA* 281 (1999): 2189–2197.

47. Dorgan JF, Hunsberger S, A., McMahon RP, et al. "Diet and sex hormones in girls: findings from a randomized controlled clinical trial." *J. Nat. Cancer Inst.* 95 (2003): 132–141.

48. Ornish D, Scherwitz LW, Billings JH, et al. "Intensive lifestyle changes for reversal of coronary heart disease." *JAMA* 280 (1998): 2001–2007.

49. Esselstyn CB, Ellis SG, Medendorp SV, et al. "A strategy to arrest and reverse coronary artery disease: a 5-year longitudinal study of a single physician's practice." *J. Family Practice* 41 (1995): 560–568.

50. Ornish D, Weidner G, Fair WR, et al. "Intensive lifestyle changes may affect the progression of prostate cancer." *J. Urol.* 174 (2005): 1065–1069; discussion 1069–1070.

51. Hildenbrand GLG, Hildenbrand LC, Bradford K, et al. "Five-year survival rates of melanoma patients treated by diet therapy after the manner of Gerson: a retrospective review." *Alternative Therapies in Health and Medicine* 1 (1995): 29–37.

52. Youngman LD, and Campbell TC. "Inhibition of aflatoxin B_1-induced gamma-glutamyl transpeptidase positive (GGT+) hepatic preneoplastic foci and tumors by low protein diets: evidence that altered GGT+ foci indicate neoplastic potential." *Carcinogenesis* 13 (1992): 1607–1613.

53. Ronai Z, Gradia S, El-Bayoumy K, et al. "Contrasting incidence of ras mutations in rat mammary and mouse skin tumors induced by anti-benzo[c]phenanthrene-3,4-diol-1,2-epoxide." *Carcinogenesis* 15 (1994): 2113–2116.

54. Jeffy BD, Schultz EU, Selmin O, et al. "Inhibition of BRCA-1 expression by benzo[a]pyrene and diol epoxide." *Mol. Carcinogenesis* 26 (1999): 100–118.

55. Gammon MD, Santella RM, Neugut AI, et al. "Environmental toxins and breast cancer on Long Island. I. Polycyclic aromatic hydrocarbon DNA adducts." *Cancer Epidemiol. Biomarkers Prev.* 11 (2002): 677–685.

56. Gammon MD, Wolff MS, Neugut AI, et al. "Environmental toxins and breast cancer on Long Island. II. Organochlorine compound levels in blood." *Cancer Epidemiol. Biomarkers Prev.* 11 (2002): 686–697.

57. Gray J, Evans N, Taylor B, Rizzo J, and Walker M. "State of the evidence: the connection between breast cancer and the environment." *Int. J. Occup. Environ. Health* 15 (2009): 43–78; Brophy JT, et al. "Breast cancer risk in relation to occupations with exposure to carcinogens and endocrine disruptors: a Canadian case-control study." *Environ. Health* 11 (2012): 1–17.

58. Brophy JT, et al. "Breast cancer risk in relation to occupations with exposure to carcinogens and endocrine disruptors: a Canadian case-control study." *Environ. Health* 11 (2012): 1–17.

59. Gray J, Evans N, Taylor B, Rizzo J, and Walker M. "State of the evidence: the connection between breast cancer and the environment." *Int. J. Occup. Environ. Health* (2009): 15, 43–78.

60. Michels KB, Mohllajee AP, Roset-Bahmanyar E, Beehler GP, and Moysich KB. "Diet and breast cancer. A review of the prospective observational studies." *Cancer* 109 (2007): 2712–2749.

61. Campbell TC, and Hayes JR. "Role of nutrition in the drug metabolizing system." *Pharmacol. Revs.* 26 (1974): 171–197; Campbell TC, and Hayes JR. "The effect of quantity and quality of dietary protein on drug metabolism." *Fed. Proc.* 35 (1976): 2470–2474.

62. Weatherholz WM, Campbell TC, and Webb RE. "Effect of dietary protein levels on the toxicity and metabolism of heptaclor." *J. Nutr.* 98 (1969): 90–94.

63. Mgbodile MUK, Hayes JR, and Campbell TC. "Effect of protein deficiency on the inducibility of the hepatic microsomal drug-metabolizing enzyme system. II. Effect on enzyme kinetics and electron transport system." *Biochem. Pharmacol.* 22 (1973): 1125–1132; Hayes JR, and Campbell TC. "Effect of protein deficiency on the inducibility of the hepatic microsomal drug-metabolizing enzyme system. III. Effect of 3-methylcholanthrene induction on activity and binding kinetics." *Biochem. Pharmacol.* 23 (1974): 1721–1732.

64. Huang HH, Hawrylewicz EJ, Kissane JQ, and Drab EA. "Effect of protein diet on release of prolactin and ovarian steroids in female rats." *Nutr. Rpts. Int.* 26 (1982): 807–820.

65. Rose DP, Goldman M, Connolly JM, and Strong LE. "High-fiber diet reduces serum estrogen concentrations in premenopausal women." *Am. J. Clin. Nutr.* 54 (1991): 520–525.

66. Rose DP, Boyar AP, Cohen L, and Strong, LE. "Effect of a low-fat diet on hormone levels in women with cystic breast disease. I. Serum steroids and gonadotropins." *J. Natl. Cancer Inst.* 78 (1987): 623–626.

67. Humphries KH, and Gill S. "Risks and benefits of hormone replacement therapy: the evidence speaks." *Canadian Med. Assoc. J.* 168 (2003): 1001–1010.

68. Writing Group for the Women's Health Initiative Investigators. "Risks and benefits of estrogen plus progestin in healthy postmenopausal women: principal results from the Women's Health Initiative Randomized Controlled Trial." *JAMA* 288 (2002): 321–333.

69. Hulley S, Grady D, Bush T, et al. "Randomized trial of estrogen plus progestin for secondary prevention of coronary heart disease in postmenopausal women. Heart and Estrogen/progestin Replacement Study (HERS) Research Group." *JAMA* 280 (1998): 605–613.

70. While this finding is not statistically significant, its consistency with the WHI finding is striking.

71. Ravdin PM, et al. "The decrease in breast-cancer incidence in 2003 in the United States." *New Engl. J. Med.* 356 (2007): 1670–1674.

72. International Agency for Cancer Research. "Globocan." Accessed 18 October 2002 at http://www-dep.iarc/globocan.html.

73. Kinzler KW, and Vogelstein B. "Lessons from Heredity. Colorectal Cancer." *Cell* 87 (1996): 159–170.

74. Ferlay J, Bray F, Pisani P, et al. GLOBOCAN 2000: *Cancer Incidence, Mortality and Prevalence Worldwide, Version 1.0.* Lyon, France: IARCPress, 2001.

75. Limited version of Ferlay et al. document available at http://www-dep.iarc/globocan.html.

76. Expert Panel. *Food, Nutrition and the Prevention of Cancer, a Global Perspective.* Washington, DC: American Institute for Cancer Research/World Cancer Research Fund, 1997.

77. Armstrong D, and Doll R. "Environmental factors and cancer incidence and mortality in different countries, with special reference to dietary practices." *Int. J. Cancer* 15 (1975): 617–631.

78. Burkitt DP. "Epidemiology of cancer of the colon and the rectum." *Cancer* 28 (1971): 3–13.

79. Jansen MCJF, Bueno-de-Mesquita HB, Buzina R, et al. "Dietary fiber and plant foods in relation to colorectal cancer mortality: The Seven Countries Study." *Int. J. Cancer* 81 (1999): 174–179.

80. Whiteley LO, and Klurfeld DM. "Are dietary fiber-induced alterations in colonic epithelial cell proliferation predictive of fiber's effect on colon cancer?" *Nutr. Cancer* 36 (2000): 131–149.

81. Most of these associations were not statistically significant, but the consistency of the inverse association between fiber and colorectal cancer was impressive.

82. Campbell TC, Wang G, Chen J, et al. "Dietary fiber intake and colon cancer mortality in The People's Republic of China." In: D. Kritchevsky, C. Bonfield, and J. W. Anderson (eds.), *Dietary Fiber*, pp. 473–480. New York: Plenum Publishing Corporation, 1990.

83. Trock B, Lanza E, and Greenwald P. "Dietary fiber, vegetables, and colon cancer: critical review and meta-analysis of the epidemiologic evidence." *J. Nat. Cancer Inst.* 82 (1990): 650–661.

84. Howe GR, Benito E, Castelleto R, et al. "Dietary intake of fiber and decreased risk of cancers of the colon and rectum: evidence from the combined analysis of 13 case-control studies." *J. Nat. Cancer Inst.* 84 (1992): 1887–1896.

85. Bingham SA, Day NE, Luben R, et al. "Dietary fibre in food and protection against colorectal cancer in the European Prospective Investigation into Cancer and Nutrition (EPIC): an observational study." *Lancet* 361 (2003): 1496–1501.

86. O'Keefe SJD, Ndaba N, and Woodward A. "Relationship between nutritional status, dietary intake patterns and plasma lipoprotein concentrations in rural black South Africans." *Hum. Nutr. Clin. Nutr.* 39 (1985): 335–341.

87. Sitas F. "Histologically diagnosed cancers in South Africa, 1988." *S. African Med. J.* 84 (1994): 344–348.

88. O'Keefe SJD, Kidd M, Espitalier-Noel G, et al. "Rarity of colon cancer in Africans is associated with low animal product consumption, not fiber." *Am. J. Gastroenterology* 94 (1999): 1373–1380.

89. McKeown-Eyssen G. "Epidemiology of colorectal cancer revisited: are serum triglycerides and/or plasma glucose associated with risk?" *Cancer Epidemiol Biomarkers Prev* 3 (1994): 687–695.

90. Giovannucci E. "Insulin and colon cancer." *Cancer Causes and Control* 6 (1995): 164–179.

91. Bruce WR, Giacca A, and Medline A. "Possible mechanisms relating diet and risk of colon cancer." *Cancer Epidemiol. Biomarkers Prev.* 9 (2000): 1271–1279.

92. Kono S, Honjo S, Todoroki I, et al. "Glucose intolerance and adenomas of the sigmoid colon in Japanese men (Japan)." *Cancer Causes and Control* 9 (1998): 441–446.

93. Schoen RE, Tangen CM, Kuller LH, et al. "Increased blood glucose and insulin, body size, and incident colorectal cancer." *J. Nat. Cancer Inst.* 91 (1999): 1147–1154.

94. Bruce WR, Wolever TMS, and Giacca A. "Mechanisms linking diet and colorectal cancer: the possible role of insulin resistance." *Nutr. Cancer* 37 (2000): 19–26.

95. Lipkin M, and Newmark H. "Development of clinical chemoprevention trials." *J. Nat. Cancer Inst.* 87 (1995): 1275–1277.

96. Holt PR, Atillasoy EO, Gilman J, et al. "Modulation of abnormal colonic epithelial cell proliferation and differentiation by low-fat dairy foods. A randomized trial." *JAMA* 280 (1998): 1074–1079.

97. Mobarhan S. "Calcium and the colon: recent findings." *Nutr. Revs.* 57 (1999): 124–126.

98. Alberts DS, Ritenbuagh C, Story JA, et al. "Randomized, double-blinded, placebo-controlled study of effect of wheat bran fiber and calcium on fecal bile acids in patients with resected adenomatous colon polyps." *J. Nat. Cancer Inst.* 88 (1996): 81–92.

99. Chen J, Campbell TC, Li J, et al. *Diet, Life-style and Mortality in China. A Study of the Characteristics of 65 Chinese Counties.* Oxford, UK; Ithaca, NY; Beijing, PRC: Oxford University Press; Cornell University Press; People's Medical Publishing House, 1990.

100. Jass JR. "Colon cancer: the shape of things to come." *Gut* 45 (1999): 794–795.

101. Burt RW. "Colon cancer screening." *Gastroenterology* 119 (2000): 837–853.

102. Winawer SJ, Zauber AG, Ho MN, et al. "Prevention of colorectal cancer by colonoscopic polypectomy." *New Engl. J. Med.* 329 (1993): 1977–1981.

103. Pignone M, Rich M, Teutsch SM, et al. "Screening for colorectal cancer in adults at average risk: a summary of the evidence for the U.S. Preventive Services Task Force." *Ann. Internal Med.* 137 (2002): 132–141.

104. Scott RJ, and Sobol HH. "Prognostic implications of cancer susceptibility genes: Any news?" *Recent Results in Cancer Research* 151 (1999): 71–84.

105. Lee ML, Wang R-T, Hsing AW, et al. "Case-control study of diet and prostate cancer in China." *Cancer Causes and Control* 9 (1998): 545–552.

106. Villers A, Soulie M, Haillot O, et al. "Prostate cancer screening (III): risk factors, natural history, course without treatment." *Progr. Urol.* 7 (1997): 655–661.

107. Stanford JL. "Prostate cancer trends 1973–1995." Bethesda, MD: SEER Program, National Cancer Institute, 1998.

108. Chan JM, and Giovannucci EL. "Dairy products, calcium, and vitamin D and risk of prostate cancer." *Epidemiol. Revs.* 23 (2001): 87–92.

109. Giovannucci E. "Dietary influences of 1,25 (OH)2 vitamin D in relation to prostate cancer: a hypothesis." *Cancer Causes and Control* 9 (1998): 567–582.

110. Chan JM, Stampfer MJ, Ma J, et al. "Insulin-like growth factor-I (IGF-I) and IGF binding protein-3 as predictors of advanced-stage prostate cancer." *J Natl Cancer Inst* 94 (2002): 1099–1109.

111. Doi SQ, Rasaiah S, Tack I, et al. "Low-protein diet suppresses serum insulin-like growth factor-1 and decelerates the progression of growth hormone-induced glomerulosclerosis." *Am. J. Nephrol.* 21 (2001): 331–339.

112. Heaney RP, McCarron DA, Dawson-Hughes B, et al. "Dietary changes favorably affect bond remodeling in older adults." *J. Am. Diet. Assoc.* 99 (1999): 1228–1233.

113. Allen NE, Appleby PN, Davey GK, et al. "Hormones and diet: low insulin-like growth factor-I but normal bioavailable androgens in vegan men." *Brit. J. Cancer* 83 (2000): 95–97.

114. Cohen P, Peehl DM, and Rosenfeld RG. "The IGF axis in the prostate." *Horm. Metab. res.* 26 (1994): 81–84.

115. Ornish D, Weidner G, Fair WR, et al. "Intensive lifestyle changes may affect the progression of prostate cancer. *J. Urol.* 174 (2005): 1065–1069; discussion 1069–1070.

116. Ornish D, Magbanua MJ, Weidner G, et al. "Changes in prostate gene expression in men undergoing an intensive nutrition and lifestyle intervention." *Proc. Natl. Acad. Sci. USA.* 105 (2008): 8369–8374.

117. Frattaroli J, Weidner G, Dnistrian AM, et al. "Clinical events in prostate cancer lifestyle trial: results from two years of follow-up." *Urol.* 72 (2008): 1319–1323.

118. Yang M, Kenfield SA, Van Blarigan EL, et al. "Dietary patterns after prostate cancer diagnosis in relation to disease-specific and total mortality." *Cancer Prev. Res.* 8 (2015): 545–551.

119. Yang M, Kenfield SA, Van Blarigan EL, et al. "Dairy intake after prostate cancer diagnosis in relation to disease-specific and total mortality." *Int. J. Cancer* 137 (2015): 2462–2469.

Chapter 9

1. Mackay IR. "Tolerance and immunity." *Brit. Med. J.* 321 (2000): 93–96.

2. Jacobson DL, Gange SJ, Rose NR, et al. "Short analytical review. Epidemiology and estimated population burden of selected autoimmune diseases in the United States." *Clin. Immunol. Immunopath.* 84 (1997): 223–243.

3. Cooper GS, Bynum ML, Somers EC. "Recent insights in the epidemiology of autoimmune diseases: improved prevalence estimates and understanding of clustering of diseases." *J. Autoimmun.* 33 (2009): 197–207.

4. Davidson A, and Diamond B. "Autoimmune diseases." *New Engl. J. Med.* 345 (2001): 340– 350.

5. Aranda R, Sydora BC, McAllister PL, et al. "Analysis of intestinal lymphocytes in mouse colitis mediated by transfer of CD4+, CD45RBhigh T cells to SCID recipients." *J. Immunol.* 158 (1997): 3464–3473.

6. Folgar S, Gatto EM, Raina G, et al. "Parkinsonism as a manifestation of multiple sclerosis." *Movement Disorders* 18 (2003): 108–113.

7. Cantorna MT. "Vitamin D and autoimmunity: is vitamin D status an environmental factor affecting autoimmune disease prevalence?" *Proc. Soc. Exp. Biol. Med.* 223 (2000): 230–233.

8. DeLuca HF, and Cantorna MT. "Vitamin D: its role and uses in immunology." *FASEB J.* 15 (2001): 2579–2585.

9. Winer S, Astsaturov I, Cheung RK, et al. "T cells of multiple sclerosis patients target a common environmental peptide that causes encephalitis in mice." *J. Immunol.* 166 (2001): 4751–4756.

10. Davenport CB. "Multiple sclerosis from the standpoint of geographic distribution and race." *Arch. Neurol. Psychiatry* 8 (1922): 51–58.

11. Alter M, Yamoor M, and Harshe M. "Multiple sclerosis and nutrition." *Arch. Neurol.* 31 (1974): 267–272.

12. Carroll M. "Innate immunity in the etiopathology of autoimmunity." *Nature Immunol.* 2 (2001): 1089–1090.

13. Karjalainen J, Martin JM, Knip M, et al. "A bovine albumin peptide as a possible trigger of insulin-dependent Diabetes Mellitus." *New Engl. J. Med.* 327 (1992): 302–307.

14. Akerblom HK, and Knip M. "Putative environmental factors and Type 1 diabetes." *Diabetes/Metabolism Revs.* 14 (1998): 31–67.

15. Naik RG, and Palmer JP. "Preservation of beta-cell function in Type 1 diabetes." *Diabetes Rev.* 7 (1999): 154–182.

16. Virtanen SM, Rasanen L, Aro A, et al. "Infant feeding in Finnish children less than 7 yr of age with newly diagnosed IDDM. Childhood diabetes in Finland Study Group." *Diabetes Care* 14 (1991): 415–417.

17. Savilahti E, Akerblom HK, Tainio V-M, et al. "Children with newly diagnosed insulin dependent diabetes mellitus have increased levels of cow's milk antibodies." *Diabetes Res.* 7 (1988): 137–140.

18. Yakota A, Yamaguchi T, Ueda T, et al. "Comparison of islet cell antibodies, islet cell surface antibodies and anti-bovine serum albumin antibodies in Type 1 diabetes." *Diabetes Res. Clin. Pract.* 9 (1990): 211–217.

19. Hammond-McKibben D, and Dosch H-M. "Cow's milk, bovine serum albumin, and IDDM: can we settle the controversies?" *Diabetes Care* 20 (1997): 897–901.

20. Akerblom HK, Vaarala O, Hyoty H, et al. "Environmental factors in the etiology of Type 1 diabetes." *Am. J. Med. Genet. (Semin. Med. Genet.)* 115 (2002): 18–29.

21. Gottlieb MS, and Root HF. "Diabetes mellitus in twins." *Diabetes* 17 (1968): 693–704.

22. Barnett AH, Eff C, Leslie RDG, et al. "Diabetes in identical twins: a study of 200 pairs." *Diabetologia* 20 (1981): 87–93.

23. Borch-Johnsen K, Joner G, Mandrup-Poulsen T, et al. "Relation between breast feeding and incidence rates of insulin-dependent diabetes mellitus: a hypothesis." *Lancet* 2 (1984): 1083–1086.

24. Perez-Bravo F, Carrasco E, Gutierrez-Lopez MD, et al. "Genetic predisposition and environmental factors leading to the development of insulin-dependent diabetes mellitus in Chilean children." *J. Mol. Med.* 74 (1996): 105–109.

25. Kostraba JN, Cruickshanks KJ, Lawler-Heavner J, et al. "Early exposure to cow's milk and solid foods in infancy, genetic predisposition, and risk of IDDM." *Diabetes* 42 (1993): 288–295.

26. Pyke DA. "The genetic perspective: putting research into practice." In: *Diabetes* 1988, Amsterdam, 1989, pp. 1227–1230.

27. Kaprio J, Tuomilehto J, Koskenvuo M, et al. "Concordance for Type 1 (insulin-dependent) and Type 2 (non-insulin-dependent) diabetes mellitus in a population-based cohort of twins in Finland." *Diabetologia* 35 (1992): 1060–1067.

28. Dahl-Jorgensen K, Joner G, and Hanssen KF. "Relationship between cow's milk consumption and incidence of IDDM in childhood." *Diabetes Care* 14 (1991): 1081–1083.

29. The proportion of Type 1 diabetes due to the consumption of cow's milk, the r^2 value, is 96%.

30. LaPorte RE, Tajima N, Akerblom HK, et al. "Geographic differences in the risk of insulin-dependent diabetes mellitus: the importance of registries." *Diabetes Care* 8(Suppl. 1) (1985): 101–107.

31. Bodansky HJ, Staines A, Stephenson C, et al. "Evidence for an environmental effect in the aetiology of insulin dependent diabetes in a transmigratory population." *Brit. Med. J.* 304 (1992): 1020–1022.

32. Burden AC, Samanta A, and Chaunduri KH. "The prevalence and incidence of insulin-dependent diabetes in white and Indian children in Leicester city (UK)." *Int. J. Diabetes Dev. Countries* 10 (1990): 8–10.

33. Elliott R, and Ong TJ. "Nutritional genomics." *Brit. Med. J.* 324 (2002): 1438–1442.

34. Onkamo P, Vaananen S, Karvonen M, et al. "Worldwide increase in incidence of Type 1 diabetes—the analysis of the data on published incidence trends." *Diabetologia* 42 (1999): 1395–1403.

35. Gerstein HC. "Cow's milk exposure and Type 1 diabetes mellitus: a critical overview of the clinical literature." *Diabetes Care* 17 (1994): 13–19.

36. Kimpimaki T, Erkkola M, Korhonen S, et al. "Short-term exclusive breastfeeding predisposes young children with increased genetic risk of Type 1 diabetes to progressive beta-cell autoimmunity." *Diabetologia* 44 (2001): 63–69.

37. Virtanen SM, Laara E, Hypponen E, et al. "Cow's milk consumption, HLA-DQB1 genotype, and Type 1 diabetes." *Diabetes* 49 (2000): 912–917.

38. Monetini L, Cavallo MG, Stefanini L, et al. "Bovine beta-casein antibodies in breast- and bottle-fed infants: their relevance in Type 1 diabetes." *Diabetes Metab. Res. Rev.* 17 (2001): 51–54.

39. Visser JTJ et al. "Potential mechanisms explaining why hydrolyzed casein-based diets outclass single amino acid-based diets in the prevention of autoimmune diabetes in diabetes-prone BB rats." *Diabetes Metab. Res. Rev.* 28 (2012): 505–513.

40. Stankov K, Benc D, and Draskovic D. "Genetic and epigenetic factors in etiology of diabetes mellitus type 1." *Pediatr.* 132 (2013): 1112–1122.

41. The EURODIAB Substudy 2 Study Group. "Vitamin D supplement in early childhood and risk of type I (insulin-dependent) diabetes mellitus." *Diabetiolgia* 42 (1999): 51–54; Hypponen E, Laara E, Jarvelin MR, and Virtanen SM. "Intake of vitamin D and risk of type I diabetes." *Lancet* 358 (2001): 1500–1504.

42. Knip M, Virtanen SM, and Akerblom HK. "Infant feeding and the risk of type 1 diabetes." *Am. J. Clin. Nutr.* 91 (2010): 1506S–1513S; Kondrashova A., et al. "A sixfold gradient in the incidence of type 1 diabetes at the eastern border of Finland." *Ann. Med.* 37 (2005): 67–72.

43. Norris JM, and Pietropaolo M. "Review article. Controversial topics series: milk proteins and diabetes." *J. Endocrinol. Invest.* 22 (1999): 568–580.

44. Borchers AT, Uibo R, and Gershwin ME. "The geoepidemiology of type 1 diabetes." *Autoimmun. Rev.* 9 (2010): A355–A365; Stankov K, Benc D, and Draskovic D. "Genetic and epigenetic factors in etiology of diabetes mellitus type 1." *Pediatr.* 132 (2013): 1112–1122.

45. Carroll KK. "Dietary proteins and amino acids—their effects on cholesterol metabolism." In: MJ Gibney, and D. Kritchevsky (eds.), *Current Topics in Nutrition and Disease, Volume 8: Animal and Vegetable Proteins in Lipid Metabolism and Atherosclerosis*, pp. 9–17. New York: Alan R. Liss, 1983; Terpstra AHM, Hermus RJJ, and West CE. "Dietary protein and cholesterol metabolism in rabbits and rats." In: MJ Gibney & D Kritchevsky (eds.), *Current Topics in Nutrition and Disease, Volume 8: Animal and Vegetable Proteins in Lipid Metabolism and Atherosclerosis,* pp. 19–49. New York: Alan R. Liss, 1983.

46. Newburgh LH, and Clarkson S. "The production of arteriosclerosis in rabbits by feeding diets rich in meat." *Arch. Intern. Med.* 31 (1932): 653–676; Meeker DR, and Kesten HD. "Experimental atherosclerosis and high protein diets." *Proc. Soc. Exp. Biol. Med.* 45 (1940): 543–545; Meeker DR, and Kesten HD. "Effect of high protein diets on experimental atherosclerosis of rabbits." *Arch. Pathol.* 31 (1941): 147–162.

47. Appleton BS, and Campbell TC. "Effect of high and low dietary protein on the dosing and postdosing periods of aflatoxin B1-induced hepatic preneoplastic lesion development in the rat." *Cancer Res.* 43 (1983): 2150–2154; Appleton BS, and Campbell TC. "Dietary protein intervention during the post-dosing phase of aflatoxin B1-induced hepatic preneoplastic lesion development." *J. Natl. Cancer Inst.* 70 (1983): 547–549.

48. Reingold SC. "Research Directions in Multiple Sclerosis." National Multiple Sclerosis Society, November 25, 2003. Accessed at http://www.nationalmssociety.org/%5CBrochures-Research.asp.

49. Ackermann A. "Die multiple sklerose in der Schweiz." *Schweiz. Med. Wchnschr.* 61 (1931): 1245–1250.

50. Swank RL. "Multiple sclerosis: correlation of its incidence with dietary fat." *Am. J. Med. Sci.* 220 (1950): 421–430.

51. Dip JB. "The distribution of multiple sclerosis in relation to the dairy industry and milk consumption." *New Zealand Med. J.* 83 (1976): 427–430.

52. McDougall JM. 2002. Multiple sclerosis stopped by McDougall/Swank Program. http://www.nealhendrickson.com/McDougall/McDnewannouncementSwank021112.htm. Accessed Nov. 16, 2002.

53. McLeod JG, Hammond SR, and Hallpike JF. "Epidemiology of multiple sclerosis in Australia. With NSW and SA survey results." *Med. J. Austr.* 160 (1994): 117–122.

54. Lawrence JS, Behrend T, Bennett PH, et al. "Geographical studies of rheumatoid arthritis." *Ann. Rheum. Dis.* 25 (1966): 425–432.

55. Keen H, and Ekoe JM. "The geography of diabetes mellitus." *Brit. Med. J.* 40 (1984): 359–365.

56. Swank RL. "Effect of low saturated fat diet in early and late cases of multiple sclerosis." *Lancet* 336 (1990): 37–39.

57. Swank RL. "Treatment of multiple sclerosis with low fat diet." *A.M.A. Arch. Neurol. Psychiatry* 69 (1953): 91–103.

58. Swank RL, and Bourdillon RB. "Multiple sclerosis: assessment of treatment with modified low fat diet." *J. Nerv. Ment. Dis.* 131 (1960): 468–488.

59. Swank RL. "Multiple sclerosis: twenty years on low fat diet." *Arch. Neurol.* 23 (1970): 460–474.

60. Agranoff BW, and Goldberg D. "Diet and the geographical distribution of multiple sclerosis." *Lancet* 2(7888) (November 2 1974): 1061–1066.

61. Malosse D, Perron H, Sasco A, et al. "Correlation between milk and dairy product consumption and multiple sclerosis prevalence: a worldwide study." *Neuroepidemiology* 11 (1992): 304–312.

62. Malosse D, and Perron H. "Correlation analysis between bovine populations, other farm animals, house pets, and multiple sclerosis prevalence." *Neuroepidemiology* 12 (1993): 15–27.

63. Lauer K. "Diet and multiple sclerosis." *Neurology* 49 (Suppl. 2) (1997): S55–S61.

64. Swank RL, Lerstad O, Strom A, et al. "Multiple sclerosis in rural Norway. Its geographic distribution and occupational incidence in relation to nutrition." *New Engl. J. Med.* 246 (1952): 721–728.

65. Dalgleish AG. "Viruses and multiple sclerosis." *Acta Neurol. Scand. Suppl.* 169 (1997): 8–15.

66. McAlpine D, Lumsden CE, and Acheson ED. *Multiple sclerosis: a reappraisal.* Edinburgh and London: E&S Livingston, 1965.

67. Alter M, Liebowitz U, and Speer J. "Risk of multiple sclerosis related to age at immigration to Israel." *Arch. Neurol.* 15 (1966): 234–237.

68. Kurtzke JF, Beebe GW, and Norman JE, Jr. "Epidemiology of multiple sclerosis in U.S. veterans: 1. Race, sex, and geographic distribution." *Neurology* 29 (1979): 1228–1235.

69. Ebers GC, Bulman DE, Sadovnick AD, et al. "A population-based study of multiple sclerosis in twins." *New Engl. J. Med.* 315 (1986): 1638–1642.

70. Yadav V, Marracci G, Kim E, et al. "Effects of a low fat plant based diet in multiple sclerosis (MS): Results of a 1-year long randomized controlled (RC) study." *Neurol.* 82 (2014): supp. P6.152.

71. Acheson ED, Bachrach CA, and Wright FM. "Some comments on the relationship of the distribution of multiple sclerosis to latitude solar radiation and other variables." *Acta Psychiatrica Neurologica Scand.* 35 (Suppl. 147) (1960): 132–147.

72. Warren S, and Warren KG. "Multiple sclerosis and associated diseases: a relationship to diabetes mellitus." *J. Canadian Sci. Neurol.* 8 (1981): 35–39.

73. Wertman E, Zilber N, and Abransky O. "An association between multiple sclerosis and Type 1 diabetes mellitus." *J. Neurol.* 239 (1992): 43–45.

74. Marrosu MG, Cocco E, Lai M, et al. "Patients with multiple sclerosis and risk of Type 1 diabetes mellitus in Sardinia, Italy: a cohort study." *Lancet* 359 (2002): 1461–1465.

75. Buzzetti R, Pozzilli P, Di Mario U, et al. "Multiple sclerosis and Type 1 diabetes." *Diabetologia* 45 (2002): 1735–1736.

76. Lux WE, and Kurtzke JF. "Is Parkinson's disease acquired? Evidence from a geographic comparison with multiple sclerosis." *Neurology* 37 (1987): 467–471.

77. Prahalad S, Shear ES, Thompson SD, et al. "Increased prevalence of familial autoimmunity in simplex and multiplex families with juvenile rheumatoid arthritis." *Arthritis Rheumatism* 46 (2002): 1851–1856.

78. Cantorna MT, Munsick C, Bemiss C, et al. "1,25-dihydroxycholecalciferol prevents and ameliorates symptoms of experimental murine inflammatory bowel disease." *J. Nutr.* 130 (2000): 2648–2652.

79. Cantorna MT, Woodward WD, Hayes CE, et al. "1,25-Dihydroxyvitamin D_3 is a positive regulator for the two anti-encephalitogenic cytokines TGF-B1 and IL-4." *J Immunol.* 160 (1998): 5314–5319.

80. Cantorna MT, Humpal-Winter J, and DeLuca HF. "Dietary calcium is a major factor in 1,25-dihydroxycholecalciferol suppression of experimental autoimmune encephalomyelitis in mice." *J. Nutr.* 129 (1999): 1966–1971.

81. Multiple Sclerosis International Federation. "Alternative Therapies." November 25, 2003. Accessed at http://www.msif.org/en/symptoms_treatments/treatment_overview/alternative.html.

Chapter 10

1. Frassetto LA, Todd KM, Morris C, Jr., et al. "Worldwide incidence of hip fracture in elderly women: relation to consumption of animal and vegetable foods." *J. Gerontology* 55 (2000): M585–M592.

2. Abelow BJ, Holford TR, and Insogna KL. "Cross-cultural association between dietary animal protein and hip fracture: a hypothesis." *Calcif. Tissue Int.* 50 (1992): 14–18.

3. Wachsman A, and Bernstein DS. "Diet and osteoporosis." *Lancet* May 4 (1968): 958–959.

4. Barzel U.S. "Acid loading and osteoporosis." *J. Am. Geriatr. Soc.* 30 (1982): 613.

5. Sherman HC. "Calcium requirement for maintenance in man." *J. Biol. Chem.* 39 (1920): 21–27.

6. Animal protein includes more of the sulfur-containing amino acids. When digested and metabolized, these amino acids produce the acid-forming sulfate ion, which must be excreted by the kidney. A recent report showed a remarkable 84% correlation between animal protein consumption and urinary acid excretion of sulfate.

7. Brosnan JT, and Brosnan ME. "Dietary protein, metabolic acidosis, and calcium balance." In: H. H. Draper (ed.), *Advances in Nutritional Research*, pp. 77–105. New York: Plenum Press, 1982.

8. Frassetto LA, Todd KM, Morris RC, Jr., et al. "Estimation of net endogenous noncarbonic acid production in humans from diet potassium and protein contents." *Am. J. Clin. Nutri.* 68 (1998): 576–583.

9. Margen S, Chu J-Y, Kaufmann NA, et al. "Studies in calcium metabolism. I. The calciuretic effect of dietary protein." *Am. J. Clin. Nutr.* 27 (1974): 584–589.

10. Hegsted M, Schuette SA, Zemel MB, et al. "Urinary calcium and calcium balance in young men as affected by level of protein and phosphorus intake." *J. Nutr.* 111 (1981): 553–562.

11. Kerstetter JE, and Allen LH. "Dietary protein increases urinary calcium." *J. Nutr.* 120 (1990): 134–136.

12. Westman EC, Yancy WS, Edman JS, et al. "Carbohydrate Diet Program." *Am. J. Med.* 113 (2002): 30–36.

13. Sellmeyer DE, Stone KL, Sebastian A, et al. "A high ratio of dietary animal to vegetable protein increases the rate of bone loss and the risk of fracture in postmenopausal women." *Am. J. Clin. Nutr.* 73 (2001): 118–122.

14. Hegsted DM. "Calcium and osteoporosis." *J. Nutr.* 116 (1986): 2316–2319.

15. Heaney RP. "Protein intake and bone health: the influence of belief systems on the conduct of nutritional science." *Am. J. Clin. Nutr.* 73 (2001): 5–6.

16. Cummings SR, and Black D. "Bone mass measurements and risk of fracture in Caucasian women: a review of findings for prospective studies." *Am. J. Med.* 98 (Suppl 2A) (1995): 2S–24S.

17. Marshall D, Johnell O, and Wedel H. "Meta-analysis of how well measures of bone mineral density predict occurrence of osteoporotic fractures." *Brit. Med. J.* 312 (1996): 1254–1259.

18. Lips P. "Epidemiology and predictors of fractures associated with osteoporosis." *Am. J. Med.* 103(2A) (1997): 3S–11S.

19. Lane NE, and Nevitt MC. "Osteoarthritis, bone mass, and fractures: how are they related?" *Arthritis Rheumatism* 46 (2002): 1–4.

20. Lucas FL, Cauley JA, Stone RA, et al. "Bone mineral density and risk of breast cancer: differences by family history of breast cancer." *Am. J. Epidemiol.* 148 (1998): 22–29.

21. Cauley JA, Lucas FL, Kuller LH, et al. "Bone mineral density and risk of breast cancer in older women: the study of osteoporotic fractures." *JAMA* 276 (1996): 1404–1408.

22. Mincey BA. "Osteoporosis in women with breast cancer." *Curr. Oncol. Rpts.* 5 (2003): 53–57.

23. Riis BJ. "The role of bone loss." *Am. J. Med.* 98 (Suppl 2A) (1995): 2S–29S.

24. Ho SC. "Body measurements, bone mass, and fractures: does the East differ from the West?" *Clin. Orthopaed. Related Res.* 323 (1996): 75–80.

25. Aspray TJ, Prentice A, Cole TJ, et al. "Low bone mineral content is common but osteoporotic fractures are rare in elderly rural Gambian women." *J. Bone Min. Res.* 11 (1996): 1019–1025.

26. Tsai K-S. "Osteoporotic fracture rate, bone mineral density, and bone metabolism in Taiwan." *J. Formosan Med. Assoc.* 96 (1997): 802–805.

27. Wu AH, Pike MC, and Stram DO. "Meta-analysis: dietary fat intake, serum estrogen levels, and the risk of breast cancer." *J. Nat. Cancer Inst.* 91 (1999): 529–534.

28. UCLA Kidney Stone Treatment Center. "Kidney Stones—Index." March, 1997. Accessed at http://www.radsci.ucla.edu:8000/gu/stones/kidneystone.html.

29. Stamatelou KK, Francis ME, Jones CA, et al. "Time trends in reported prevalence of kidney stones." *Kidney Int.* 63 (2003): 1817–1823.

30. This genetically rare type of kidney stone results from an inability of the kidney to reabsorb cysteine, an amino acid.

31. Ramello A, Vitale C, and Marangella M. "Epidemiology of nephrolothiasis." *J. Nephrol.* 13(Suppl 3) (2000): S65–S70.

32. Robertson WG, Peacock M, and Hodgkinson A. "Dietary changes and the incidence of urinary calculi in the U.K. between 1958 and 1976." *Chron. Dis.* 32 (1979): 469–476.

33. Robertson WG, Peacock M, Heyburn PJ, et al. "Risk factors in calcium stone disease of the urinary tract." *Brit. J. Urology* 50 (1978): 449–454.

34. Robertson WG. "Epidemiological risk factors in calcium stone disease." *Scand. J. Urol. Nephrol. Suppl.* 53 (1980): 15–30.

35. Robertson WG, Peacock M, Heyburn PJ, et al. "Should recurrent calcium oxalate stone formers become vegetarians?" *Brit. J. Urology* 51 (1979): 427–431.

36. This information was shown in Dr. Robertson's seminar in Toronto.

37. Robertson WG. "Diet and calcium stones." *Miner Electrolyte Metab.* 13 (1987): 228–234.

38. Cao LC, Boeve ER, de Bruijn WC, et al. "A review of new concepts in renal stone research." *Scanning Microscopy* 7 (1993): 1049–1065.

39. Scales CDJ, Smith AC, Hanley JM, Seigal CS, and Urologic Diseases in America Project. "Prevalence of kidney stones in the United States." *Eur. Urol.* 62 (2012): 160–165.

40. Broghi L. et al. "Urinary volume, water and recurrences in idiopathic calcium nephrolithiasis: a 5-year randomized prospective study." *J Urol.* 155 (1996): 839–843.

41. Turney BW et al. "Diet and risk of kidney stones in the Oxford cohort of the European Prospective Investigation into Cancer and Nutrition (EPIC)." *Eur. J. Epidemiol.* 29 (2014): 363–369.

42. Friedman DS, Congdon N, Kempen J, et al. "Vision problems in the U.S.: prevalence of adult vision impairment and age-related eye disease in America." Bethesda, MD: Prevent Blindness in America. National Eye Institute, 2002.

43. Foote CS. *Photosensitized Oxidation and Singlet Oxygen: Consequences in Biological Systems. Vol. 2* New York: Academic Press, 1976.

44. Seddon JM, Ajani UA, Sperduto RD, et al. "Dietary carotenoids, vitamins A, C, and E, and advanced age-related macular degeneration." *JAMA* 272 (1994): 1413–1420.

45. Eye Disease Case-Control Study Group. "Antioxidant status and neovascular age-related macular degeneration." *Arch. Ophthalmol.* 111 (1993): 104–109.

46. The other four food groups were broccoli, carrot, sweet potato, and winter squash, showing disease reductions of 53%, 28%, 33%, and 44%, respectively. Each reduction was only approaching or was marginally statistically significant.

47. Berman ER. *Biochemistry of the Eye. (Perspectives in Vision Research)*. New York: Plenum Publishing Corporation, 1991.

48. Lyle BJ, Mares-Perlman JA, Klein BEK, et al. "Antioxidant intake and risk of incident age-related nuclear cataracts in the Beaver Dam Eye Study." *Am. J. Epidemiol.* 149 (1999): 801–809.

49. Bates CJ, Chen SJ, Macdonald A, et al. "Quantitation of vitamin E and a carotenoid pigment in cataracterous human lenses, and the effect of a dietary supplement." *Int. J. Vitam. Nutr. Res.* 66 (1996): 316–321.

50. Varma SD, Beachy NA, and Richards RD. "Photoperoxidation of lens lipids: prevention by vitamin E." *Photochem. Photobiol.* 36 (1982): 623–626.

51. Talan J. "Alzheimer's diagnoses can be two years late." *Ithaca J.*: 8A.

52. Alzheimer's Association. "2016 Alzheimer's Disease Facts and Figures." Accessed September 2, 2016 at http://www.alz.org/facts/.

53. Petersen RC, Smith GE, Waring SC, et al. "Mild cognitive impairment." *Arch. Neurol.* 56 (1999): 303–308.

54. Kivipelto M, Helkala E-L, Hanninen T, et al. "Midlife vascular risk factors and late-life mild cognitive impairment. A population based study." *Neurology* 56 (2001): 1683–1689.

55. Breteler MMB, Claus JJ, Grobbee DE, et al. "Cardiovascular disease and distribution of cognitive function in elderly people: the Rotterdam Study." *Brit. Med. J.* 308 (1994): 1604–1608.

56. Haan MN, Shemanski L, Jagust WJ, et al. "The role of APOE e4 in modulating effects of other risk factors for cognitive decline in elderly persons." *JAMA* 282 (1999): 40–46.

57. Sparks DL, Martin TA, Gross DR, et al. "Link between heart disease, cholesterol, and Alzheimer's Disease: a review." *Microscopy Res. Tech.* 50 (2000): 287–290.

58. Slooter AJ, Tang MX, van Duijn CM, et al. "Apolipoprotein E e4 and risk of dementia with stroke. A population based investigation." *JAMA* 277 (1997): 818–821.

59. Messier C, and Gagnon M. "Glucose regulation and cognitive functions: relation to Alzheimer's disease and diabetes." *Behav. Brain Res.* 75 (1996): 1–11.

60. Ott A, Stolk RP, Hofman A, et al. "Association of diabetes mellitus and dementia: the Rotterdam Study." *Diabetologia* 39 (1996): 1392–1397.

61. Kannel WB, Wolf PA, Verter J, et al. "Epidemiologic assessment of the role of blood pressure in stroke." *JAMA* 214 (1970): 301–310.

62. Launer LJ, Masaki K, Petrovitch H, et al. "The association between midlife blood pressure levels and late-life cognitive function." *JAMA* 274 (1995): 1846–1851.

63. White L, Petrovitch H, Ross GW., et al. "Prevalence of dementia in older Japanese-American men in Hawaii. The Honolulu-Asia Aging Study." *JAMA*, 276: 955–960, 1996.

64. Hendrie HC, Ogunniyi A, Hall KS, et al. "Incidence of dementia and Alzheimer Disease in 2 communities: Yoruba residing in Ibadan, Nigeria and African Americans residing in Indianapolis, Indiana." *JAMA* 285 (2001): 739–747.

65. Chandra V, Pandav R, Dodge HH, et al. "Incidence of Alzheimer's disease in a rural community in India: the Indo-U.S. Study." *Neurology* 57 (2001): 985–989.

66. Grant WB. "Dietary links to Alzheimer's Disease: 1999 Update." *J. Alzheimer's Dis* 1 (1999): 197–201.

67. Grant WB. "Incidence of dementia and Alzheimer disease in Nigeria and the United States." *JAMA* 285 (2001): 2448.

68. This recently published study is more interesting than the others because vitamin E was measured in a way that is more discriminating by considering the fact that vitamin E is carried in the blood fat. That is, a high level of blood vitamin E may, at times, be due to high levels of blood fat. *Am. J. Epidemiol.* 150 (1999): 37–44.

69. The effects of vitamin C and selenium in a study by Perkins (*Am. J. Epidemiol.* 150 [1999]: 37–44) were not statistically significant in a logistic regression model, according to the authors. I disagree with their conclusion because the inverse "dose-response" trend (high antioxidant blood levels, less memory loss) was impressive and clearly significant. The authors failed to address this finding in their analysis.

70. Ortega RM, Requejo AM, Andres P, et al. "Dietary intake and cognitive function in a group of elderly people." *Am. J. Clin. Nutr.* 66 (1997): 803–809.

71. Perrig WJ, Perrig P, and Stahelin HB. "The relation between antioxidants and memory performance in the old and very old." *J. Am. Geriatr. Soc.* 45 (1997): 718–724.

72. Gale CR, Martyn CN, and Cooper C. "Cognitive impairment and mortality in a cohort of elderly people." *Brit. Med. J.* 312 (1996): 608–611.

73. Goodwin JS, Goodwin JM, and Garry PJ. "Association between nutritional status and cognitive functioning in a healthy elderly population." *JAMA* 249 (1983): 2917–2921.

74. Jama JW, Launer LJ, Witteman JCM, et al. "Dietary antioxidants and cognitive function in a population-based sample of older persons: the Rotterdam Study." *Am. J. Epidemiol.* 144 (1996): 275–280.

75. Martin A, Prior R, Shukitt-Hale B, et al. "Effect of fruits, vegetables or vitamin E-rich diet on vitamins E and C distribution in peripheral and brain tissues: implications for brain function." *J. Gerontology* 55A (2000): B144–B151.

76. Joseph JA, Shukitt-Hale B, Denisova NA, et al. "Reversals of age-related declines in neuronal signal transduction, cognitive, and motor behavioral deficits with blueberry, spinach, or strawberry dietary supplementation." *J. Neurosci.* 19 (1999): 8114–8121.

77. Gillman MW, Cupples LA, Gagnon D, et al. "Protective effect of fruits and vegetables on development of stroke in men." *JAMA* 273 (1995): 1113–1117.

78. Kalmijn S, Launer LJ, Ott A, et al. "Dietary fat intake and the risk of incident dementia in the Rotterdam Study." *Ann. Neurol.* 42 (1997): 776–782.

79. Alzheimer's trend was not statistically significant, perhaps due to the small number of disease cases.

80. Clarke R, Smith D, Jobst KA, et al. "Folate, vitamin B_{12}, and serum total homocysteine levels in confirmed Alzheimer disease." *Arch. Neurol.* 55 (1998): 1449–1455.

81. McCully KS. "Homocysteine theory of arteriosclerosis: development and current status." In: A. M. Gotto, Jr. and R. Paoletti (eds.), *Atherosclerosis Reviews, Vol. 11*, pp. 157–246. New York: Raven Press, 1983.

82. There is a potential snag in this logic, however. Homocysteine levels are regulated in part by B vitamins, most notably folic acid and vitamin B_{12}, and people who are deficient in these vitamins may have higher homocysteine levels. People who do not consume animal-based foods are at risk for having low B_{12} levels, and thus high homocysteine levels. However, as described in chapter eleven, this has more to do with our separation from nature, and not a deficiency of plant-based diets.

PART III

1. Scelfo J. "Dieting: The Next Atkins?" *Newsweek* (2003, May 4).

Chapter 11

1. U.S. Food and Drug Administration. "What Is a Dietary Supplement?" Silver Spring, MD: U.S. Food and Drug Administration, 2015.

2. Lariviere D. "Nutritional supplements flexing muscles as growth industry." *Forbes*, April 18, 2013. Accessed at http://www.forbes.com/sites/davidlariviere/2013/04/18/nutritional-supplements-flexing-their-muscles-as-growth-industry/.

3. CodexFund. "CODEX and dietary supplements. Frequently asked questions." CodexFund, 2010.

4. U.S. Federal Trade Commission. "Complaint counsel's proposed findings of fact, conclusions of law and proposed order (Docket No. 9175)." Washington, DC: U.S. Federal Trade Commission, December 27, 1985.

5. Atkins RC. *Dr. Atkins' New Diet Revolution*. New York: Avon Books, 1999.

6. The Alpha-Tocopherol Beta Carotene Cancer Prevention Study Group. "The effect of vitamin E and beta carotene on the incidence of lung cancer and other cancers in male smokers." *New Engl. J. Med.* 330 (1994): 1029–1035.

7. Omenn GS, Goodman GE, Thornquist MD, et al. "Effects of a combination of beta carotene and vitamin A on lung cancer and cardiovascular disease." *New Engl. J. Med.* 334 (1996): 1150–1155.

8. U.S. Preventive Services Task Force. "Routine vitamin supplementation to prevent cancer and cardiovascular disease: recommendations and rationale." *Ann. Internal Med.* 139 (2003): 51–55.

9. Morris CD, and Carson S. "Routine vitamin supplementation to prevent cardiovascular disease: a summary of the evidence for the U.S. Preventive Services Task Force." *Ann. Internal Med.* 139 (2003): 56–70.

10. Kolata G. "Vitamins: more may be too many (Science Section)." *New York Times,* April 29, 2003: 1, 6.

11. de Souza A, and Moloi MW. "Involuntary movements due to the vitamin B_{12} deficiency." *Neurol. Res.* 36 (2014): 1121–1128.

12. LeBlanc E, Chou R, Zakher B, Daeges M, and Pappas M. "Screening for vitamin D deficiency: systematic review for the U.S. Preventive Services Task Force Recommendation." Rockville, MD: Agency for Healthcare Research and Quality.

13. Pines A. "Vitamin D and health issues—questioned benefits." *Climacteric* 17 (2014): 657–659.

14. Bowen R. "Vitamin D (calcitrol)." *Vitamins: Introduction and Index*. Accessed at http://www.vivo.colostate.edu/hbooks/pathphys/endocrine/otherendo/vitamind.html.

15. U.S. Department of Agriculture. "USDA Nutrient Database for Standard Reference." Washington, DC: U.S. Department of Agriculture, Agriculture Research Service, 2002. Accessed at https://ndb.nal.usda.gov/.

16. Holden JM, Eldridge AL, Beecher GR, et al. "Carotenoid content of U.S. foods: an update of the database." *J. Food Comp. Anal.* 12 (1999): 169–196.

17. The exact food listings in the database were: ground beef, 80% lean meat/20% fat, raw; pork, fresh, ground, raw; chicken, broilers or fryers, meat and skin, raw; milk, dry, whole; spinach, raw; tomatoes, red, ripe, raw, year-round average; lima beans, large, mature seeds, raw; peas, green, raw; potatoes, russet, flesh and skin, raw.

18. Mozafar A. "Enrichment of some B-vitamins in plants with application of organic fertilizers." *Plant and Soil* 167 (1994): 305–311.

19. Brand D, and Segelken R. "Largest scientific effort in Cornell's history announced." *Cornell Chronicle,* May 9, 2002.

20. Ashrafi K, Chang FY, Watts JL, et al. "Genome-wide RNAi analysis of *Caenorhabitis elegans* fat regulatory genes." *Nature* 421 (2003): 268–272.

21. Shermer M. "Skeptical sayings. Wit and wisdom from skeptics past and present." *Skeptic* 9 (2002): 28.

22. I've never really liked putting such specific cutoff points on initiation, promotion, and progression of chronic disease, because these cutoff points for each stage of chronic disease are completely arbitrary. What's important to know is that a chronic disease can be with us for most of our lives, and if it progresses, it will do so in a very fluid, continuous manner.

23. Ornish D, Weidner G, Fair WR, et al. "Intensive lifestyle changes may affect the progression of prostate cancer." *J. Urol.* 174 (2005): 1065–1069; discussion 1069–1070.

24. McDougall JA. *McDougall's Medicine, A Challenging Second Opinion*. Piscataway, NJ: New Century, 1985.

25. Swank RL. "Multiple sclerosis: twenty years on low fat diet." *Arch. Neurol.* 23 (1970): 460–474.

26. Swank RL. "Effect of low saturated fat diet in early and late cases of multiple sclerosis." *Lancet* 336 (1990): 37–39.

27. Kim, T. K., and Han, P. L. "Chronic stress and moderate physical exercise prompt widespread common activation and limited differential activation in specific brain regions." *Neurochemistry international* (2016).

28. Campbell TC (with Jacobson H). *Whole: Rethinking the Science of Nutrition*. Dallas: BenBella Books, 2013.

Chapter 12

1. Davey, G. K. et al. "EPIC-Oxford: lifestyle characteristics and nutrient intakes in a cohort of 33, 883 meat eaters and 31, 546 non meat-eaters in the UK." *Publ. Health Nutr.* 6 (2003): 259-268; Sobiecki, J. G., Appleby, P. N., Bradbury, K. E., and Key, T. J. "High compliance with dietary recommendations in a cohort of meat eaters, fish eaters, vegetarians, and vegans: results from the European Prospective Investigation into Cancer and Nutrition-Oxford study." *Nutr. Res.* 36 (2016): 464-477.

PART IV

1. Campbell TC (with Jacobson H). *Whole: Rethinking the Science of Nutrition*. Dallas: BenBella Books, 2013.

Chapter 13

1. Colen DD. "To die in Tijuana; a story of faith, hope and laetrile." *Washington Post Magazine*, September 4, 1977: 10.

2. Burros M. "The sting? America's supplements appetite; scientists are dubious, but America's appetite for food supplements keeps growing." *Washington Post*, August 2, 1979: E1.

3. Hilgartner S. *Science on Stage. Expert Advice As Public Drama*. Stanford, CA: Stanford University Press, 2000.

4. National Research Council. *Diet, Nutrition and Cancer*. Washington, DC: National Academy Press, 1982.

5. U.S. Senate. "Dietary goals for the United States, 2nd Edition." Washington, DC: U.S. Government Printing Office, 1977.

6. American Council of Science and Health. "About American Council on Science and Health." Accessed September 3, 2016 at http://acsh.org/wp admin/admin-ajax.php.

7. Mindfully.org. "American Council on Science and Health (ACSH)." Accessed September 3, 2016 at http://www.mindfully.org/Pesticide/ACSH-Koop.htm.

8. American Society for Nutrition. Accessed September 3, 2016 at http://www.nutrition.org.

Chapter 14

1. National Research Council. *Diet, Nutrition, and Cancer*. Washington, DC: National Academy Press, 1982.

2. United States Federal Trade Commission. "Complaint counsel's proposed findings of fact, conclusions of law and proposed order (Docket No. 9175)." Washington, DC: United States Federal Trade Commission, December 27, 1985.

3. Associated Press. "Company news; General Nutrition settles complaint." *New York Times*, June 14, 1988: D5.

4. Willett W. "Diet and cancer: one view at the start of the millennium." *Cancer Epi. Biom. Prev.* 10 (2001): 3–8.

5. Belanger CF, Hennekens CH, Rosner B, et al. "The Nurses' Health Study." *Am. J. Nursing* (1978): 1039–1040.

6. Marchione M. "Taking the long view; for 25 years, Harvard's Nurses' Health Study has sought answers to women's health questions." *Milwaukee Journal-Sentinel*, July 16, 2001: 01G.

7. Carroll KK. "Experimental evidence of dietary factors and hormone-dependent cancers." *Cancer Res.* 35 (1975): 3374–3383.

8. Chen J, Campbell TC, Li J, et al. *Diet, Life-style and Mortality in China. A Study of the Characteristics of 65 Chinese Counties*. Oxford, UK; Ithaca, NY; Beijing, PRC: Oxford University Press; Cornell University Press; People's Medical Publishing House, 1990.

9. Hu FB, Stampfer MJ, Manson JE, et al. "Dietary protein and risk of ischemic heart disease in women." *Am. Journ. Clin. Nutr.* 70 (1999): 221–227.

10. Holmes MD, Hunter DJ, Colditz GA, et al. "Association of dietary intake of fat and fatty acids with risk of breast cancer." *JAMA* 281 (1999): 914–920.

11. U.S. Department of Agriculture. "Agriculture Fact Book." Washington, DC: U.S. Department of Agriculture, 1998. cited in: Information Plus. *Nutrition: A Key to Good Health*. Wylie, TX: Information Plus, 1999.

12. While the average percentage of calories derived from fat has gone down slightly, average daily fat intake, in grams, has stayed the same or has gone up.

13. Information Plus. *Nutrition: A Key to Good Health*. Wylie, TX: Information Plus, 1999.

14. Wegmans.com. Accessed January 19, 2004, at http://www.wegmans.com/recipes.

15. Mardiweb.com. "Cheesecake." Accessed January 19, 2004, at http://mardiweb.com/lowfat/dessert.ht m#Recipe000857.

16. Anonymous. "Center to Coordinate Women's Health Study." *Chicago Sun-Times*, October 12, 1992: 14N.

17. Prentice RL, Kakar F, Hursting S, et al. "Aspects of the rationale for the Women's Health Trial." *J. Natl. Cancer Inst.* 80 (1988): 802–814.

18. Henderson MM, Kushi LH, Thompson DJ, et al. "Feasibility of a randomized trial of a low-fat diet for the prevention of breast cancer: dietary compliance in the Women's Health Trial Vanguard Study." *Prev. Med.* 19 (1990): 115–133.

19. Self S, Prentice R, Iverson D, et al. "Statistical design of the Women's Health Trial." *Controlled Clin. Trials* 9 (1988): 119–136.

20. Armstrong D, and Doll R. "Environmental factors and cancer incidence and mortality in different countries, with special reference to dietary practices." *Int. J. Cancer* 15 (1975): 617–631.

21. Campbell TC. "The dietary causes of degenerative diseases: nutrients vs foods." In: N. J. Temple and D. P. Burkitt (eds.), *Western Diseases: Their Dietary Prevention andReversibility*, pp. 119–152. Totowa, NJ: Humana Press, 1994.

22. White E, Shattuck AL, Kristal AR, et al. "Maintenance of a low-fat diet: follow-up of the Women's Health Trial." *Cancer Epi. Biom. Prev.* 1 (1992): 315–323.

23. Willett WC, Hunter DJ, Stampfer MJ, et al. "Dietary fat and fiber in relation to risk of breast cancer. An 8-year follow-up." *J. Am. Med. Assoc.* 268 (1992): 2037–2044.

24. Willett W. "Dietary fat and breast cancer." *Toxicol. Sci.* 52 (Suppl.) (1999): 127–146.

25. Hunter DJ, Spiegelman D, Adami H-O, et al. "Cohort studies of fat intake and the risk of breast cancer—a pooled analysis." *New Engl. J. Med.* 334 (1996): 356–361.

26. Missmer SA, Smith-Warner SA, Spiegelman D, et al. "Meat and dairy consumption and breast cancer: a pooled analysis of cohort studies." *Int. J. Epidemiol.* 31 (2002): 78–85.

27. Rockhill B, Willett WC, Hunter DJ, et al. "Physical activity and breast cancer risk in a cohort of young women." *J. Nat. Cancer Inst.* 90 (1998): 1155–1160.

28. Smith-Warner SA, Spiegelman D, Adami H-O, et al. "Types of dietary fat and breast cancer: a pooled analysis of cohort studies." *Int. J. Cancer* 92 (2001): 767–774.

29. Hunter DJ, Morris JS, Stampfer MJ, et al. "A prospective study of selenium status and breast cancer risk." *JAMA* 264 (1990): 1128–1131.

30. Smith-Warner SA, Spiegelman D, Yaun S-S, et al. "Intake of fruits and vegetables and risk of breast cancer: a pooled analysis of cohort studies." *JAMA* 285 (2001): 769–776.

31. Mukamal KJ, Conigrave KM, Mittleman MA, et al. "Roles of drinking pattern and type of alcohol consumed in coronary heart disease in men." *New Engl. J. Med.* 348 (2003): 109–118.

32. Tanasescu M, Hu FB, Willett WC, et al. "Alcohol consumption and risk of coronary heart disease among men with Type 2 diabetes mellitus." *J. Am. Coll. Cardiol.* 38 (2001): 1836–1842.

33. Smith-Warner SA, Spiegelman D, Yaun S-S, et al. "Alcohol and breast cancer in women. A pooled analysis of cohort studies." *JAMA* 279 (1998): 535–540.

34. He K, Rimm EB, Merchant A, et al. "Fish consumption and risk of stroke in men." *JAMA* 288 (2002): 3130–3136.

35. Albert CM, Hennekens CH, O'Donnell CJ, et al. "Fish consumption and risk of sudden cardiac death." *JAMA* 279 (1998): 23–28.

36. U.S. Department of Agriculture. "USDA Nutrient Database for Standard Reference." Washington, DC: U.S. Department of Agriculture, Agriculture Research Service, 2002. Accessed at http://www.nal.usda.gov/fnic/foodcomp.

37. Hu FB, Stampfer MJ, Rimm EB, et al. "A prospective study of egg consumption and risk of cardiovascular disease in men and women." *JAMA* 281 (1999): 1387–1394.

38. Hu FB, Manson JE, and Willett WC. "Types of dietary fat and risk of coronary heart disease: a critical review." *J. Am. Coll. Nutr.* 20 (2001): 5–19.

39. Mitchell S. "Eggs might reduce breast cancer risk." United Press International, February 21, 2003.

40. Steinmetz KA, and Potter JD. "Egg consumption and cancer of the colon and rectum." *Eur. J. Cancer Prev.* 3 (1994): 237–245.

41. Giovannucci E, Rimm EB, Stampfer MJ, et al. "Intake of fat, meat, and fiber in relation to risk of colon cancer in men." *Cancer Res.* 54 (1994): 2390–2397.

42. Fuchs CS, Giovannucci E, Colditz GA, et al. "Dietary fiber and the risk of colorectal cancer and adenoma in women." *New Engl. J. Med.* 340 (1999): 169–176.

43. Higginson J. "Present trends in cancer epidemiology." *Proc. Can. Cancer Conf.* 8 (1969): 40–75.

44. Burkitt DP. "Epidemiology of cancer of the colon and the rectum." *Cancer* 28 (1971): 3–13.

45. Trowell IIC, and Burkitt DP. *Western Diseases: Their Emergence and Prevention.* London: Butler & Tanner, Ltd., 1981.

46. Boyd NF, Martin LJ, Noffel M, et al. "A meta-analysis of studies of dietary-fat and breast cancer risk." *Brit. J. Cancer* 68 (1993): 627–636.

47. Campbell TC. "Animal protein and ischemic heart disease." *Am. J. Clin. Nutr.* 71 (2000): 849–850.

48. Hu FB, and Willett W. "Reply to TC Campbell." *Am. J. Clin. Nutr.* 71 (2000): 850.

49. Morris CD, and Carson S. "Routine vitamin supplementation to prevent cardiovascular disease: a summary of the evidence for the U.S. Preventive Services Task Force." *Ann. Internal Med.* 139 (2003): 56–70.

50. U.S. Preventive Services Task Force. "Routine vitamin supplementation to prevent cancer and cardiovascular disease: recommendations and rationale." *Ann. Internal Med.* 139 (2003): 51–55.

51. Nurses' Health Study. Accessed at http://www.nurseshealthstudy.org/.

52. Satija A, Yu E, Willett WC, and Hu FB. "Understanding nutritional epidemiology and its role in policy." *Adv. Nutr.* 6 (2015): 5–18.

53. "Vitamins and supplements: Miracle healers." *The Economist,* September 19, 2015. Accessed at http://www.economist.com/news/business/21665064-despite-scandals-and-scepticism-americas-supplement-industry-looks-healthy-miracle-healers.

54. Bradley J. "NBJ: 'The US supplement industry is $37 billion, not $12 billion.'" *NutraIngredients-USA.com,* June 1, 2015. Accessed at http://www.nutraingredients-usa.com/Markets/NBJ-The-US-supplement-industry-is-37-billion-not-12-billion.

55. Daniells S. "TABS Analytics vitamins & minerals study: Are heavy users in decline?" *NutraIngredients-USA.com,* May 23, 2016. Accessed at http://www.nutraingredients-usa.com/Markets/TABS-Analytics-Vitamins-Minerals-Study-Are-heavy-users-in-decline.

56. Hooper L, Thompson RL, Harrison RA, et al. "Risks and benefits of omega 3 fats for mortality, cardiovascular disease, and cancer: systematic review." *BMJ* 332 (2006): 752–760.

57. Gaziano JM, Glynn RJ, Christen WG, et al. "Vitamins E and C in the prevention of prostate and total cancer in men: the Physicians' Health Study II randomized controlled trial." *JAMA* 301 (2009): 52–62.

58. Christen WG, Glynn RJ, Sesso HD, et al. "Age-related cataract in a randomized trial of vitamins E and C in men." *Arch. Ophthalmol.* 128 (2010): 1397–1405.

59. Christen WG, Glynn RJ, Manson JE, et al. "Effects of multivitamin supplement on cataract and age-related macular degeneration in a randomized trial of male physicians." *Ophthalmol.* 121 (2014): 525–534.

60. Sesso HD, Christen WG, Bubes V, et al. "Multivitamins in the prevention of cardiovascular disease in men: the Physicians' Health Study II randomized controlled trial." *JAMA* 17 (2012): 1751–1760.

61. Gaziano JM, Sesso HD, Christen WG, et al. "Multivitamins in the prevention of cancer in men: the Physicians' Health Study II randomized controlled trial." *JAMA* 308 (2012): 1871–1880.

62. Wang L, Sesso HD, Glynn L, et al. "Vitamin E and C supplementation and risk of cancer in men: posttrial follow-up in the Physicians' Health Study II randomized trial." *Am. J. Clin. Nutr.* 100 (2014): 915–923.

63. Wang J, Eliassen AH, Spiegelman D, et al. "Plasma free 25-hydroxyvitamin D, vitamin D binding protein, and risk of breast cancer in the Nurses' Health Study II." *Cancer Causes & Control* 25 (2014): 819–827; Bertrand KA, Rosner B, Eliassen AH, et al. "Premenopausal plasma 25-hydroxyvitamin D, mammographic density, and risk of breast cancer." *Breast Cancer Res. Treat.* 149 (2015): 479–487.

64. Massa J, Cho E, Orav EJ, et al. "Long-term use of multivitamins and risk of colorectal adenoma in women." *Brit. J. Cancer* 110 (2014): 249–255.

Chapter 15

1. MRC Agricultural Marketing Resource Center. "Food consumption trends." July 2012.

2. National Dairy Council. "Our Story." Accessed September 3, 2016, at https://www.nationaldairycouncil.org/our-story.

3. Dairy Management Inc. "DMI and the Dairy Checkoff." Accessed September 3, 2016, at http://www.dairy.org/about-dmi.

4. Dairy Management Inc. Press release. "Dairy checkoff 2003 unified marketing plan budget geared to help increase demand in domestic and international markets." Accessed January 24, 2003, at http://www.dairycheckoff.com/news/release-012403.asp.

5. National Watermelon Promotion Board. Accessed January 12, 2004, at http://www. watermelon.org.

6. Dairy Management Inc. "2001 Annual Report." Dairy Management, Inc., 2001. Accessed at http://www.dairycheckoff.com/annualreport.htm/.

7. United States Department of Agriculture. "Report to Congress on the National Dairy Promotion and Research Program and the National Fluid Milk Processor Promotion Program." 2000. Accessed 2004 at http://www.ams.usda.gov/dairy/prb_intro.htm.IN.

8. United States Department of Agriculture. "Report to Congress on the National Dairy Promotion and Research Program and the National Fluid Milk Processor Promotion Program." 2003. Accessed 2004 at http://www.ams.usda.gov/dairy/prb/prb_rept_2003. htm.

9. Nutrition Explorations. July 2003. Accessed at http://www.nutritionexplorations.com.

10. Powell A. "School of Public Health hosts food fight: McDonald's, dairy industry, dietary reformers face off at symposium." *Harvard Gazette*, October 24, 2002. Accessed at http://www.news.harvard.edu/gazette/2002/10.24/09-food.html.

11. Ha YL, Grimm NK, and Pariza MW. "Anticarcinogens from fried ground beef: heat-altered derivatives of linoleic acid." *Carcinogensis* 8 (1987): 1881–1887.

12. Ha YL, Storkson J, and Pariza MW. "Inhibition of benzo(a)pyrene-induced mouse forestomach neoplasia by conjugated denoic derivatives of linoleic acid." *Cancer Res.* 50 (1990): 1097–1101.

13. Aydin R, Pariza MW, and Cook ME. "Olive oil prevents the adverse effects of dietary conjugated linoleic acid on chick hatchability and egg quality." *J. Nutr.* 131 (2001): 800–806.

14. Peters JM, Park Y, Gonzalez FJ, et al. "Influence of conjugated linoleic acid on body composition and target gene expression in peroxisome proliferator-activated receptor alpha-null mice." *Biochim. Biophys. Acta* 1533 (2001): 233–242.

15. Ntambi JM, Choi Y, Park Y, et al. "Effect of conjugated linoleic acid (CLA) on immune responses, body composition and stearoyl-CoA desaturase." *Can. J. Appl. Physiol.* 27 (2002): 617–627.

16. Ip C, Chin SF, Scimeca JA, et al. "Mammary cancer prevention by conjugated dienoic derivative of linoleic acid." *Cancer Res.* 51 (1991): 6118–6124.

17. Ip C, Cheng J, Thompson HJ, et al. "Retention of conjugated linoleic acid in the mammary gland is associated with tumor inhibition during the post-initiation phase of carcinogenesis." *Carcinogenesis* 18 (1997): 755–759.

18. Yaukey J. "Changing cows' diets elevates milks' cancer-fighting." *Ithaca Journal* November 12, 1996: 1.

19. Belury MA. "Inhibition of carcinogenesis by conjugated linoleic acid: potential mechanisms of action." *J. Nutr.* 132 (2002): 2995–2998.

20. Ip C, Banni S, Angioni E, et al. "Conjugated linoleic acid-enriched butter fat alters mammary gland morphogenesis and reduces cancer risk in rats." *J. Nutr.* 129 (1999): 2135–2142.

21. Griinari JM, Corl BA, Lacy SH, et al. "Conjugated linoleic acid is synthesized endogenously in lactating dairy cows by D⁹-desaturase." *J. Nutr.* 130 (2000): 2285–2291.

22. Ip C, Dong Y, Thompson HJ, et al. "Control of rat mammary epithelium proliferation by conjugated linoleic acid." *Nutr. Cancer* 39 (2001): 233–238.

23. Ip C, Dong Y, Ip MM, et al. "Conjugated linoleic acid isomers and mammary cancer prevention." *Nutr. Cancer* 43 (2002): 52–58.

24. Giovannucci E. "Insulin and colon cancer." *Cancer Causes and Control* 6 (1995): 164–179.

25. Mills PK, Beeson WL, Phillips RL, et al. "Cohort study of diet, lifestyle, and prostate cancer." *Cancer* 64 (1989): 598–604.

26. Search for keyword "lycopene" at http://www.ncbi.nlm.nih.gov.

27. Christian MS, Schulte S, and Hellwig J. "Developmental (embryo-fetal toxicity/teratogenecity) toxicity studies of synthetic crystalline lycopene in rats and rabbits." *Food Chem. Toxicol.* 41 (2003): 773–783.

28. Giovannucci E, Rimm E, Liu Y, et al. "A prospective study of tomato products, lycopene, and prostate cancer risk." *J. Nat. Cancer Inst.* 94 (2002): 391–398.

29. Gann PH, and Khachik F. "Tomatoes or lycopene versus prostate cancer: is evolution anti-reductionist?" *J. Nat. Cancer Inst.* 95 (2003): 1563–1565.

30. Tucker G. "Nutritional enhancement of plants." *Curr. Opin.* 14 (2003): 221–225.

31. He Y. *Effects of carotenoids and dietary carotenoid extracts on aflatoxin B_1-induced mutagenesis and hepatocarcinogenesis.* Ithaca, NY: Cornell University, PhD Thesis, 1990.

32. He Y, and Campbell TC. "Effects of carotenoids on aflatoxin B_1-induced mutagenesis in S. typhimurium TA 100 and TA 98." *Nutr. Cancer* 13 (1990): 243–253.

33. Kotecha R, Takami A, and Espinoza JL. Dietary phytochemicals and cancer chemoprevention: a review of the clinical evidence. *Oncotarget* (2016, May 25).

34. Gontero, P., et al. A randomized double-blind placebo controlled phase I-II study on clinical and molecular effects of dietary supplements in men with precancerous prostatic lesions. Chemoprevention or "chemopromotion"? *Prostate* 75 (2015): 1177–1186.

35. U.S. Department of Agriculture. "USDA Nutrient Database for Standard Reference." Washington, DC: U.S. Department of Agriculture, Agriculture Research Service, 2002. Accessed at https://ndb.nal.usda.gov/.

36. Eberhardt MV, Lee CY, and Liu RH. "Antioxidant activity of fresh apples." *Nature* 405 (2000): 903–904.

Chapter 16

1. Food and Nutrition Board, and Institute of Medicine. "Dietary reference intakes for energy, carbohydrates, fiber, fat, fatty acids, cholesterol, protein, and amino acids (macronutrients)." Washington, DC: National Academy Press, 2002. Accessed at http://www.nap.edu/catalog/10490/dietary-reference-intakes-for-energy-carbohydrate-fiber-fat-fatty-acids-cholesterol-protein-and-amino-acids-macronutrients.

2. National Academy of Sciences. Press Release. "Report offers new eating and physical activity targets to reduce chronic disease risk." September 5, 2002. Washington, DC: National Research Council, Institute of Medicine. Accessed at http://www8.nationalacademies.org/onpinews/newsitem.aspx?RecordID=10490.

3. Wegmans Company. "Recipe and nutrient facts." Accessed 2003. Available from http://www.wegmans.com.

4. U.S. Department of Agriculture. "USDA Nutrient Database for Standard Reference." Washington, DC: U.S. Department of Agriculture, Agriculture Research Service, 2002. Accessed at http://www.nal.usda.gov/fnic/foodcomp.

5. The RDA has been expressed as a singular quantity of protein, as 0.8 grams of protein per kilogram of body weight. Assuming a daily intake of 2,200 calories for a 70 kg person, this 0.8 grams is equivalent to about 10–11% of total calories: 70 kg × 0.8 gm/kg × 4 cal/gm × 1/2200 cal × 100 = 10.2%.

6. Wright JD, Kennedy-Stephenson J, Wang CY, et al. "Trends in Intake of Energy and Macronutrients—United States, 1971–2000." *MMWR* 53 (2004, February 6): 80–82.

7. Boseley S. "Sugar industry threatens to scupper WHO." *The Guardian* April 21, 2003.

8. Brundtland GH. "Sweet and sour; The WHO is accused by the sugar industry of giving unscientific nutrition advice. But its recommendations are based on solid evidence, says Gro Harlem Brundtland." *New Scientist*, May 3, 2003: 23.

9. International Life Sciences Institute. ILSI North America. Accessed September 3, 2016. Available from http://www.ilsina.org.

10. Kursban M. "Commentary: conflicted panel makes for unfit guidelines." Physicians Committee for Responsible Medicine. Accessed June 2003. Available from http://www.pcrm.org/health/commentary/commentary0004.html.

11. Chaitowitz S. "Court rules against USDA's secrecy and failure to disclose conflict of interest in setting nutrition policies." Physicians Committee for Responsible Medicine. Accessed January 27, 2004. Available from http://www.pcrm.org/news/health001002.html.

12. For several years I have been on the science advisory board of PCRM.

13. National Academy of Sciences, and Institute of Medicine. "Dietary Reference Intakes for Energy, Carbohydrates, Fiber, Fat, Fatty Acids, Cholesterol, Protein, and Amino Acids [summary statement]." Washington, DC: National Academy Press, September, 2002.

14. U.S. Department of Agriculture, Food and Nutrition Service. "Summary of Major Programs for Latest Available Month." Alexandria, VA: Food and Nutrition Service, August 5, 2016. Accessed at http://www.fns.usda.gov/sites/default/files/pd/currentsum.xls.

15. U.S. Department of Agriculture, Food and Nutrition Service. "WIC Program: Monthly Data—State Level Participation by Category and Program Costs, FY 2014 (Final)." Alexandria, VA: Food and Nutrition Service, August 5, 2016. Accessed at http://www.fns.usda.gov/sites/default/files/pd/WICAgencies2014ytd.xls.

16. National Institutes of Health. February 2004. Accessed at http://www.nih.gov.

17. National Institutes of Health. "Operating Plan for FY 2016." Accessed September 3, 2016, at https://officeofbudget.od.nih.gov/pdfs/FY17/FY%202016%20NIH%20Operating%20Plan%20Posting.pdf.

18. National Institutes of Health. "Estimates of Funding for Various Research, Condition, and Disease Categories (RCDC)." Bethesda, MD: National Institutes of Health, February 10, 2016. Accessed at https://report.nih.gov/categorical_spending.aspx.

19. Calculated from data in table accessed in note 18.

20. National Cancer Institute. "FY 1999 Questions and Answers provided for the record for the FY 1999 House Appropriations Subcommitee." July 15, 2003. Accessed at http://www3.cancer.gov/admin/fmb/1999QAs.htm.

21. National Cancer Institute. FY 2001 Congressional Justification. Accessed March 2, 2004. Available from http://www3.cancer.gov/admin/fmb/index.html.

22. Angell M. "The pharmaceutical industry—to whom is it accountable?" *New Engl. J. Med.* 342 (2000): 1902–1904.

23. National Cancer Institute. FY 2004 Congressional Justification. Accessed 2003. Available from http://www3.cancer.gov/admin/fmb/index/html.

24. Demas A. *Food Education in the Elementary Classroom as a Means of Gaining Acceptance of Diverse Low Fat Foods in the School Lunch Program* [PhD Dissertation]. Ithaca, NY: Cornell University, 1995: 325pp.

25. Dietary Guidelines Advisory Committee. "Scientific Report of the 2015 Dietary Guidelines Advisory Committe: Part A. Executive Summary." Rockville, MD: Office of Disease Prevention and Health Promotion. Accessed August 27, 2016. Available from https://health.gov/dietaryguidelines/2015-scientific-report/02-executive-summary.asp.

26. Thune J, et al. Letter to The Honorable Sylvia Matthews Burwell and The Honorable Thomas J. Vilsack. March 12, 2015. Available from http://www.agri-pulse.com/Uploaded/DietaryGuidelinesLetter03122015.pdf.

27. Hartzler V. Letter to The Honorable Thomas J. Vilsack and The Honorable Sylvia Matthews Burwell. March 31, 2015. Available from https://health.gov/dietaryguidelines/2015/resources/2015-2020_Dietary_Guidelines.pdf.

28. Center for Science in the Public Interest. "Congressional Catering: How Big Food and Agricultural Special Interests Wield Influence in Congress and Undermine Public Health." June 2015. Available from https://cspinet.org/new/pdf/riders-dga-campaign-analysis-report.pdf.

29. U.S. Department of Health and Human Services and U.S. Department of Agriculture. *2015–2020 Dietary Guidelines for Americans* (8th ed.). Washington, DC: Author, December 2015. Available from https://health.gov/dietaryguidelines/2015/resources/2015-2020_Dietary_Guidelines.pdf.

Chapter 17

1. Austoker J. "The 'treatment of choice': breast cancer surgery 1860–1985." *Soc. Soc. Hist. Med. Bull (London)* 37 (1985): 100–107.

2. Naifeh SW. *The Best Doctors in America, 1994–1995*. Aiken, SC: Woodward & White, 1994.

3. McDougall JA, and McDougall MA. *The McDougall Plan*. Clinton, NJ: New Win Publishing, Inc., 1983.

4. Committee on Nutrition in Medical Education. "Nutrition Education in U.S. Medical Schools." Washington, DC: National Academy of Sciences, 1985.

5. White PL, Johnson OC, and Kibler MJ. "Council on Foods and Nutrition, American Medical Association—its relation to physicians." *Postgraduate Med.* 30 (1961): 502–507.

6. Lo C. "Integrating nutrition as a theme throughout the medical school curriculum." *Am. J. Clin. Nutr.* 72 (Suppl) (2000): 882S–889S.

7. Pearson TA, Stone EJ, Grundy SM, et al. "Translation of nutrition science into medical education: the Nutrition Academic Award Program." *Am. J. Clin. Nutr.* 74 (2001): 164–170.

8. Kassler WJ. "Appendix F: Testimony of the American Medical Student Association." Washington, DC: National Academy of Sciences, 1985.

9. Zeisel SH, and Plaisted CS. "CD-ROMs for Nutrition Education." *J. Am. Coll. Nutr.* 18 (1999): 287.

10. Two or three reputable agencies have also sponsored this program, but I suspect that the administrators of these agencies felt it necessary to associate with a project in medical education for their own purposes, regardless of the dubious list of other organizations.

11. Nutrition in Medicine. Accessed September 30, 2016, at http://nutritioninmedicine.org/portal/.

12. Weinsier RL, Boker JR, Brooks CM, et al. "Nutrition training in graduate medical (residency) education: a survey of selected training programs." *Am. J. Clin. Nutr.* 54 (1991): 957–962.

13. Young EA. "National Dairy Council Award for Excellence in Medical/Dental Nutrition Education Lecture, 1992: perspectives on nutrition in medical education." *Am. J. Clin. Nutr.* 56 (1992): 745–751.

14. Kushner RF. "Will there be a tipping point in medical nutrition education?" *Am. J. Clin. Nutr.* 77 (2003): 288–291.

15. Angell M. "Is academic medicine for sale?" *New Engl. J. Med.* 342 (2000): 1516–1518.

16. Moynihan R. "Who pays for the pizza? Redefining the relationships between doctors and drug companies 1: Entanglement." *BMJ* 326 (2003): 1189–1192.

17. Moynihan R. "Who pays for the pizza? Redefining the relationships between doctors and drug companies. 2. Disentanglement." *BMJ* 326 (2003): 1193–1196.

18. Avorn J, Chen M, & Hartley R. "Scientific versus commercial sources of influence on the prescribing behavior of physicians." *Am. J. Med.* 73 (1982): 4–8.

19. Lurie N, Rich EC, Simpson DE, et al. "Pharmaceutical representatives in academic medical centers: interaction with faculty and housestaff." *J. Gen. Intern. Med.* 5 (1990): 240–243.

20. Steinman MA, Shlipak MG, & McPhee SJ. "Of principles and pens: attitudes and practices of medicine housestaff toward pharmaceutical industry promotions." *Am. J. Med.* 110 (2001): 551–557.

21. Lexchin J, "Interactions between physicians and the pharmaceutical industry: what does the literature say?" *Can. Med. Assoc. J.* 149 (1993): 1401–1407.

22. Lexchin J. "What information do physicians receive from pharmaceutical representatives?" *Can. Fam. Physician* 43 (1997): 941–945.

23. Baird P. "Getting it right: industry sponsorship and medical research." *Can. Med. Assoc. Journ.* 168 (2003): 1267–1269.

24. Smith R. "Medical journals and pharmaceutical companies: uneasy bedfellows." *BMJ* 326 (2003): 1202–1205.

25. Chopra SS. "Industry funding of clinical trials: benefit or bias?" *JAMA* 290 (2003): 113–114.

26. Healy D. "In the grip of the python: conflicts at the university-industry interface." *Sci. Engineering Ethics* 9 (2003): 59–71.

27. Olivieri NF. "Patients' health or company profits? The commercialization of academic research." *Sci. Engineering Ethics* 9 (2003): 29–41.

28. Johnson L. "Schools report research interest conflicts." *Ithaca Journal,* October 24, 2002: 3A.

29. Agovino T. "Prescription use by children multiplying, study says." *Ithaca Journal,* September 19, 2002: 1A.

30. Associated Press. "Survey: many guidelines written by doctors with ties to companies." *Ithaca Journal,* February 12, 2002.

31. Weiss R. "Correctly prescribed drugs take heavy toll; millions affected by toxic reactions." *Washington Post,* April 15, 1998: A01.

32. Lasser KE, Allen PD, Woolhandler SJ, et al. "Timing of new black box warnings and withdrawals for prescription medications." *JAMA* 287 (2002): 2215–2220.

33. Lazarou J, Pomeranz B, and Corey PN. "Incidence of adverse drug reactions in hospitalized patients." *JAMA* 279 (1998): 1200–1205.

34. Adams KM, Kohlmeier M, Zeisel SH. "Nutrition education in U.S. medical schools: latest update of a national survey." *Acad. Med.* 85 (2010): 1537–1542.

35. Giocomino B, Cram P, Vaughan-Sarrazin M, Girotra S. "Abstract 208: Association of hospital prices for coronary artery bypass graft surgery with hospital quality and reimbursement." *Circulation: Cardiovascular Quality and Outcomes* 8 (2015): A208 (poster session).

36. Shanafelt TD, Hasan O, Dyrbye LN, et al. "Changes in Burnout and Satisfaction With Work-Life Balance in Physicians and the General US Working Population Between 2011 and 2014." *Mayo Clin. Proc.* 90 (2015): 1600–1613.

Chapter 18

1. National Center for Education Statistics. "Fast Facts." Accessed September 3, 2016, at https://nces.ed.gov/fastfacts/.

2. National Institutes of Health. "About NIH: What We Do: Budget." April 4, 2016. Accessed September 3, 2016, at https://www.nih.gov/about-nih/what-we-do/budget.

3. U.S. Department of Agriculture, National Institute of Food and Agriculture. "Extension." Accessed September 3, 2016, at https://nifa.usda.gov/extension.

4. Center for Media and Democracy. "SourceWatch: Physicians Committee for Responsible Medicine: Court Rules against USDA Secrecy & Conflicts of Interest." Last modified March 12, 2015. Accessed September 3, 2016, at http://www.sourcewatch.org/index.php/Physicians_Committee_for_Responsible_Medicine#Court_rules_against_USDA_secrecy_.26_conflicts_of_interest.

5. National Research Council. *Diet, Nutrition, and Cancer.* Washington, DC: National Academy Press, 1982.

6. Kingkade T. "Tenure decline: Inside Higher Ed survey finds provosts relying on non-tenured faculty." *Huffington Post,* January 23, 2013. Accessed at http://www.huffingtonpost.com/2013/01/23/tenure-decline_n_2537418.html.

7. Pankin R, and Weiss C. "Part-time faculty in higher education: a selected annotated bibliography." DigitalCommons@Providence, Sociology Department Faculty Publications, October 1, 2011. Accessed at http://digitalcommons.providence.edu/cgi/viewcontent.cgi?article=1000&context=sociology_fac.

8. Washburn J. "Science's worst enemy: corporate funding." *DiscoverMagazine.com,* October 11, 2007. Accessed at http://discovermagazine.com/2007/oct/sciences-worst-enemy-private-funding.

9. Association of American Colleges & Universities. "Academic freedom and educational responsibility." January 6, 2006. Accessed at https://www.aacu.org/about/statements/academic-freedom.

Chapter 19

1. Macilwain G. *The General Nature and Treatment of Tumors.* London: John Churchill, 1845.

2. Williams H. *The Ethics of Diet. A Catena of Authorities Deprecatory of the Practice of Flesh-Eating.* London: F. Pitman, 1883.

3. U.S. Census Bureau. "U.S. Popclock Projection." March, 2004. Accessed at http://www.census.gov/cgi-bin/popclock.

4. Centers for Disease Control. "Prevalence of adults with no known risk factors for coronary heart disease—behavioral risk factor surveillance system, 1992." *MMWR* 43 (February 4, 1994): 61–63, 69.

5. Kaufman DW, Kelly JP, Rosenberg L, et al. "Recent patterns of medication use in the ambulatory adult population of the United States: the Slone survey." *JAMA* 287 (2002): 337–344.

6. Flegal KM, Carroll MD, Ogden CL, et al. "Prevalence and trends in obesity among U.S. adults, 1999–2000." *JAMA* 288 (2002): 1723–1727.

7. American Heart Association. "High blood cholesterol and other lipids—statistics." March, 2004. Accessed at http://www.americanheart.org/presenter.jhtml?identifier=2016.

8. Wolz M, Cutler J, Roccella EJ, et al. "Statement from the National High Blood Pressure Education Program: prevalence of hypertension." *Am. J. Hypertens.* 13 (2000): 103–104.

9. Lucas JW, Schiller JS, and Benson V. "Summary health statistics for U.S. Adults: National Health Interview Survey, 2001." National Center for Health Statistics. *Vital Health Stat.* 10 (218). 2004

10. Robbins J. *The Food Revolution.* Berkeley, CA: Conari Press, 2001.

11. I strongly recommend reading John Robbins' *The Food Revolution*, which convincingly details the connection between your diet and the environment.

12. World Health Organization. "The World Health Report 1997: Press Release. Human and social costs of chronic diseases will rise unless confronted now, WHO Director-General says." Geneva, Switzerland: World Health Organization, 1997. Accessed at http://www.who.int/ whr2001/2001/archives/1997/presse.htm.

13. Ornish D, Brown SE, Scherwitz LW, et al. "Can lifestyle changes reverse coronary heart disease?" *Lancet* 336 (1990): 129–133; Esselstyn CB, Ellis SG, Medendorp SV, and Crowe TD. "A strategy to arrest and reverse coronary artery disease: a 5-year longitudinal study of a single physician's practice." *J. Family Practice* 41 (1995): 560–568.

14. Vegetarian Resource Group. "How Many Vegetarians Are There?" March 2004. Accessed at http://www.vrg.org/journal/vj2003issue3/vj2003issue3poll.htm.

15. Herman-Cohen V. "Vegan revolution." *Ithaca Journal* (reprinted from *LA Times*), August 11, 2003: 12A.

16. Sabate J, Duk A, and Lee CL. "Publication trends of vegetarian nutrition articles in biomedical literature, 1966–1995." *Am. J. Clin. Nutr.* 70 (Suppl) (1999): 601S–607S.

Appendix A

1. Boyd JN, Misslbeck N, Parker RS, et al. "Sucrose enhanced emergence of aflatoxin B$_1$ (AFB1) induced GGt positive rat hepatic cell foci." *Fed. Proc.* 41 (1982): 356 Abst.

2. Tannenbaum A, and Silverstone H. "Nutrition in relation to cancer." *Adv. Cancer Res.* 1 (1953): 451–501.

3. Youngman LD. *The growth and development of aflatoxin B$_1$-induced preneoplastic lesions, tumors, metastasis, and spontaneous tumors as they are influenced by dietary protein level, type, and intervention.* Ithaca, NY: Cornell University, PhD Thesis, 1990.

4. Youngman LD, and Campbell TC. "Inhibition of aflatoxin B$_1$-induced gamma-glutamyl transpeptidase positive (GGT+) hepatic preneoplastic foci and tumors by low protein diets: evidence that altered GGT+ foci indicate neoplastic potential." *Carcinogenesis* 13 (1992): 1607–1613.

5. Horio F, Youngman LD, Bell RC, et al. "Thermogenesis, low-protein diets, and decreased development of AFB1-induced preneoplastic foci in rat liver." *Nutr. Cancer* 16 (1991): 31–41.

6. Bell RC, Levitsky DA, and Campbell TC. "Enhanced thermogenesis and reduced growth rates do not inhibit GGT+ hepatic preneoplastic foci development." *FASEB J.* 6 (1992): 1395 Abs.

7. Miller DS, and Payne PR. "Weight maintenance and food intake." *J. Nutr.* 78 (1962): 255–262.

8. Stirling JL, and Stock MJ. "Metabolic origins of thermogenesis by diet." *Nature* 220 (1968): 801–801.

9. Donald P, Pitts GC, and Pohl SL. "Body weight and composition in laboratory rats: effects of diets with high or low protein concentrations." *Science* 211 (1981): 185–186.

10. Rothwell NJ, Stock MJ, and Tyzbir RS. "Mechanisms of thermogenesis induced by low protein diets." *Metabolism* 32 (1983): 257–261.

11. Rothwell NJ, and Stock MJ. "Influence of carbohydrate and fat intake on diet-induced thermogenesis and brown fat activity in rats fed low protein diets." *J Nutr* 117 (1987): 1721–1726.

12. Krieger E, Youngman LD, and Campbell TC. "The modulation of aflatoxin (AFB1) induced preneoplastic lesions by dietary protein and voluntary exercise in Fischer 344 rats." *FASEB J.* 2 (1988): 3304 Abs.

Appendix B

1. Chen J, Campbell TC, Li J, et al. *Diet, Life-style and Mortality in China. A Study of the Characteristics of 65 Chinese Counties.* Oxford, UK; Ithaca, NY; Beijing, PRC: Oxford University Press; Cornell University Press; People's Medical Publishing House, 1990.

2. There were eighty-two mortality rates, but about a third of these rates were duplicates of the same disease for people of different ages.

3. This also means that very little or no useful information is obtained by including the values of all the individuals in the county. There is only one disease rate for each county; thus it is only necessary to have one number for any of the variables being compared with the disease rate.

4. Piazza A. *Food Consumption and Nutritional Status in the People's Republic of China.* London: Westview Press, 1986.

5. Messina M, and Messina V. *The Dietitian's Guide to Vegetarian Diets. Issues and Applications.* Gaithersburg, MD: Aspen Publishers, Inc., 1996.

Appendix C

1. Holick MF. In: ME Shils, JA Olson, M Shike, and AC Ross (eds.). *Modern Nutrition in Health and Disease*, 9th ed., pp. 329–345. Baltimore: Williams and Wilkins, 1999.

2. Barger-Lux MJ, Heaney R, Dowell S, et al. "Vitamin D and its major metabolites: serum levels after graded oral dosing in healthy men." *Osteoporosis Int.* 8 (1998): 222–230.

3. The biological half-life of storage vitamin D is 10–19 days, the time it takes for half of it to disappear.

4. Colston KW, Berger U, and Coombes RC. "Possible role for vitamin D in controlling breast cancer cell proliferation." *Lancet* 1 (1989): 188–191.

5. Nieves J, Cosman F, Herbert J, et al. "High prevalence of vitamin D deficiency and reduced bone mass in multiple sclerosis." *Neurology* 44 (1994): 1687–1692.

6. Al-Qadreh A, Voskaki I, Kassiou C, et al. "Treatment of osteopenia in children with insulin-dependent diabetes mellitus: the effect of 1-alpha hydroxyvitamin D_3." *Eur. J. Pediatr.* 155 (1996): 15–17.

7. Cantorna MT, Hayes CE, and DeLuca HF. "1,25-Dihydroxyvitamin D_3 reversibly blocks the progression of relapsing encephalomyelitis, a model of multiple sclerosis." *Proc. National Acad. Sci.* 93 (1996): 7861–7864.

8. Rozen F, Yang X-F, Huynh H, et al. "Antiproliferative action of vitamin D-related compounds and insulin-like growth factor-binding protein 5 accumulation." *J. Nat. Cancer Inst.* 89 (1997): 652–656.

9. Cosman F, Nieves J, Komar L, et al. "Fracture history and bone loss in patients with MS." *Neurology* 51 (1998): 1161–1165.

10. Giovannucci E, Rimm E, Wolk A, et al. "Calcium and fructose intake in relation to risk of prostate cancer." *Cancer Res.* 58 (1998): 442–447.

11. Peehl DM, Krishnan AV, and Feldman D. "Pathways mediating the growth-inhibitory action of vitamin D in prostate cancer." *J. Nutr.* 133 (Suppl) (2003): 2461S–2469S.

12. Zella JB, McCary LC, and DeLuca HF. "Oral administration of 1,25-dihydroxyvitamin D_3 completely protects NOD mice from insulin-dependent diabetes mellitus." *Arch. Biochem Biophys.* 417 (2003): 77–80.

13. Davenport CB. "Multiple sclerosis from the standpoint of geographic distribution and race." *Arch. Neurol. Psychiatry* 8 (1922): 51–58.

14. Alter M, Yamoor M, and Harshe M. "Multiple sclerosis and nutrition." *Arch. Neurol.* 31 (1974): 267–272.

15. Van der Mei IA, Ponsonby AL, Blizzard L, et al. "Regional variation in multiple sclerosis prevalence in Australia and its association with ambivalent ultraviolet radiation." *Neuroepidemiology* 20 (2001): 168–174.

16. McLeod JG, Hammond SR, and Hallpike JF. "Epidemiology of multiple sclerosis in Australia. With NSW and SA survey results." *Med. J. Austr.* 160 (1994): 117–122.

17. Holick MF. "Vitamin D: a millennium perspective." *J. Cell. Biochem.* 88 (2003): 296–307.

18. MacLaughlin JA, Gange W, Taylor D, et al. "Cultured psoriatic fibroblasts from involved and uninvolved sites have a partial, but not absolute resistance to the proliferation-inhibtion activity of 1,25-dihydroxyvitamin Ds." *Proc. National Acad. Sci.* 52 (1985): 5409–5412.

19. Goldberg P, Fleming MC, and Picard EH. "Multiple sclerosis: decreased relapse rate through dietary supplementation with calcium, magnesium and vitamin D." *Med. Hypoth.* 21 (1986): 193–200.

20. Andjelkovic Z, Vojinovic J, Pejnovic N, et al. "Disease modifying and immunomodulatory effects of high dose 1a(OH)D$_3$ in rheumatoid arthritis patients." *Clin. Exp. Rheumatol.* 17 (1999): 453–456.

21. Hypponen E, Laara E, Reunanen A, et al. "Intake of vitamin D and risk of Type 1 diabetes: a birth-cohort study." *Lancet* 358 (2001): 1500–1503.

22. Breslau NA, Brinkley L, Hill KD, et al. "Relationship of animal protein-rich diet to kidney stone formation and calcium metabolism." *J. Clin. Endocrinol. Metab.* 66 (1988): 140–146.

23. Langman CB. "Calcitriol metabolism during chronic metabolic acidosis." *Semin. Nephrol.* 9 (1989): 65–71.

24. Chan JM, Giovannucci EL, Andersson S-O, et al. "Dairy products, calcium, phosphorus, vitamin D, and risk of prostate cancer (Sweden)." *Cancer Causes and Control* 9 (1998): 559–566.

25. Byrne PM, Freaney R, and McKenna MJ. "Vitamin D supplementation in the elderly: review of safety and effectiveness of different regimes." *Calcified Tissue Int.* 56 (1995): 518–520.

26. Agranoff BW, and Goldberg D. "Diet and the geographical distribution of multiple sclerosis." *Lancet* 2 (November 2 1974): 1061–1066.

27. Akerblom HK, Vaarala O, Hyoty H, et al. "Environmental factors in the etiology of Type 1 diabetes." *Am. J. Med. Genet.* (*Semin. Med. Genet.*) 115 (2002): 18–29.

28. Chan JM, Stampfer MJ, Ma J, et al. "Insulin-like growth factor-I (IGF-I) and IGF binding protein-3 as predictors of advanced-stage prostate cancer." *J. Natl. Cancer Inst.* 94 (2002): 1099–1109.

29. Cohen P, Peehl DM, and Rosenfeld RG. "The IGF axis in the prostate." *Horm. Metab. res.* 26 (1994): 81–84.

30. Doi SQ, Rasaiah S, Tack I, et al. "Low-protein diet suppresses serum insulin-like growth factor-1 and decelerates the progression of growth hormone-induced glomerulosclerosis." *Am. J. Nephrol.* 21 (2001): 331–339.

31. Heaney RP, McCarron DA, Dawson-Hughes B, et al. "Dietary changes favorably affect bond remodeling in older adults." *J. Am. Diet. Assoc.* 99 (1999): 1228–1233.

32. Allen NE, Appleby PN, Davey GK, et al. "Hormones and diet: low insulin-like growth factor-I but normal bioavailable androgens in vegan men." *Brit. J. Cancer* 83 (2000): 95–97.

INDEX

ABOUT THE AUTHORS

For more than forty years, **Dr. T. Colin Campbell** has been at the forefront of nutrition research. His legacy, the China Study, is the most comprehensive study of health and nutrition ever conducted. Dr. Campbell is Jacob Gould Schurman Professor Emeritus of Nutritional Biochemistry at Cornell University. He has received more than seventy grant-years of peer-reviewed research funding and authored more than 300 research papers. The China Study was the culmination of a twenty-year partnership of Cornell University, Oxford University, and the Chinese Academy of Preventative Medicine.

Thomas M. Campbell II, MD is the co-founder and clinical director of the University of Rochester Program for Nutrition in Medicine. A board certified family physician, Dr. Campbell is also medical director of the T. Colin Campbell Center for Nutrition Studies. A graduate of Cornell University, Thomas is also the author of *The China Study Solution* (*The Campbell Plan* in hardcover).

Online Certificate in Plant-Based Nutrition

"The science is there and it must be made known. We cannot let the status quo go unchallenged and watch our loved ones suffer unnecessarily. It is time to stand up, clear the air and take control of our health."
The China Study, p. 18

Learn more at nutritionstudies.org/certificate

· Highly acclaimed program with thousands of international graduates

· Ivy League course content offered in partnership with eCornell

· World-class lecturers, featuring Dr. T. Colin Campbell

· Self-paced, 5-7 hours per week with 24/7 access

· Continuing Education credits available

· Complete in as little as 6 weeks

· Interactive instructor team

Contact eCornell to enroll

     info@ecornell.com   1-866-eCornell

From the author of the groundbreaking
bestseller, *The China Study*, comes the much-anticipated ...

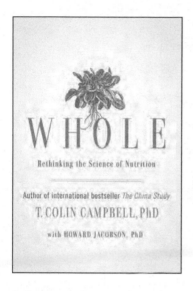

WHOLE
Rethinking the Science of Nutrition

By T. COLIN CAMPBELL, PhD
and HOWARD JACOBSON, PhD

Whole picks up where *The China Study* left off. *The China Study* revealed what we should eat and provided the powerful empirical support for this answer. *Whole* answers *why* a whole-food, plant-based diet provides optimal nutrition. *Whole* demonstrates how far the scientific reductionism of the nutrition orthodoxy has gotten off track and reveals the elegant holistic workings of nutrition, from the cellular level to the operation of the entire organism. *Whole* is a marvelous journey through cutting-edge thinking on nutrition, led by one of the masters of the science.

For more than 40 years, T. COLIN CAMPBELL, PhD, has been at the forefront of nutrition research. His legacy, the China Study, is the most comprehensive study of health and nutrition ever conducted. Dr. Campbell is the coauthor of the bestselling book, *The China Study*, and the Jacob Gould Schurman Professor Emeritus of Nutritional Biochemistry at Cornell University. He has received more than 70 grant-years of peer-reviewed research funding and authored more than 300 research papers. The China Study was the culmination of a 20-year partnership of Cornell University, Oxford University, and the Chinese Academy of Preventive Medicine.

Visit **THECHINASTUDY.COM** to learn more!

"I have often been asked—a few hundred times, I think—what do my family and I eat? ...Now I am happy to say that there is a cookbook that comes about as close to the real deal for our family as I can imagine it. This is it."
—T. COLIN CAMPBELL, PhD, coauthor of *The China Study*

LeAnne Campbell, daughter of *The China Study's* T. Colin Campbell, delivers easily prepared and delicious recipes that support optimal nutrition in ...

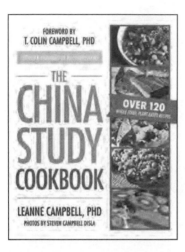

The China Study Cookbook

Over 120 Whole Food, Plant-Based Recipes

By LEANNE CAMPBELL, PhD

The China Study Cookbook takes the vital scientific findings from *The China Study* and puts the science into action. Written by LeAnne Campbell, PhD, daughter of *The China Study* coauthor T. Colin Campbell, PhD, and mother of two hungry teenagers, *The China Study Cookbook* features delicious, easily prepared plant-based recipes. From her Fabulous Sweet Potato Enchiladas to No-Bake Peanut Butter Bars, all of LeAnne's recipes have no added fat and minimal sugar and salt to promote optimal health. Filled with helpful tips on substitutions, keeping foods nutrient-rich, and transitioning to a plant-based diet, *The China Study Cookbook* shows how to transform individual health and the health of the entire family.

LEANNE CAMPBELL, PhD, has been preparing meals based on a whole food, plant-based diet for almost 20 years. Campbell has raised two sons—Steven and Nelson, now 18 and 17—on this diet. As a working mother, she has found ways to prepare quick and easy meals without using animal products or adding fat.

Visit **THECHINASTUDY.COM** and **THECHINASTUDYCOOKBOOK.COM** to learn more!

More than 100,000 copies sold in the series ...

The Happy Herbivore Series
By LINDSAY S. NIXON

  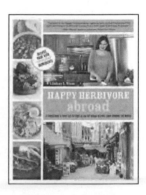

Lindsay S. Nixon's website, HappyHerbivore.com, topped over five million page views in 2012 alone with her sought-after, plant-based diet tips, delicious recipes, and cooking how-tos. True to her creed, Nixon's vegan dishes in her cookbooks are simple and refreshing for your palate.

LINDSAY S. NIXON is author of the bestselling Happy Herbivore vegan cookbook series: *The Happy Herbivore Cookbook, Everyday Happy Herbivore*, and *Happy Herbivore Abroad*, which have sold more than 100,000 copies combined. Nixon has been featured on The Food Network and *Dr. Oz*, and she has spoken at Google. Her recipes have also been featured in *The New York Times, Vegetarian Times, Shape Magazine, Bust, Women's Health*, WebMD, and countless other online publications. A rising star in the culinary world, Nixon is praised for her ability to use everyday ingredients to create healthy, low-fat recipes that are easy to make and light on your wallet.

Visit HAPPYHERBIVORE.COM to learn more!

"It turns out that if we eat the way that promotes the best health for ourselves, we also promote the best health for the planet."
—T. COLIN CAMPBELL, PhD, coauthor of *The China Study*

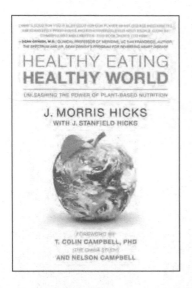

Healthy Eating, Healthy World
Unleashing the Power of Plant-Based Nutrition
By J. MORRIS HICKS
with J. STANFIELD HICKS

This powerful book explains exactly why a plant-based diet is the best choice you can make for yourself and for the planet. Simply incorporating more whole plant food and fewer animal products into your regular diet, you can enjoy vibrant health while greatly reducing your risk for ailments such as diabetes, cancer, and heart disease. And, if everyone adopted this diet, we would see improvement in poverty levels, health care costs, the energy crisis, and many environmental problems. While this sounds too good to be true, it's not. *Healthy Eating, Healthy World* arms you with the knowledge you need to make better food and lifestyle choices. It is a comprehensive yet accessible guide to incorporating healthy and delicious foods into your diet, so you can improve your life and your world.

A former senior corporate executive with Ralph Lauren in New York, J. MORRIS HICKS has always focused on the "big picture" when analyzing any issue. In 2002, after becoming curious about our "optimal diet," he began an intensive study of what we eat from a global perspective. Leveraging his expertise in making complex things simple, he is now delivering his powerful message in his book, on his daily blog, and in public speaking engagements—embarking on his new career as a writer, speaker, blogger, and consultant—promoting health, hope, and harmony on planet Earth.

Visit THECHINASTUDY.COM to learn more!

New York Times bestselling author of *Forks Over Knives— The Cookbook* writes *Better Than Vegan*, a cookbook of healthy, low-fat, and no-oil vegan recipes . . .

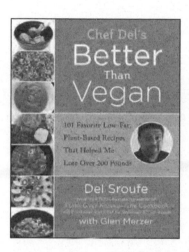

Better Than Vegan

101 Favorite Low-Fat, Plant-Based Recipes That Helped Me Lose Over 200 Pounds

By CHEF DEL SROUFE

The science is very clear. A whole food, plant-based diet is the healthiest possible way to eat—but veganism itself doesn't mean health, as Chef Del Sroufe, author of the bestselling *Forks Over Knives—The Cookbook*, knows better than anyone. Sroufe managed to reach 475 pounds while eating a vegan diet rich in pastries, peanut butter, and potato chips. After converting to a vegan diet with minimal processed foods, sugars, and added oils, he lost more than 240 pounds without giving up great food.

In *Better Than Vegan*, Sroufe tells his remarkable personal journey of how he went on to lose hundreds of pounds on a healthy vegan diet and then shares the kinds of meals (with no oil and low in fat and sugar) that restored him to health. He provides 101 delicious, mouth-watering recipes that prove that the healthiest diet can also be the most delicious, including Portobello Wraps with Spicy Asian Slaw , Gnocchi, Three Sisters Enchiladas, and Lemon Berry Sorbet.

Better Than Vegan offers healthy and professional cooking tips with nutritional advice to help you achieve the optimal vegan diet.

Visit **THECHINASTUDY.COM** to learn more!

An important conversation on how we can reduce instances of disease and symptoms through diet . . .

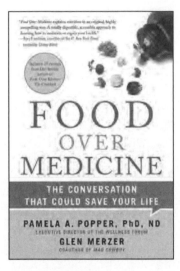

Food Over Medicine

By PAMELA A. POPPER, PhD, ND
and GLEN MERZER

Recipes by CHEF DEL SROUFE

Nearly half of Americans take at least one prescription medicine, with almost a quarter taking three or more, as diseases such as diabetes, obesity, and dementia grow more prevalent than ever. The problem with medicating common ailments, such as high blood pressure or elevated cholesterol, is that drugs treat symptoms—and may even improve test results—without addressing the cause: diet.

Overmedicated, overfed, and malnourished, most Americans fail to realize the answer to lower disease rates doesn't lie in more pills but in the foods we eat.

In *Food Over Medicine*, Pamela A. Popper, PhD, ND, and Glen Merzer invite the reader into a conversation about the dire state of American health—the result of poor nutrition choices stemming from food politics and medical misinformation. But, more important, they share the key to getting and staying healthy for life.

Includes recipes from CHEF DEL SROUFE, author of the bestselling *Forks Over Knives—The Cookbook* and *Better Than Vegan*

Visit THECHINASTUDY.COM to learn more!

WHOLE FOODS FOR A WHOLE LIFETIME OF HEALTH

THE SIMPLE WAY TO LOSE WEIGHT AND REVERSE ILLNESS, USING A WHOLE-FOOD, PLANT-BASED DIET

THE CHINA STUDY SOLUTION

THOMAS CAMPBELL, MD
CO-AUTHOR OF *THE CHINA STUDY*
FOREWORD BY T. COLIN CAMPBELL, PhD

The groundbreaking, influential bestseller *The China Study* explained why a plant-based, whole-food diet is linked to lower rates of obesity and chronic disease. Now, *China Study* co-author Thomas Campbell, MD, shows you how to make the transition—and enjoy the journey—with a 2-week whole-food, plant-based diet plan. Featuring 55 delicious recipes and answers to the most frequently asked nutrition questions, *The China Study Solution* makes healthy eating easy and sustainable for your entire family.

TheChinaStudySolution.com

~ **On sale now wherever books and e-books are sold** ~